DISCLAIMER!

This book is intended as an educational tool to acquaint the reader with alternative methods of preventing and treating cancer. Nexus Publishing hopes the book will enable you to improve your well-being and to better understand, assess, and choose the appropriate course of treatment.

Because the methods described in this book are for the most part alternative methods, by definition, many of them have not been investigated and/or approved by any government or regulatory agency. National, state, and local laws vary regarding the use and application of many of the treatments that are discussed. Accordingly, this book schould not be substituted for the advice and treatment of a physician or other licensed healthcare professional. Pregnant women in particular are especially urged to consult witht their physician before using any therapy.

Your health is important. Use this book wisely. Discuss the alternative treatment options that are described with your doctor. Ulitmately, you, the reader, must take full responsibility for your health an how you use this book. Nexus Publishing and the author expressly disclaim responsibility for any adverse effects resulting from your use of the information that is contained in this book.

It is not only for what we do that we are held responsible, but also for what we do not do!

Molière

Impressions

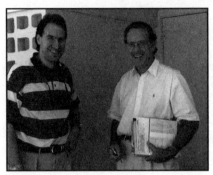

Klaus Pertl and Dr. John Clement 1998 at the IAT clinic in Freeport / Bahamas.

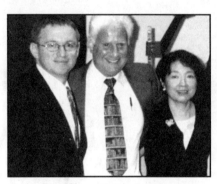

Together with Dr. Michael Schachter and Prof. Sophie Chen in Dubai / Saudi Arabia

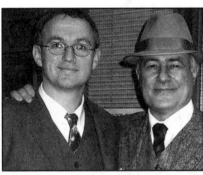

Together with Dr. Giancarlo Pizza, the italian founder of the Transfer Faktor-Therapy in Bologna.

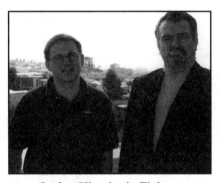

Lothar Hirneise in Tiujana together with Dan Rogers from the CHIPSA-clinic

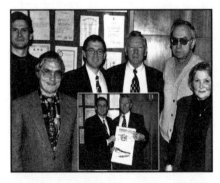

Research in Moscow about the Nentzi, native Russians who do not know cancer.

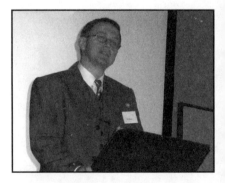

Lothar Hirneise is a well respected speaker all over europe. Here at the WDDTY conference in London.

Impressions

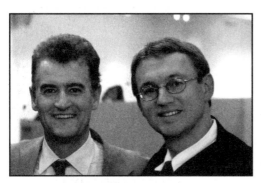

Together with Jack Black, founder of Mindstore and one of Europe`s most success-full personal development trainer.

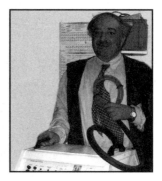

Together with Prof. Dr. Dr. P. Pappas in Athen (PapImi-Therapie)

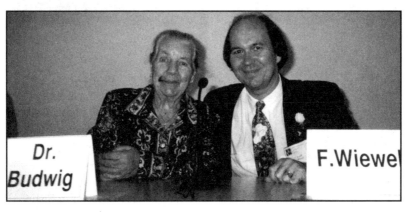

Dr. Johanna Budwig and Frank Wiewel,
President of *People against Cancer* Amerika, Stuttgart 1998

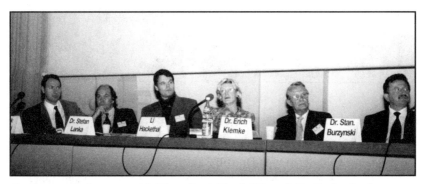

Conference in Stuttgart with Klaus Pertl, Frank Wiewel, Dr. Stefan Lanka, Li Hackethal, Dr. Erich Klemke, Dr. Stanislav Burzynski and many others.

Impressions

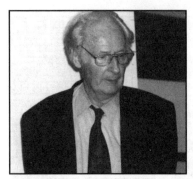

Together with Dr. Pekar,
founder of the Galvano-Therapy

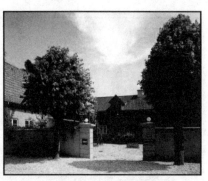

In Humlegaarden / Denmark
with Dr. Finn Skött Andersen

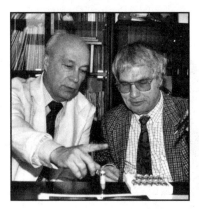

Prof. Kikko and Dr. Willy
Blumenschein in Moscow

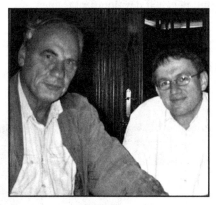

Together with
Dr. Ryke Geerd Hamer in Spain

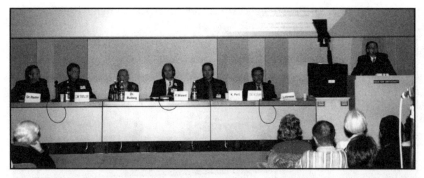

Conference in Stuttgart with Dr. Bill Raider, Dr. Jack Taylor, Dr. Johanna
Budwig, Frank Wiewel, Klaus Pertl, Dr. Nikolaus Klehr und many more.

Impressions

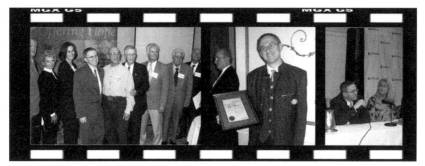

Left (middle): Lothar Hirneise, Bernie Siegel, Congressman Berkley Bedell...

NFAM award ceremony in Washington D.C. 2002

Lothar Hirneise received on the 16th of November 2002 in Washington D.C. the **Founders Award for Alternative and Complementary Medicine**. Other winners have been f.e. Bernie Siegel, author of *Love, Medicine & Miracles*.

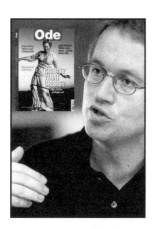

Articles, interviews or where Lothar Hirneise will speak you can find here: www.hirneise.de

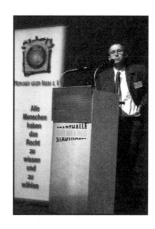

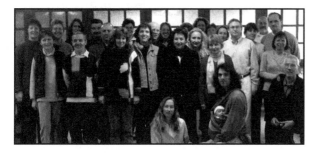

Together with the 1. group of *Holistic Cancer Consultants* from Germany, Austria and Spain. More informations under: www.hcc-usa.com www.hcc-uk.com

If
nothing
changes,
nothing
changes

Chemotherapy
heals cancer
and the world is flat

Lothar Hirneise

Translation:
Sprachendienste Holtz-Stosch GmbH
www.ho-st.de

ISBN 3-9810502-0-7

October 2005

Original:
Chemotherapie heilt Krebs und die Erde ist eine Scheibe
Sensei Verlag Kernen / Germany
www.sensei.de

Nexus GmbH Germany
Cannstatterstr. 13 * 71394 Kernen
www.nexus-book.com

Contents:

3. Diagnosis Cancer

4. Chemotherapy and radiation

5. Conventional therapies 185

6. The 3E Program

7. Non-Conventional Cancer Therapies

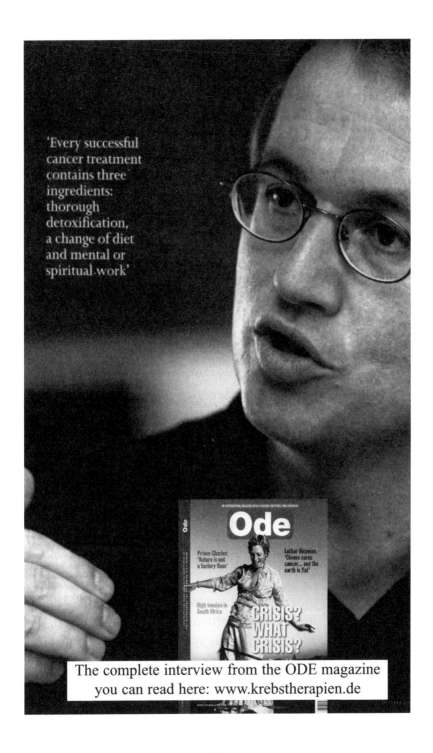

'Every successful cancer treatment contains three ingredients: thorough detoxification, a change of diet and mental or spiritual work'

The complete interview from the ODE magazine you can read here: www.krebstherapien.de

Foreword to the English edition

In recent years my work has taken me to numerous countries and I can honestly say that I have many friends on this globe. When these friends learned that I had written a book, and that after a few months it had become a bestseller in Germany, naturally I started to feel some "gentle pressure" to at least publish the book in English, as well. However in spite of this pleasant pressure, it has taken me two years to get to this point. The main reason was clearly my permanent lack of time. Particularly the work involved in establishing the first German holistic cancer center, which will be open in early 2006 in Buoch near Stuttgart, claimed a lot of my time (www.dgk-buoch.com). However this one reason why I am even more pleased that this book is now finally appearing in English, and that I can thus show cancer patients and therapists outside of German-speaking countries, how cancer can be treated successfully.

I am often asked to describe the main differences in treating cancer patients in the various countries, and my response is: "Do you have two days to spare for the answer, because there are enormous differences?" With conventional medicine just about everything is the same. With conventional medicine it makes no difference whether you receive chemotherapy in Dubai, London, Hong Kong, or San Diego, and it precisely for this reason that conventional medicine presents such a strong front.

The situation is totally different within non-conventional medicine. In this area the primary issue is how well the indigenous natural medicine has survived. In America natural medicine is almost completely dead, and in the Arabic countries, unfortunately, it currently in the process of being killed. In Europe natural medicine has at least survived to some extent, and in Asia and Africa it is indeed attempted. However in these countries the pharmaceutical companies are the least successful, because on these continents energetic processes and words are part of daily life.

Unfortunately the country, which has been affected more catastrophically than any other, is the USA. In America financial interests, even in alternative medicine, have gained the upper hand, and I experience on a daily basis, that particularly cancer patients only worry about therapies that are fourth or fifth in importance, instead of: First things first! You don't believe me? Then just visit an Internet forum about alternative cancer therapies, or talk to patients who have been treated by alternative physicians. You will quickly realize that virtually the entire discussion is based on miracle cures: they range from vitamin C to enzymes and minerals, to secret preparations from China or South America. In addition you will notice that even in those groups where important things like nutrition or detoxification are discussed, so much superficial knowledge is being diffused that I can well understand why allopathic practitioners just shake their heads. The reason this development is so frightening is that cancer patients thus remain passive based on this superficial information. However if I have learned anything in all these years, I have learned that cancer patients must actively change their lives, and merely taking medications, regardless whether allopathic or alternative is not enough.

Moreover there is the negative trend of complementary medicine, which is not just a trend in the United States. In my opinion, what originally started with good intentions, namely to combine "the best that allopathy had to offer with natural healing processes" has developed into a moneymaking machine. Today we have a situation that is similar to driving a car with one foot on the gas pedal and the other foot on the brake, in the hope to better control the car. Not to mention the fact that usually it is only the rich who can afford these therapies. Complementary medicine lies to its patients by leading them to believe that a person can do two different things at the same time with the result that the patient once again remains in a state of passivity, instead of dealing with the changes that are really necessary. Once I thought that there really was such a thing as a combination of allopathy and natural healing methods. Unfortunately many years and thousands of cancer patients later, I had to recognize that this is a lie. It is a lie that a lot people use to earn a lot of money!

I know that I am not making any friends with these statements, particularly in the "alternative camp", but I would like to say at the very beginning of this book, that I have not written this book to make myself popular with alternative physicians and unpopular with allopathic physicians. My only intent with this book is to show CANCER PATIENTS paths that lead to healing to. People with cancer motivate me each day anew to continue on in spite of the negative global trends in medicine, and these are the people who teach me on a daily basis that the impossible is doable.

There is still so much to change, let's do it together!

Lothar Hirneise

We believe people with cancer have two very fundamental rights - the right to know and the right to choose

Frank Wiewel
President of People against Cancer USA

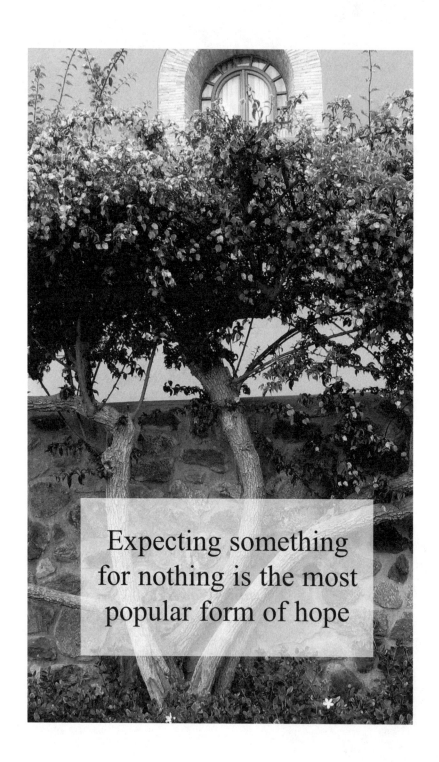

Expecting something for nothing is the most popular form of hope

Here is what you can expect from this book and what you should not expect from this book!

Almost without exception people view the diagnosis of cancer as a type of punishment and injustice, which they initially confront with a sense of powerlessness. This sense of powerlessness however is primarily due to false reports in the press and the consequent lack of information on the part of patients. To a great extent cancer is not a terminal illness to which one is helplessly surrendered.

How have I come to this conclusion, which certainly may appear as "quite presumptive" in the light of the many deaths attributed to cancer each year? Unfortunately I cannot provide you with an answer to this question in just a few words; and this is precisely the reason that this detailed book has been written. If you have read it carefully then you will understand for yourself, why I have come to the firm conviction that by no means is cancer the dangerous illness that it is always made out to be, even though so many people die of cancer.

In the following pages I will explain to you how allopathic medicine normally treats your type of cancer, and why its practitioners believe that they must do it this way. This is very important because it will enable you to better communicate with your doctor. I want to make it clear from the very beginning that it is very important to me that you conduct a satisfying dialog with your doctors, alternative practitioners, and other professional helpers. I am an absolute proponent of close collaboration with therapists (here I mean to all helpers, regardless of whether alternative practitioner, psychologist, etc.) and I am an opponent of the attitude, "I'll get through this on my own".

On the other hand, my experience has shown me that it is very difficult to find therapists with whom you can really conduct the necessary dialog. I would also like to explain an additional bias at the beginning of the book. I am neither for nor against conventional medicine and I am neither for nor against non-conventional medicine. I am exclusively concerned with people's welfare, and whatever contributes to regaining their health is all the same to me. If I have become more and more interested in non-conventional medicine in recent years, then this has nothing to do with any prejudices or personal interests, rather it is due to the results of my own research which have convinced me that conventional medicine is not nearly as successful in treating chronic illnesses like cancer, as many patients, unfortunately, still believe.

It is very important to me that you understand this, because if an author writes positively about non-conventional therapies and exposes errors of conventional medicine, then that author is happily relegated to an "esoteric corner", or even worse, that author is considered a "doctor hater". Believe me, nothing is further from my intent and interests, and anyone who knows me, understands that I am a man who thinks quite logically, and that I prefer to move on diplomatic, rather than revolutionary, paths.

Naturally it is a tactic of allopathic medicine to present me as an enemy of physicians who are not used to entering into a dialog with those who do not share their views, and instead dismiss all people with different opinions as crackpots. To apply the title of crackpot to people who think differently has some great advantages. In the first place you can always play the role of one who knows better, and secondly you do not have to change, because everything is all right (comfortably right).

We all know from our own experience that nothing in life is more difficult than changing ourselves. Naturally this also applies to doctors, or perhaps it would be better to say, this primarily applies to doctors. And I can understand this. A person has studied at the university for 5-6 years, then spent 2-4 years in specialization, and perhaps a few more years in a hospital to gain experience, and here comes Mr. Hirneise, who does not even have a doctor's degree, and maintains that this knowledge gained over years is at least in part, if not entirely, wrong.

It takes genuine greatness of character for a person to question his knowledge and thus a portion of his personality over and over again in the course of his life; and the number of people who are capable of doing this is very small. I thank God for the privilege of becoming acquainted with some of these people, and I am eternally grateful to these people that they have shared so much of their priceless knowledge with me. Without their input I would never have thought so much about why people become ill, or how they can be restored to health. In this book I would like to share with you in a brief form the unifying theme I have found as to why people who are most seriously ill have become healthy again.

In order for you to learn as much from this book as possible, unfortunately it is also necessary to refer to circumstances, which on first glance appear to have nothing to do with your illness. However only if you understand that political and financial interests can contribute to a medicine has being prescribed for you, which perhaps will harm you more than it will help you, can you conduct an open dialog with your doctor; a dialog that could determine whether you live or die.

In almost every case this dialog will determine whether you will live or not. You should be clear about this for yourself, and you should prepare for this discussion. I am always amazed again and again at how little patients know about their illness. Every woman browses through catalogs before she purchases a new kitchen, not to mention men and cars. However when it comes to purchasing a therapy, very few patients inform themselves in detail about their illness, rather they rely on statements from neighbors and acquaintances, or on the statements of a doctor. If you are wondering about my choice of words, "purchasing a therapy", then this may be because you have not yet considered that medicine is a business just like other enterprises.

Even if payment is organized somewhat differently through the health insurance system, than it is for other businesses, nevertheless in the final analysis it comes down to buying and selling. As patient you must always remind yourself of this fact, because you never have to accept an "unfriendly therapy salesperson" again.

This is no appeal to haggle over a discount, but rather an appeal to speak to a doctor like one grown-up speaks to another grown-up, and to place at least the same minimum requirements on this business transaction that are placed on the purchase of a car. Would you deal with a car salesman who would respond to your question as to whether the car that you are interested in is also available in a special paint finish, with the following statement: "Either you take it or go to a different dealership"? You would certainly leave immediately and take your business elsewhere. However when a doctor responds with insult or with arrogance to a patient's questions, then this is accepted by many patients without so much as a murmur, because they are not aware that they are paying the doctor's salary with their monthly insurance premium.

Another point: patients believe that if they are not nice to their doctor they will have disadvantages in their treatment as a consequence. No doubt this can be true, on the other hand, every patient should ask himself whether he really wants to be treated by this kind of therapist. If these lines should give rise to the impression that I am not fond of doctors, then this is 100% incorrect as good friends of mine are doctors. However I feel that my primary responsibility rests with patients, and in my more than 10 years of clinical experience, and principally through my experience with cancer patients, I have learned that it is the "uncomfortable patients" who return to health. By uncomfortable, I do not mean arrogant or loud, but rather

demanding. Demand that which is your due of your doctor –
namely that he helps you to the full extent possible.

Good doctors are never irritated with legitimate questions,
and they know how unsure patients are, particularly right after
the diagnosis. If your doctor does not take the necessary time,
then find a therapist for whom you are valuable enough that
he will take the necessary time.

By the way, if I write "somewhat more" in this book about
non-conventional cancer therapies, than I do about allopathic
applications, there two reasons why. First, those who purchase
this book expect to learn something about successful therapies
other than chemotherapy and radiation, and second, it is simply a fact that is not easy to write about conventional cancer
therapies if you want to describe them independently of pharmaceutical funding and career thinking.

Another tip: Use this book as a workbook. This book is
structured in such a manner that when you have completed it
you will know what is important for you. Moreover it is
important that you understand that even in holistic therapy
there are things that are necessary, things that are important,
and things that are not-so-important. I say this because I know
there are many books and reports in which hundreds of therapies are listed, and after reading all this material the patient
neither remembers what he has read, nor does know how he
should then begin "his" therapy. Thus I recommend that you
take notes while you are reading and do not leave any question open. Your life and the happiness of your family are at
stake. Do not put yourself under time pressure; at this point
just think about your future. Everything else is secondary.

However I do not want to conceal from you what this book
cannot do. It will not tell you which therapy you should start
today, it cannot relieve you of the responsibility of perhaps
speaking with various therapists; and more than anything else
there is one other thing it cannot do: It cannot change you.
From the bottom of my heart my desire for you is that you will

start to view your future today (again) in an extremely positive light, and that you will create your future yourself through visualization and activities. Whatever you have hoped for up to this point – it is possible!

1

The medical status quo

Why this book and the 3E Program are so vitally needed!

In recent years I have traveled the world over to find and investigate successful cancer therapies. At first I did this for personal reasons, later I did it as director of research for the National Foundation for Alternative Medicine in Washington, and today I do it as president of People Against Cancer Germany. Whether in Mexico, Russia, or Italy, it quickly became clear to me that medicine is no science. No doubt you or one of your acquaintances has experienced a situation wherein three doctors have been consulted for their opinion, and you have come home with three different opinions. That has absolutely nothing to do with science, and if we leave out surgery and emergency medicine, this "non-science" pervades all areas of medicine.

My travels through the oncology literature were not any better. Here as well contradictory statements are the order of the day, and discussions with doctors relative to how the test results of the studies in all the books should be evaluated end in total confusion. The same study will produce statements such as, "this is a new medical breakthrough", or "Forget this study, just look at who financed it". As a logical thinking person, conventional medicine, as practiced today, is nothing more than a pool of contradictory statements, from which anybody may take what he wants, protected by health insurance organizations, governments, and many medical associations. At a point when I had long admitted to myself that I could still spend many years in listening to the most widely varying opinions about what cancer is, how it starts, and above all, how it should be treated, I began to look more closely at the material that I had collected, and I spent several months evaluating it. The most important element in the initial evaluation of my travels at that time was that there were compelling similarities in people who had survived cancer in a so-called "final stage".

This brought me to the point of viewing oncology correctly for the first time – namely from the patients' perspective and not from the perspective of doctors and scientists. From this perspective it was finally possible for me to again consider oncology logically. First I could put previously collected knowledge into an understandable system and precisely order all theories about origin and treatment of cancer in the proper category. Second, all the different propositions of conventional and non-conventional therapies were no longer confusing to me, rather they became ever clearer aids in establishing the truth.

T wo results were quickly apparent. First I found out that patients in a final stage of cancer can be treated much more successfully if they did not have to subject themselves to any massive conventional therapies. Unfortunately such people are found only rarely in western countries, since standard medical practice, (and unfortunately legislation as well), almost exclusively permit, (i.e. pay for) conventional therapies only. The second thing I found out is that people who are seriously ill with cancer are never healed through specific

31

medications; rather they are healed through solitary mental or spiritual work, and/or through a combination therapy with detoxification or nutritional measures. And something else was noticeable in my evaluations. None of the patients had used therapies in the advanced stage that had serious side effects in any shape or form (although naturally this had frequently occurred during the first therapy or therapies).

The old law: Primum non nocere (first, do no harm), which unfortunately was forgotten in 19th and 20th century medicine, put people on the road to health, more directly and with fewer complications, than does modern medicine. Now perhaps you are thinking, "OK but this is nothing new". Why then are no conclusions or consequences drawn from this fact? Why hasn't anybody started to put this knowledge into a system for Everyman? Why does everyone believe that he can sell his piece of the larger oncological puzzle as the total picture? I quickly found the answer to all of these questions. I was simply not "caught" in any of the systems, where all those who have at least a part of this knowledge are normally stuck. I did not have to earn my living "selling" therapies or medications. I was not compelled, for political or financial reasons, to promote my career. I had never before publicly maintained what I would have to retract or which would have lead to a loss of face.

On first glance this may not seem so significant to you. But if you take a closer look at who is maintaining what today, and why, then you will quickly learn that this point always plays a significant role. Thus I was that which one could term in good English as "independent". Of course my psychoanalytical training and my mathematical/logical way of thinking helped later to integrate the collected knowledge in the 3E Program. However when I let the recent years pass by in review, then I realize that more than anything else it was my (financial and intellectual) independence that enabled me to bring my oncological experiences into a system.

After all these "revelations" I started to view oncology in its entirety from "my" scientific position, and consider my future experiences always and exclusively from my critical perspective. Seeing therapies from the empirical point of view (theory of experiences) does not mean leaving the scientific path, on the contrary.

Today I am more of a scientist than I was when I still believed in all the unproven medical "facts". Today if I think about how much vitamin C a person requires or whether the "non-vitamin C production" of our body is really a gene defect, as many "scientists" still believe, then my "systematic 3E thinking" helps me to quickly find an answer. If, with this book, I should be successful in initiating you into this systematic thinking, and if I can make clear to you why this is so important for your health, then I have achieved my goal.

Origination of the 3E Program

After evaluating all the data available to me, and after countless interviews with patients and therapists in many countries, I started to ask other questions of patients who had survived a final stage of cancer. And for the first time all the answers made sense, and they could be explained in "my" system. It was immediate, from this point on there were no more unexplainable "spontaneous remissions" or "miracle healings", but rather just people, who for the most part allowed themselves to be led by a feeling (this is also referred to as unconscious) instead of by their understanding, and who thus found the right path to a new health.

If we want to understand why people are healthy, we must first deal with the issue of energy. Have you ever wondered what the difference is between a person who is dead, and the same person a thousandth of a second before he is dead. Under the microscope or during a CT scan everything would appear the same; yes even the hemogram would be the same and yet in spite of this the difference could not be any greater. Many would say the difference is that between a person with a soul, or a person without a soul. I call it an energy difference. To better understand what I mean when I refer to energy in this book, I would first like to define this word more precisely. For me energy is an invisible life force that neither was created nor can it be destroyed, but which can either flow or not flow. Thus we can create conditions in which this energy can flow, such as generation of a new life, or we can destroy structures, which disturbs the flow of this energy (what we usually term illness) or allows it to completely flow out (death). Between these two points there are millions of intermediate steps (illnesses, love, faith, sympathy, etc.) that determine our daily life. In addition to the word energy, the word order likewise plays a super-ordinate role. The higher the order in a system, the better energy can flow into this system. As an example let's consider our aging process. The highest order exists on the day of our birth (provided we view this day as the first day of a person's life, and not its conception). From this point on we move inexorably into entropy (the opposite of order), i.e. into a chaos. Everything that we undertake until our death serves order and works against entropy.

For people, but also for animals and plants, this means that one of our main tasks consists in daily getting order into our life. We deal with this mainly via light, nutrition, and our thoughts, or what religion would call spirituality. The older we get, the more effort is devoted to this area, and the more important it becomes. You have certainly experienced the fact that older people become "stubborn" and "increasingly obsessive". They eat lunch and dinner at exactly the same time and require daily schedules that are increasingly regulated. Behind this is nothing more than a well thought-out system against the permanent increase of entropy in old age. Thus entropy is the attempt to transform ordered structures into unordered structures.

We age because after birth the forces of entropy win the upper hand over our body, as homeostasis (balance) is no longer capable of conquering these destructive forces.

The law of order

Just consider with open eyes what Americans, and also many Europeans, eat and you will quickly determine that in their "plastic food", the number of worthwhile ingredients is virtually nil, and in addition many toxins are present. But how is it then that people can eat junk food for decades without becoming seriously ill?

The "scientific" answer to this question is usually: it's just due to healthy genes. The truth however is that at this point we cannot even begin to read the language of the gene, and such statements are nothing more than words of despair from people who cannot admit that in reality they have no idea why something is the way it is. Or consider all the smart books about nutrition. If what was written in these books about vitamins, enzymes, hormones etc. were true, then many of my friends would have long been dead due to scurvy (through the destruction of vitamin C through smoking) or a chronic illness (because they hardly ever eat anything healthy). Likewise, alcoholics, anorexics, and millions of people in India or Africa prove to this author how "important" vitamins, enzymes, minerals etc. really are.

OK, then why don't all these "undernourished" people die?

Think of the human body as a large barrel, into which energy must be filled daily, similar to the gas tank of a car. However as opposed to a car there are at least three main energy sources that we can "tap" (nutrition, light, and our thoughts). Thus, if one energy source should fail, then we can always fall back on the other two. This also provides an explanation for our previous example, as to why people who live on junk food, and who also smoke, do not necessarily become ill. As long as a person is capable of using the other energy sources, he can maintain his life order.

33 % Energy Light	33 % Energy Nutrition	33 % Energy Mind	1 % God

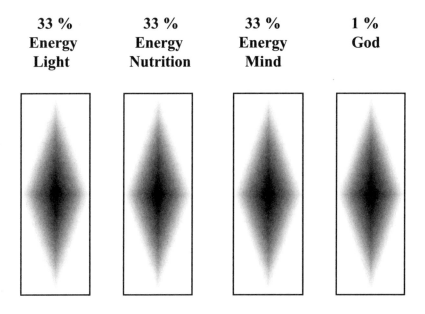

Unfortunately all three energy sources do not generate the same (necessary) life energy, in the same manner for all people. Not every person is capable of letting so much energy flow through a prayer or through meditation that he can get by on the food intake of an Indian Yoga master. By the same token, not everyone is successful in spending so much time outdoors that instead of healthy food he can eat just eat food in which the nutrients have been boiled away, and hamburgers; and even the best diet cannot help a person who is no longer capable of making the power of the other energy sources accessible to him. Only if we are capable of using all three energy sources in our striving for order, can we ensure that we will not be ill, or that a recovery process will start.

To live (survive) many people need only 40% of the attainable energy, others in turn need 70%. As long as they are capable of obtaining the energy that is necessary for their life they also will not become ill. However through the normal aging process and associated accumulation of toxins and "consumable materials" it becomes increasingly difficult to retain the necessary energy as a person ages. The same problem occurs if one has an illness that robs him of energy. Since almost all illnesses rob energy, a person must basically take responsibility and ensure that he avoids energy robbers, like poor nutrition, negative people, and negative thoughts. Thus you see that you can become old with poor nutrition, but at the moment you become sick, you can no longer afford poor nutrition if you want to return to health.

By the way this also explains the "folklore mistakes". You have certainly heard a sentence such as, "Yes but my grandfather was still smoking at age 90 and never got lung cancer," or "My grandmother only ate butter and fatty sausage and was healthy her entire life. It just cannot be all that bad". Undoubtedly all of these people are correct. Many people can smoke for 60 years and do not get lung cancer. Others can eat poorly for decades and still remain healthy. However what is not mentioned is what these people have done CORRECTLY. Most observers only see the cigarettes, and do not understand that other energy givers compensated for the consumption of cigarettes, which certainly were energy robbers. However if you have cancer, then you already have changed cells as energy robbers and cannot afford any additional energy robbers. If you believe that you can continue to smoke as a cancer patient, or continue on with a poor diet, then you must read this chapter again.

Do illnesses really exist?

Doctors have been speaking for thousands of years about the importance of the unity of body (nutrition), soul (light), and spirit (thoughts-faith). However this unity has become more and more forgotten in 20ᵗʰ century and 21ˢᵗ century medicine. Due to the hunger for profit over the last two centuries so many illnesses have come about that even medical professionals cannot name them all. However the great question of this century is: Do illnesses really exist, or that which we call an illness nothing more than a hand-selected grouping of symptoms? Let this question run through your mind for a while, before you reject it as crazy (i.e. push it out of your world). Name any illness and just consider for a moment if it really exists? Multiple sclerosis, cancer, rheumatism, high blood pressure or whatever you call it, in the final analysis they are syndromes (various symptoms) and not illnesses.

Considered at first glance one could say that it does not matter whether it is termed an illness or syndrome. However on second glance there is a significant difference. When a patient with an illness comes into a doctor's practice, his illness is treated. When a patient with a syndrome comes to the doctor, the syndrome or individual symptoms will be treated but the doctor never gets around to researching the cause and causally (aetiologically) treating the patient, because it is clear to the doctor hat symptoms always have a cause.

However if I as a doctor start by assuming that cancer, MS, rheumatism, etc. are illnesses, then I do not even begin to search for the cause. Today doctors even go so far that they high blood pressure, a high cholesterol level, or migraines illnesses and treat them with medications. No one considers today why our body generates the high blood pressure, whether pains makes sense, or whether they are perhaps even part of an important self-healing program. We have complete-ly lost faith in evolution and instead believe in the idols named gene technology and randomized double blind studies. To this day we do not know how our memory functions or why beards grow on men. Not to mention the fact that there is "machine" that you can one throw water and grass into and it will pro-duce milk and meat. Do you know this machine? It is also referred to as a cow in the vernacular. We do not even begin to understand the "daily things" like hunger, thirst, anger, dreams, joy, sympathy, and antipathy (at the same time how-ever we believe that we are able to decipher the language of genes). All of these things however have something to do with energy.

Hunger and thirst we usually call feelings, just like anger or love. But what is really behind the term feeling? Here we are actually speaking of flowing energy and the central ques-tion is: What influence does this flowing energy have on our health? Let me explain it this way: This energy is the all-deciding influence on your health and just because doctors do not learn anything about this during their studies, does not mean for a minute that these energies are not important in medicine.

Just think about how you feel when you have a full blad-der. Sooner or later this feeling will dominate everything in your life. Regardless of whether you are driving a car, swim-ming, or eating. The pressure to empty your bladder will rule your life. This energy is even capable of influencing your dreams. Most likely you have dreamt that you had to urinate, and then woke up with a full bladder. The feeling of a full bladder however is only one example. Love and particularly here being in love, anger, hate, hunger, faith, fear, etc. are at least every bit as important and rule our daily life. Doesn't it seem crazy that precisely these important things do not play a role in today's medicine? In my own clinical work, I have pre-cisely experienced this for years. Everything was centered on the illness and treatment with medication. I never doubted that this system was right, I was 100% sure that everything had its reason. Perhaps this is why I can understand doctors so well today. Most of them are very good people, who work however in an inhuman system that they can only break out of with significant personal and financial penalties. Nevertheless we cannot avoid the confession that today's treatment of chronic illnesses has reached a dead-end.

Modern oncology
or why patients and doctors know so little!

If a person studies the subject of cancer as a non-oncologist, then he will rarely be taken seriously, when expressing his opinion. Sooner or later something astonishing will occur. You quickly learn that there are many doctors who do not know very much about what cancer actually is or how it should be treated. You may think, "Correct, my doctor sent me to an oncologist precisely for this reason, because he is a specialist in the treatment of cancer". However oncologists have also specialized in something else, namely they have specialized in three cancer therapies, more precisely known as, chemotherapy, radiation, and surgery. In a few cases we could add hormonal therapy to this list, and everything else is categorized as study. "But they treat cancer patients every day, they must certainly know what they are doing".

If we consider this sentence more precisely, then we will note that it was not all that long ago that doctors sold heroin as cough medicine, and promoted contergan and other medicines as harmless. For decades they have told us that cancer can be healed thanks to chemotherapy, radiation, interleukin, interferon, etc. and that vaccines are effective and safe, - not to mention the AIDS dilemma. In addition we are supposed to be thankful that pharmaceutical companies have developed more than 70,000 medicines for our health, (and not perhaps for their wallets).

Human reason and comfort
Most cancer patients are quite healthy when they go to the doctor. They seldom have pain and do not feel particularly sick. The patient only starts to feel bad after the doctor has pronounced the word cancer. Then there is an increase in the

drama when the doctor explains that he must first make the patient very sick through conventional therapy like chemotherapy, radiation, or with a sharp knife, so that the patient can then return to health. At the latest our healthy human capacity to reason should come into play at this point and question the whole procedure. But no, since pharmaceutical companies in recent decades have spent billions in explaining to us that a medicine is only as effective as its side-effects, we also take this as a given and believe that everything is correct. This type of "medical self-concept" is now every bit as much of our daily life as is surfing the Internet. Or just think of amalgam, which for the most part consists of 52% mercury, a substance that is extremely toxic for humans. The rest is copper, tin, silver, and zinc. Perhaps you have broken a thermometer and you had to clean up of the mercury that flowed out. You were certainly very careful that you did not come into close contact with this substance.

On the other hand we pack the same substance into our teeth and hope that nothing negative will happen to us, and then discuss how much of this toxin can escape from the inlays and how many milligrams of mercury are really harmful. We are only too happy to hear the phrases of the pharmaceutical industry that mercury is absolutely harmless. Of course, the alternative would be to have the fillings removed and telling the dentist how he should proceed so that not too much mercury gets into our body in the removal process. Not to mention the high costs. Here it is certainly easier to turn off our understanding and to believe others – right? Are you aware that amalgam would never, ever, receive approval from the German Federal Institute for Drugs and Medical Devices or from the FDA!

Please do not misunderstand me. I do not want to get into the countless discussions about what is healthy for us, but rather demonstrate to you with this example how easy it is for us to place the responsibility for our health in the hands of others, whether they are doctors, insurance companies, or the media. Not only when we are very sick, (this is the latest point), but rather from youth on we must learn to engage our understanding, where our health or our happiness in life are involved.

While I am writing these lines, I hear on the news that the latest long-term English study on the birth control pill has found out that this pill is absolutely harmless for women. Honestly how dumb do these "scientists" think that we really are? Can it really be true that millions of women and their gynecologists believe that chemical intervention in the female hormonal balance does not bring disadvantages? Doesn't anyone consider anymore what happens to our ground water that daily must handle quantities of hormones that get into the wastewater system through the urine of women taking the pill? Are all the studies, which have previously proven that the additional taking of estrogen and progesterone clearly increases the risk of cancer and thrombosis, as ephemeral as yesterday's snow?

The answer unfortunately is a clear YES, then otherwise millions of young women would not have birth control pills prescribed, and millions of gynecologists would not break their oath, and there would not be so many young women taking urine from pregnant mares (from which in part estrogen is extracted) in the menopausal years In this case as well our comfort zone shuts such things out. It is certainly easier to swallow a pill every day as a pregnancy prevention measure, than it is to expend the additional effort which natural family planning involves.

But even at the risk that you view these comments as a general attack on the pharmaceutical industry or doctors, I will describe to you how things could reach the point that too many doctors treat cancer with just a few therapies, even though there are many successful therapies, as this book proves.

A doctor's career

In order to better understand why doctors are not aware of very successful cancer therapies, or dismiss them as quackery, we must better understand how a person becomes a doctor, by whom they are taught, from whom the doctor obtains most of his information, and what role is played by politics. If you have cancer and believe that this has nothing to do with your illness, then unfortunately I must disappoint you. If you do not know the next lines then it will be difficult to understand why the doctor treating you is perhaps using a therapy that he knows will not help you very much, if it will help you at all, or that the entire treatment is just a single experiment (also called studies in universities) with you.

You are most likely well aware that Germany is not the only country where a person must study for many years before he can call himself a doctor. But have you ever thought about what the students actually learn (must learn), and by whom they are taught? Have you ever considered what a doctor in the clinic or at the university must say so in order to become a professor?

The field of oncology is handled in a few hours, and in these hours medical students learn that the illness of cancer is equal to the problem of tumor, and the tumor must be conquered in order to conquer cancer. This fits in well with Louis Pasteur's statements that microbes are the cause of everything. However when we take a look around the world in the 21st century then we see that it is still only the perspective of Louis Pasteur that is being taught at all universities. When we go to our family doctor, we do ourselves a favor if we remember that he will not be treating us, he will be treating our tumor. Consequently we must not forget that our tumor is a part of us, just as the tumor is also only a symptom of our illness, and not the illness itself.

Because the doctor believes that he understands my illness so precisely, he also requires little time to deal with me as a person. This is an important point, which is forgotten time and again. All illnesses are listed worldwide according to a standardized system, and at the university doctors learn what they should do with this illness or that illness precisely in accordance with this scheme. But this is not all. Doctors must use this system if they do not want legal problems, or if they do not want be relegated to the ranks of the outsiders. Let me use an example to explain all this more in more detail.

Let's assume that your doctor diagnoses increased cholesterol in your case. According to the usual university system it will be recommended that you avoid food with a high portion of cholesterol, and if he recommends that you even more strictly adhere to the scheme (often in spite of knowing better), then he will also prescribe a cholesterol-reducing medication. Since he naturally does not want to lose you as a customer (patient), he will most likely not tell you anything about the hazard, or the proven uselessness of many of these medications, (both the hazard and uselessness have been demonstrated in many studies – in this regard see the book: What Doctors Don't Tell You, by Lynne McTaggart, for example). However in my view this is still the secondary problem. The main problem is that many doctors have apparently "forgotten" that they learned at the university how closely the cholesterol level is linked to the health of our liver, or with our lipometabolism.

Thus the problem is not the high cholesterol level, but rather the problem is in the question: Why does our body produce so much cholesterol (is it perhaps to equalize the acid base balance, or as a necessary antioxidant – which for starters would be very intelligent)? You see, when doctors proceed in accordance with the usual: "Let's fight the symptoms" system, then this can be a step backwards. With the exceptions of antibiotics and Zovirax (antivirus medication), there is not one out of 70,000! medications that treats an illness. All of the other medications concentrate on symptoms.

Patrick Kingsley, an English doctor who mainly treats people with cancer and multiple sclerosis takes a lot of time for each initial discussion: "How can I treat someone with such a serious diagnosis as cancer or MS, without knowing what this patient eats, what he does for work, how happy he is, etc. There is a significant difference whether a woman with breast cancer who shares the attitude with her husband: "This cancer is not going to kill me" comes to my practice or whether the same woman is going through a divorce and works in a flower shop where she is in daily contract with flowers that are contaminated with pesticides."

Consider for a moment which woman has the greater chance of survival. It's logical; naturally the first woman in the example is what you are probably thinking. Unfortunately it is not logical at all to assume that doctors will form a complete picture of a person. Why not? This is because they know precisely who has which illness and they also known how this illness, (please notice, I do not say this person), should be treated. For example did you know that the average time that a doctor spends with his patient per appointment is approximately 6 minutes. In 99% of all cases an oncologist is more interested in your tumor than he is in you. Consequently he will try to cut out the tumor, or he will attempt to destroy it with chemotherapy or radiation. But will he explain to you what other cancer therapies are also on this planet and:

* What getting radiation will mean to your body and spirit? (In this regard I am not just referring to losing hair and throwing up, rather I am referring to serious side effects and main effects like heart and kidney problems, nerve damage, billions of new free radicals, collapsed intestine, impotence etc.!) Moreover, did he take a cell culture or an EVA test to determine which chemotherapy preparations

are even effective for you. Were you prepared for chemotherapy or what was undertaken to limit the side effects? Most likely they gave you even more chemicals in the form of so-called antiemetics (against vomiting).

* By the same token neither is the following paradox considered:
While you are taking medication that strongly suppresses the immune system, of all places you are sent to a place where there is the highest concentration of viruses and bacteria – the hospital. Most likely the majority of patients do not consider this to be important because they don't know how many patients die through this type of treatment. While I have been writing this book, I have been confronted with precisely such a case. A few days ago a patient, I know, received his first chemotherapy and died shortly thereafter from a so-called "uncontrollable infection" that he contracted in the hospital.

* What successes the doctor has experienced with this type of medication for this type of illness? Did you also get his statistics or did you only get those of his colleagues? You must request these results in writing. Do not allow yourself to be fobbed off with words like: "I have had 20 years of experience in this area". Often it is namely 1-2 years experience and 18-19 years of repetition. Please believe me, if a professor has had good results with any medication or with a certain therapy, then he has published the results in at least two medical journals.

* How you should eat? If your doctor tells you that you can continue as you are presently doing, then get out of there as fast as you can. (If he himself understands nothing about nutrition then at least he should introduce you to someone who knows about nutrition and cancer.)

* That cancer can be cured and what YOU can contribute to keeping the tumor from returning?

* What you can do to strengthen your immune system?

* How important the psyche is in cancer illnesses? This has nothing to do with you being emotionally ill or "cracked". Cancer patients do not have a psychic defect but rather they must be offered counsel on how important meditation, visualization, or generally stated "going into yourself" is for recovery, and above all how important it is as a prophylactic against metastases.

It is not just my experiences that demonstrate that a lot is discussed in the hospital about how extensively you are being treated. Daily life however is totally different. A holistic approach does not take place. The word extensive is used only for the diagnosis; in this regard we are the absolute world champions. Another x-ray, another blood test, another CT etc., with no consideration of the enormous costs involved, the person is totally forgotten in this regard. This focus is purely on tables, numbers, measured values and no longer on what actually triggered the illness. And just how certain is this diagnosis anyway? Can a doctor really tell which lymph node is affected during an operation? What does this little shadow on the x-ray image tell us? Now are these cells under the microscope from a benign tumor, or from a malignant tumor?

Many years ago I was in a neurological department due to a harmless "sciatic pain syndrome" and was run through the diagnostic mill. Routine procedure called for a contrast CT (the equipment had just recently been purchased) and I was diagnosed with a "space occupying process" in the brain, in English: a brain tumor. And while I was still considering what this diagnosis meant for my future, the head physician of the department checked the diagnoses of his senior physicians a few days later and explained to me that the diagnosis of his colleague was that of a novice, and that my space occupying process was nothing more than the fact that one of my brain ventricle was simply larger at birth than the other three. The thought of what would have happened if the head physician of the department had been on vacation at the time haunts me to this day.

Watch out – people are concerned about you!

It is not just the doctors who make mistakes. As soon as the world learns that you have cancer many people will try to help you out with counsel and acts of kindness. At first this is something positive and getting so much attention is helpful for a lot of cancer patients. But watch out, as soon as someone utters the sentence: "This doctor (this therapy) is the best for you", you need to be very careful. I must have heard this sentence hundreds of times: "Dr. XY is an absolute specialist in his field." Usually I don't respond to this remark because I value my precious time, but whenever I hear this sentence I should really ask the following questions: "How do you know that"? Have you personally verified this statement? Which criteria serve as the basis for the statement that he is the best doctor in his field? Do his colleagues say this? "What do his opponents say about this etc."?

Often my hair stands on edge, when I hear what people tell me about "experts". If I take the time to respond, I often say: "Did you know that the best experts at the five largest publishing houses in England rejected the Harry Potter book"? Here as well I must remove misunderstandings from the very outset. Naturally there are bad, good, and very good doctors. Unfortunately there is no evaluation scale like there is in athletics or in the stock market.

In Germany there are many, many doctors. Just estimate for yourself what percent of a profession is really good, and considering your own estimate, what is the chance that you will encounter a "not so good" doctor. Or what actually characterize a good oncologist? Set up a few criteria for yourself. Intuition or scientist? Great knowledge or gifted craftsman? Small or large practice? University clinic or city hospital?

Family doctor or specialist? The answers to these questions will quickly help you determine that it is almost impossible to find out which doctor is good or not so good. Do you really want to depend on the statement of your neighbor, a friend, or your doctor, when something as important as your life is involved. On the other hand, you "must" rely on someone. Do it conscientiously – there can only be one person and you are this person.

Naturally you can also gamble and rely on someone who you do not know very well, but if you do this you should be honest with yourself and your loved ones and do it knowingly. It is better to learn as much as possible about what cancer is or could be; what it means for your life and which changes and therapies are necessary, so that you can (again) live in the way that you desire. Reading this book is certainly one part of this path and will help you in the process of finding your path.

In order to feel secure on your path over time, it is very important that you not always let other people get you off your path. This sounds a lot easier than it really is. Particularly where cancer is concerned, many helpers believe to know your path better than you do yourself. If you discuss this book with a conventional doctor, you will determine that there are usually 4 different reactions to it. It is important to be familiar with these reactions before you discuss this book with a doctor, alternative practitioner, or another therapist, in order to tell during the dialog, who is sitting across from you to better classify the answers.

Naturally I am aware that is not quite fair to classify doctors into 4 categories, as every doctor is unique and a I conscientious risk the fact that many physicians may not be particularly fond of me because of this classification. On the other hand I consider it to be very important to enlighten you in this regard, as I experience time and again that a professional helpers can say almost anything and he will be believed, if he has a title or if he can present himself in a convincing manner. But it is YOUR life and I feel responsible to cancer patients (by the way some of my good friends are doctors). For the sake of simplicity I have given the following names to the four groups:

Bessis

Bessis are people who basically know everything better than everyone else. A Bessi will tell you directly that if you do not avail yourself of the therapy suggested by the Bessi then you will experience significant harm; in the case of cancer you will hear words like: "In this case I cannot assume any responsibility for you". Have you ever considered the responsibility a doctor actually assumes when he has you radiated 30-40 times. If you survive then he ascribes it to his therapy, and if you die then the cancer was stronger. With Bessis it is not too hard to be thrown out of the room if you ask uncomfortable questions.

Unfortunately from my daily practice I must tell you that there are a lot of Bessis among oncologists. The advantage associated with Bessis is that they represent a clear line, and as patient you know precisely where you stand. While good dialogs seldom take place, Bessis however express themselves clearly and the patient can easily verify the arguments and make his decision. Naturally, Bessis will not discuss a book like this one with you, and they will dismiss almost everything as alternative nonsense, quackery, and non-scientific.

Gallis

Gallis usually are very popular with patients, journalists, and organizations, as they have great empathy (intuition) and conduct a dialog (albeit short) with the patient. They listen to the anxieties of the patients and the patient feels accepted by the doctor. However where concrete suggestions for the therapy are involved, they always represent the same conventional therapies as the Bessis.

The difference however is that they act very understanding relative to the patient and are pleased to give out counsel like: "Eat healthy, avoid too much stress", or "If you think that a mistletoe therapy will work....", or "While I don't believe in this, I don't have anything against it, as long as you take the chemotherapy and/or radiation". Gallis are the helpers who are the most difficult for me and for you to evaluate and who are that main contributors to the fact that there is nothing going on in the entire field of oncology. Externally they present themselves as promoters of complementary medicine, in truth however, they fight oncological progress a lot more than do the Bessis, because they do it diplomatically.

Gallis will dismiss this book as quite interesting but not really scientific, not written by a doctor, or "If this would help you then we would have been using these therapies for a long time in our clinic", and they will not go into more detailed questions with you.

Kappis

Kappis are doctors who, expressed in good English, do not give a hoot about your well-being. They will not mince words in telling you which conventional therapies there are for your illness and that you must waste no time. In daily work they are better lawyers than doctors because they always only do the "in" thing, career promotion, or what is most convenient at the time, in order not to deal with their own personal problems. By the way this is an important point. Many patients do not understand that doctors are also people with their daily psychic fluctuations, and moreover behind the white doctor's smock often there are just people who may have more problems than you do yourself. The fact that they do not want to deal with patients often has nothing to do with a non-professional attitude, but rather has a lot to do with personally protecting the physician's psyche. Naturally I am aware that this may not be what a patient expects from a doctor. However this knowledge helps you to the extent that you don't have to get so irritated with your doctor when he hides behind the next appointment, or only deals superficially with your important questions. Unfortunately Kappis come across as being very competent in discussion, they use a lot of foreign words, and continuously refer to the latest research, so that usually patients are very impressed.

Kappis will dismiss this book as not up to date, and will explain to you why none of this could be true using a lot of Latin. As an alternative to the information in this book they will naturally suggest a conventional cancer therapy and often even explain in detail why non-conventional therapies (although they do not even know any of these) can't function.

Dokkies

Dokkies are doctors who first take time for their patients, and second understand that cancer therapy means more than just destroying a tumor. They will discuss all areas of a cancer therapy with you and never come across as know-it-alls. It is not easy to find doccies as unfortunately insurance companies do not pay enough for the necessary time with patients, and even doctors have to earn money. Should you be acquainted with such a doctor or alternative practitioner, then you are certainly numbered among the happier patients. In addition, this book will help you to find such therapists. Dokkies will take this book seriously and explain to you what they think is wrong in the book and what they think is right in the book. Both aspects will be explained to you in understandable terms.

For the most part you will recognize Dokkies because they will not act insulted or oversensitive should you ever be of a contrary opinion, rather they will discuss the matter with you briefly. The problems associated with doccies is basically the lack of payment and misunderstanding of patients who expect therapies and not just discussions. But it is precisely these discussions that allow a good oncologist to determine how he can help you. It is only a doctor who believes through a pathological report to know in advance which illness he must treat, who does not need to speak with his patient in detail. In my opinion this catastrophic direction of medicine has assumed such proportions today that insurance companies are prepared to spend more than 100,000 Euros for a chemotherapy, and at the same time reject, holistic oriented therapies that only cost a fraction of this amount.

Unfortunately the chance that this picture will change in coming years is virtually nil. Naturally you are free to sue your insurance company, and thankfully there have been some positive judgments in the meantime. However my job is to tell you how to gain energy, not how to lose it. This is precisely what will happen if you go against the insurance companies or the establishment, as long as you have tumors in the body. Naturally this does not mean that you should sit back and take everything complacently, but from my experience I cannot recommend going to court against your insurance company as long as you are seriously ill. The inhuman correspondence with insurance company case workers or their attorneys will certainly block a lot of energy, this is why you should save this type of activity for later, whenever that may turn out to be.

I have often experienced, mainly in Germany, that even people who can afford it are not prepared to spend money for their health or for their life happiness. Phrases like "what have I been giving money to the insurance company for all these years?, or "I am not touching my hard-earned money", I have heard more than once. There is no doubt that these people are right in what they say.

However when they have a tumor in the body the issue is not being right or not, but rather becoming well as soon as possible, and this does not happen when you are always fighting. Please take these words to heart. I have become acquainted with far too many people who took these words lightly and then were no longer able to concentrate on the essential elements of a cancer therapy.

The because – in-spite of therapy

This book is not designed to just enlighten you about which successful cancer therapies are available, but rather I also hope that it will motivate you to reflect on your past life. This applies to you when you read this book, because you yourself are affected, whether you read this book as a lay person, or as a professional helper. To be involved with cancer, and that independently, whether as patient or as helper, also means always confronting death and the meaning of life.

Many authors justifiably call cancer the turning point of life. The question however is a turning point in which direction. I am firmly convinced that it is not so important what we decide for, but rather it is much more important, to make a decision and then to live this decision as best as possible. This also means never to look back, and to love the present. To make this possible we must create our future on a daily basis and this also includes reflecting about our world, about our fellow beings, and about their thought systems. Don't be alarmed, I am not going to make a philosophic presentation, but rather simply communicate to you that I have noticed that people who have survived a final stage of cancer, in every case have also thought about the philosophic aspects of life.

Many people believe that it is very strenuous always dealing with those that are terminally ill. I have never found this to be the case, quite the contrary. To talk with people who are free of material interests, is incredibly instructive, funny (usually very funny) and one receives many positive waves from the other side. Haven't you always wanted to speak with the Dalai Lama or with the Pope? These two people have or had made themselves free of material interests, and for decades they have been busy with religious and philosophic aspects of life – just like the terminally ill – only longer. I have always viewed it as a privilege to be able to speak with such people, and if I can say today that I am a much happier person, then all these people have contributed to this. To learn new things, to feel new things, to reflect and to make decisions, isn't that what we call life? Without such a process I would never have sat down and taken all the effort to write this book to help you. Instead I would again manage a company – and again earn a lot more money than I am doing today.

But only when one has cancer, or when one comes to another turning point in life, does one understand how important money really is. For each of us money probably has a different value – from unimportant – to selling your own grandmother for it. In the process we forget again and again that the real important things in our life usually do not depend on money. Love for our children and partners, sex, friendship, the smell of flowers or meadow, joy in eating and much much more. This does not mean that the purchase of new home, a car or a first class plane ticket cannot also bring joy, but none of this is comparable with the feeling of watching your child while he or she is asleep. On the next pages I would like to communicate an idea to you, a theory: The because / in spite of theory.

This idea should motivate you to think about your illness and about your recovery in a way that perhaps you have not done before. When reading this book it is not so important to whether I am right with this idea or not, but rather that you know that there is much more that you can do for your cure than you are aware of.

The theory

Let's say that 10 people injure their back because they have lifted something that was too heavy. Each of them will treat this "illness" in a different way in the next three weeks. One goes in for acupuncture, another gets a prescription for Voltaren (an anti-inflammatory medication), another gets a prescription for 20 massages, and another gets homeopathic drops. After 3 weeks all 10 patients are again free of pain. Now if you were to ask each of these patients individually, which therapy he would take the next time he injures his back, then you would get a different answer from each patient. But not only this, every one of them would also recommend his therapist to others.

Let's assume further that of the 10 patients, after another 20 days, 1 patient still had pains and would want to swap with the other 9 patients. You can be sure that he would no longer recommend his doctor and would start immediately with one of the therapies that the other patients used.

Let's say in addition, that 1 of the 9 patients, who today are free of pain, threw his medication into the waste basket, instead of taking it. Which doctor would he actually recommend and which therapy direction would he present to a medical conference? You certainly understand now where I am headed and why this chapter is entitled the because / in spite of theory – because there are very few people who are not afraid to ask the following question:

"Has the patient returned to health BECAUSE he has followed this therapy or INSPITE OF THE FACT that he has followed this therapy."

I was first confronted with this question more than 20 years ago in my hospital work and later I ran into it again and again in books and medical discussions. However each time I discussed this question briefly and then again set it aside. I am grateful to Dr. Budwig that I thought more about this important question. In a discussion with her, I said that chemotherapies in the final analysis had also demonstrated successes, e.g. with testicular cancer or for Morbus Hodgkin. She asked me how I knew this and I answered that I personally knew patients who had returned to health thanks to chemotherapy for these types of cancer, and in addition this could also be found in many books. To this she answered: "I also know patients who have received chemotherapy and then had no more tumor. However I consider it to be non-scientific and premature to maintain that these patients survived because of the chemotherapy."

I must confess that at the time I did not go into more detail with Dr. Budwig but something inside of me did not forget this sentence and it has often found its path in my cerebral cortex. Now there is hardly a day that passes in my work in which this sentence does not play a role, as most patients still believe that they have been healed through medication. Many patients swear that this or that medication, or that this or that therapy helped them. At the same time, the same therapy, the same medicine did not help other patients. There are not too many people today who would come up with the idea and would maintain that a child died because of chemotherapy. But let's take a look at this point from a "neutral" perspective.

Please take a look at the side effects listed on the information sheet that comes with most chemotherapeutic medications that are prescribed for children with cancer. Now ask yourself: "How long could you give your child this medication before he or she would die?

You have read correctly: How long until he or she would die. It is one hundred percent certain that every child would die on any kind of chemotherapy – if given the medication over a long enough period of time. The question is not whether people (can) die due to chemotherapy, rather the question is: "How long can a person withstand chemotherapy, without dying from it. Doctors always assume that all children, all people will immediately respond to the chemotherapy or radiation treatment. But we all know that many people are allergic to pollen and many are not, many can drink milk, and many can't... - I could continue this list for many pages.

Now are we supposed to believe that it is only with the strongest poisons medicine has to offer that all people respond the same? If this were not so serious, we would have to laugh at such nonsense.

Now let's consider the second part of the theory. In the first part of the theory, the issue is that we never hold chemotherapy responsible for the fact that people die. In the second part of the theory the issue is that we basically consider chemotherapy responsible when people get better. But no one asks the question here: "Did the patient recover in spite of getting chemotherapy or radiation?" Today we know that for flu it is better to rest a few days, eat little, and in a few days we are healthy again. No however, there are people who have no time to be sick, and instead of resting they work sweating in the office and in the evening they go to a smoke-filled restaurant with their customers. Even if it takes somewhat longer, most of these people also return to health with this office/restaurant therapy. But no one would ever come up with the idea that office work and sitting around in smoke-filled restaurants is an optimal therapy for flu. These people have become healthy in spite of the office/restaurant therapy.

Everything that is not part of allopathic practice is called alternative therapy. What is forgotten is that allopathy is really the alternative; it is an alternative to a medical tradition that developed over thousands of years and which has proven itself. The allopathic alternative has been successful in displacing all other therapies in less than half a century. We forget that it was not all that long ago that doctors offered their services on the street for little money. Then medicine got its big chance, as more and more doctors understood how they could make more and more money with their medicine. 100 years later the medical industry/medication manufacturers conglomerate has displaced everything that had proven itself. Naturally this phenomenon does not apply just to medicine, but applies generally for different areas of our life. At this point I do not want to write a political discussion of the present medical industry, but if we do not understand how we have reached the point that all the "non-scientific facts" of today's oncology, and that is what they are, all of a sudden are represented as scientific facts then neither can we make independent decisions. I would also prefer less complicated development in the medical industry, but it does not help to close our eyes to facts and act as if things were different just because we don't like the way things are.

Now does this mean that all medications are worthless and it is solely our self-healing power that returns us to health? And if yes, why do these medications fail so frequently with cancer? Instead of giving you a direct answer, I would like to describe what I have noticed in my research.

Most non-conventional therapies differ from conventional therapies in that they take the foremost principle of the "old medicine" into consideration: Primum non nocere (first do no harm). This means that unlike chemotherapy, these therapies could be given to a healthy person for years, and that person would not die of the treatment – which is something that cannot be said of radiation or chemotherapy. Thus if the lowest common denominator in all successful cancer therapies that I know of is: Primum non nocere (first do no harm) could it be possible in this case, that this and only this is the reason why people get better? Only that can exist, which is permitted to exist! It was not enough to hear this sentence once, rather I had to experience it many times over. But today I am an independent person and allow myself to think freely. You should also start with this and I would like to invite you to take a look with me at what it would mean if I were to be right.

Doctors would practice their profession mainly by talking with their patients and would no longer pull out the prescription pad. We would all have to think differently and consider what we could do to become healthy or to stay healthy. Most significant however would be the demise of the pharmaceutical companies' influence on our policies and our entire social system. I do not want to go into more detail here relative to the enormous effects that this would have on the whole world, instead I invite you to consider this, then only in this way can you really understand why nothing can exist, that is not permitted to exist.

Moreover there is another question that arises for cancer patients. To do no harm to a person is one thing, but are there other ways to help a cancer patient to get better? Homeopathy, orgone, psychology, healing hands, frequency devices, magnetic fields, spiritual accompanists etc. have already helped cancer patients according to information provided by thousands of therapists. However did they heal these people, or have they at least contributed a part to the healing? If the last question can be answered with yes, then naturally the next question is what would happen if we now combine five of these therapies. Could they jointly heal?

Questions after questions that I have been dealing with for years, and the more I speak about these things with open-minded people all over the world, the closer I get to logical answers. These answers could easily fill 2-3 books. In countless discussions however I have reached the conviction that it would not help to write down all of these answers because people only act when they are convinced of something, and people are not convinced by just reading books, they are convinced primarily when someone animates them to reflect. As in this example: How do I motivate people on an island to build a boot? With construction plans for boats? No, I tell them stories of sea voyages and ensure that they dream of distant worlds.

In the same way I hope that I can motivate you through my words to dream of your distant world of health that is still distant today, and that you trust yourself to build your boat as fast as possible.

2

Cancer – what is it?

What is a medical school graduate talking about when he uses the word cancer?

Before we discuss various theories concerning what cancer is or is not, I would like to tell you something about the importance of these theories. You will notice on the following pages that the answer to the question "What is cancer really" has two main camps. In one camp are the proponents of allopathy who naturally (must) stay with the mutation theory, and in the other camp are all the other theories. I cannot tell you 100% who is right and who is wrong, even if 99.9% percent of my research contradicts the mutation theory.

However for you as a cancer patient it is most likely vital that you make a decision. I cannot relieve you of this responsibility and the reason is: My research has clearly shown that non-conventional therapies in many cases only help if the body has not been previously damaged by aggressive therapies – through therapies not through cancer. Most cancer patients however only start with non-conventional therapies after conventional therapies have failed, in the style of: "Now let's do 3 cycles of chemotherapy and 30 radiations and if the tumor comes back then we can always try an alternative therapy." This book will help you make an informed decision and you will not be able to avoid making an informed decision.

The Beckenbauer soccer tactic: "Let's wait a while", does not work for cancer because chemotherapies and primarily radiation, cause irreparable damage. Even if many doctors still maintain the contrary – oncological experience clearly speaks a different language. It is very important that you make your own opinion, and not get involved with these theories before you decide for a therapy. You must also know that doctors in hospitals always represent the mutation theory; legally they have no other choice.

The mutation theory

First it must be stated that even in allopathy there is no real agreement on how cancer is caused. There are reports of cancer being caused through viral infections e.g. Burkitt-Lymphoma, through the Eppstein-Barr virus, liver cell cancer through hepatitis B, and T-cell leukemia through a retrovirus named HTLV-1. For the most part however the reports involve cancer-causing substances, so-called noxa in the form of radiation and chemicals. These noxa then ensure that certain genes, which normally would repair these genetic defects, are inactivated, and a malignant tumor can develop. Since our cells are exposed again and again to these attacks in the course of aging, naturally the probability of contracting cancer also increases with age in a parallel relationship. In summary we can say that cancer occurs because mutations occur in our cell nucleus, the DNA (deoxyribonucleic acid), and over years a tumor forms from this. This is why it is called the mutation theory.

Let's say that the mutation theory is correct, then we should be able to take the nucleus of a cancer cell, transfer it into a healthy cell, and this cell would then become a cancer cell. Naturally this also applies the other way around. If we were to transfer a healthy nucleus into a cancer cell, then this cancerous cell must then become healthy again. Unfortunately this is not the case, as McKinney demonstrated in 1969 and B. Mintz and Karl Illmensee published in 1975. For example McKinney replaced the nucleus of an egg cell of the leopard frog with the malignant nucleus of a cancer cell. But after fertilization completely healthy frogs were born. Please think about this for a moment. That part of a cell, which according to prevailing academic opinion, is responsible for determining whether a person develops a tumor, is transplanted, and what happens? Nothing, absolutely nothing. Also Seeger's research findings, that tumor cells, which are freed from their mitochondria and then immunized do not generate cancer, clearly contradicts the mutation theory.

How come our heart does not get cancer?

The answer to this question contains an additional argument as to why in most cases cancer in the onset stage has nothing to do with our DNA. I emphasize the word onset stage here because today we know that cells that have once degenerated through various mechanisms of activation, which I do not want to discuss in more detail at this point, invoke DNA changes. If cancer is a problem of our nucleus, then it is also logical to assume that each cell nucleus can degenerate, including the billions of cells in our heart. However the fact is that certain cells, or that almost the entire heart does not get cancer, although there are billions of cells there with a DNA. Unfortunately this fact is not explained with the mutation theory, however the mitochondria theory, which I will discuss in more detail later, does explain this.

This is just one important objection as to why the mutation theory cannot be correct, not to mention the facts that have been confirmed for years that cancer cells produce increased H_2O_2, that an increased peroxilipid production is present, that a charge reversal with potassium outflow from the changed cell takes place, that there is a shift of hydrogen concentration towards alkalosis, that an accumulation of cholesteroal ester in the cancer cell occurs, as well as various types of membrane damage, there is a depolarization (shift of electric potential) etc. etc. Just using studies from the 50s and 60s I can list more than 100 changes that cannot be brought into harmony with the mutation theory. For some time now the central issue for many holistic doctors has not been whether the mutation theory is correct or not, but rather: Why isn't there practical application of this knowledge and why, in spite of information to the contrary, in all probability, are far more than 90% of all cancer patients worldwide treated in accordance with the totally outdated mutation theory which says: Destroy the tumor and the cancer is gone. Millions of cancer fatalities prove every year that cancer is not simply a tumor that can be cut out.

Now add metastasis!
When tumors return within a short time, then it means that the tumor has metastasized, i.e. metastases are present. From the allopathic perspective metastases are tumor cells that have removed themselves from the original tumor and have settled elsewhere in the body. But before you accept this theory as a given, I would like to point out a few contradictions within this theory.

1. If metastases were really daughter cells of the primary tumor, then they would also have the characteristics of the "parents". Frequently however metastases consist of many different cell types. If they are all descendents of a degenerated cell, then how can they suddenly consist of different cell types?

2. According to conventional opinion we permanently develop cancer cells, which are destroyed daily by our immune system. Would it not then be logical after an operation to do everything in our power to strengthen our immune system, or restore it so that it can destroy the remaining tumor cells.

Instead we destroy our immune system with toxins or radiation.

3. If it were true that radiation only represents a problem for metastases, but not for our healthy cells – which is again and again maintained by all radiologists in the world – then it would certainly be logical that people who are subjected to radiation treatment several times a year, would thus support their immune system because they would be destroying existing cancer cells.

This radiation then would make cancer avoidable – naturally given the prerequisite that the statements of these radiologists would contain a bit of truth. Have you ever wondered why there is not a single oncologist has had himself radiated for preventative reasons?

4. Why are we not able to find these metastases in the blood, in spite of the most modern laboratory equipment.

5. How do we know that the circulating tumor cells that apparently can be found in the blood, come from the tumor, and are not "totally normal cancer cells" that the body apparently produces daily anyway?

6. Let's assume that a patient with a primary liver tumor develops a brain metastasis. Since these cells are supposed to be daughter cells of the liver tumor, do these patients then have a "little liver" in the brain?

7. A 1cm³ tumor has approximately 1.073.741.824 cells (over a trillion). Usually tumors can only be detected when they are 6-8mm in size. At a size of only a cubic millimeter a tumor already consists of more than a million cells. Do you really believe that a tumor which "only" has one million cells, has not already been forming metastases for some time. This would indicate that basically every tumor had been producing metastases for some time before it was diagnosed.

8. For most cancer patients, tumors return after the first treatment, or the cancer patients already have additional tumors when the primary tumor is diagnosed. In these cases allopathic practitioners then say that unfortunately the primary tumor has formed metastases. This is logical because the smallest tumor that can be detected with current diagnostic processes already consists of billions of cells. What is not logical is that when blood is donated it is not examined for micro-metastases. Wouldn't it be a compelling necessity to examine blood for cancer cells? If it is true (which I personally do not believe) that these cancer cells are responsible for new tumors, then every doctor runs the risk of transferring cancer with every blood transfusion. Because we are using blood that was donated in other countries for transfusion, naturally any logically thinking person may ask the question, "What role does the government play in this regard"? The lapidary answers such as: "The blood is previously treated or cleaned are not satisfactory from a microbiological standpoint.

9. If it is true that metastases wander through the body and settle elsewhere, then why does this almost always occur in the liver, the lungs, in the head, and in the bones? Isn't it odd that these cells never settle in the pancreas, the spleen, the kidneys, or in the left ring finger?

I am aware that this may sound somewhat sarcastic, but no one today talks about why for instance there is so much metastases in the liver. Everyone knows that the liver is our most important detoxifying organ (next to our lungs, which many people do not know) and every doctor, who thinks, also knows that detoxification therapies play an important role in any chronic illness. And although this association so to speak is presented on a silver platter, conventional doctors still dispute that there is a connection. The reason for this is quite simple. If doctors were to finally admit that there is a connection here, then they could no longer sustain the outdated metastasis theory. At the same time there is not even an approach to a theory in any textbook as to why cancer cells always settle in just a few places. Either I am the only person that has thought about this, or there are very good reasons why this is never discussed.

10. Nor does the mass of tumor cells seem to be important. As part of their study, researchers associated with the US scientist, Michael F. Clarke, investigated cells that they had isolated from the cancerous tissue obtained from nine women who had breast cancer. With special antibodies the researchers were successful in isolating the different types of cancer cells within a tumor, in individual populations. The different cell populations were subsequently injected into mice with deficient immune systems.

What was interesting in this regard was that for many cell types, just 100 to 200 of the newly discovered cells formed malignant tumors, while thousands of other isolated cancer cell types did not cause any new tumors. All of the cancer stem cells discovered in this manner had a certain protein marker (CD44). And they had either just a small amount of another marker (CD24), or it was not present at all.

In lay terms this means that we can forget the oft-cited argument: "You better have an operation soon, before the tumor spreads", because neither the quantity of cancer cells, nor even the size of the tumor are significant.

Summary:
Even if there are many different viewpoints about metastasis, we cannot avoid one fact: The whole issue of micro-metastases remains a theory to this day, and as long as this theory is

not proven, all therapists and patients should not act as if micro-metastases really exist. Here we must consider what would happen to today's oncology, if the metastases theory would be dismissed. 90% of oncologists would then become just surgeons, because without chemotherapies and radiation against metastases there would only be a little work for the rest.

Again and again I am surprised that oncologists who are involved with cancer on a daily basis know so little about these scientific facts. The answers to the question why would unfortunately fill an entire book, and cannot be discussed in more detail here. Direct answers, which have to do with money, satisfying egos, and building up a power base are most likely familiar to you.

But we should not go so easy on ourselves and ascribe the total blame to doctors; we are the ones who still believe that the doctor makes us healthy. As long as we do not work on ourselves collectively, and finally come to understand, that only we can heal ourselves, there will be doctors who satisfy a market where healing is sought through third-parties or through medication.

The mutation theory approach to therapy:

Destruction of the tumor and the metastasis. As a patient of a conventional doctor, you must be aware of how your doctor thinks; namely: Tumor = cancer and tumor gone = cancer gone.

Mistaking cause and effect

Or why cancer-causing therapies are prescribed for so many people due to the mutation theory

Imagine that an extraterrestrial visitor comes to earth and by chance sees several houses on fire within a few days. Each time the extraterrestrial visitor sees the firefighters, and after the 10th fire he thinks: "Hmm whenever there is a fire the firefighters are there, thus the firefighters must also be responsible for the fire". For this reason he calls his extraterrestrial colleagues for help and they attack the firefighters.

Now perhaps this anecdote brings a smile, but this is precisely what happens every day in the field of oncology. The fire (the tumor) is put out by the firefighters (regulation programs). This is not a simple job and it is very strenuous (fever, pain, fatigue, etc.). But instead of supporting the firefighters, the extraterrestrials now show up in white outfits and fight the firefighters with the most deadly weapons available (chemotherapy, irradiation, etc.)

If this situation were not so serious it would laughable. However the people who suffer most from this confusion of cause for effect are innocent physicians and patients, and I simply cannot accept the fact that all the substantiating evidence that is suppressed on a daily basis. This is why I would like to explain what is wrong here, in more detail.

Under the microscope, pathologists observe changes in the degree of differentiation of a cell. Differentiation is a medical term and it refers to cells transforming into cells in more mature structures with specialized tasks. Now we basically assume that the more immature a tumor tissue is, (i.e. how little its structure and function resemble structure and function of the host tissue), the more undifferentiated, and at the same time, the more malignant the cell is. But is this really the case? Let's consider a normal cell in the process of becoming a cancer cell. Long before the genetic changes take place, there are changes in the cell membrane, the enzyme formation, the respiration chain etc. Only AFTER these changes, do we observe cell adaptations (regulation system) to the changed situation (milieu), in the form of genetic adaptations of the DNA and RNA. There are hundreds of studies in this area and they can be verified in the laboratory at any time. These genetic or morphological adaptations have now been made visible by pathologists e.g. through dyes (Feulgen, MGG AgNOr etc.). Easily visible characteristics such as nucleus size, form, and size of the cell membrane or cell, are further characteristics that pathologists use to determine whether a cell is a cancer cell. The more changed a cell appears under the microscope, the more malignant will be its classification. But a so-called highly differentiated cell is not a very malignant cell; rather it is a cell that is extremely adapted to the dominant (ill) milieu. It is logical to conclude that milieu changes have an influence on cells. The only alternative to adaptation is death of the cell. And now decide for yourself: "Which do you prefer? Dead cells or adapted cells?"

The crucial error made by conventional medicine is to now declare these cell adaptations to be the CAUSE of cancer, even though better information is available. This is like playing dominos and maintaining that the seventh domino has fallen because the sixth domino fell. However the fact that the sixth domino fell because of the fifth domino, or that its falling could have anything to do with the first domino, is denied. In allopathy the cause for everything is attributed to the sixth domino (genes, toxins, etc.). In the view of holistically thinking people, this is a small but crucial conceptual error that costs the lives of thousands of people every day.

WHY?

The reason why this catastrophic scientific misinterpretation is still being taught can be easily answered with a counter-question: "What would happen if the truth were taught?" The effects on our society would be so enormous that even I have wondered whether there might be a better way, a better alternative to unsparing enlightenment. Virtually the entire medical industry is stuck in just such catastrophic dead-end. It is a dead-end that they can no longer get out of without revolutionary changes.

However we cannot just blame others. Are we not ourselves to blame? We who permanently close our eyes to facts, just because we desire a different world? Germany is not the only country where publications appear on a daily and weekly basis offering reports about politics, but primarily about the elite, the rich, and the beautiful, that are known to "not quite" correspond to the truth, (to put it mildly for legal reasons). But it is precisely these magazines that have the greatest number of readers in the market. This means that millions of people buy these magazines every day and read lies DELIBERATE-LY because it is the only way that they can deal with the world. A different example. Do you believe that the war in Iraq took place because America felt threatened by Iraq's weapons of mass destruction? No, you don't believe that? However this means then that you do believe that people are deliberately being killed in Iraq for other reasons. But where medical issues are involved, a market that can easily take on the oil and weapons markets of this world, then most people believe that life and health are the top priorities. I am sorry to say that this is not the case, and that it is very important that you understand these interrelationships. If you do not understand them, then you will not understand why even when knowing better, the outdated mutation theory is still being taught at universities, with all its attendant catastrophic effects on our lives.

The mitochondrial theory

or why our heart and
our brain cannot get cancer.

Even in the non-conventional scene, there is no agreement on what cancer is. The most popular theory is certainly however the mitochondrial theory. This theory says that our cells switch their metabolism over to fermentation. Let me explain this to you in more detail. As we know from our biology class, for example sugar ($C_6H_{12}O_6$) in our mitochondria is broken down into water and carbon-dioxide via multiple intermediate steps. The intermediate steps are important because otherwise we would develop so much heat in the breakdown process that we would burn up. On one hand our cells are energy producers, in order to maintain our body heat of 37 degrees C, and on the other hand each of has the most intelligent cooling system that can be imagined. Now why our cells at the end of this breaking down process do not build up more water and carbon dioxide is still disputed by the individual theorists.

The only area where there is some unity is that cytochrome oxidases (enzymes) and/or an excessive consumption of glutathione plays a significant role, as described by Dr. Heinrich Kremer in his German book: The Quiet Revolution of Cancer and AIDS Medicine. In summary this means that our cells produce only 192 Joule instead of 2814 Joule and consequently we have a real energy problem in our body, with the most widely varying effects on our organism such as tumors for instance. The most important single effect however consists of lowered tension of our cell membrane. This lowered cell membrane tension plays a significant role because the cell membrane decides what comes into a cell and what comes out of a cell. Due to this changed tension it can be the case that no more oxygen gets into the cell. In this case there are only two possibilities left for cell. Either it decides to die, or it starts to live without oxygen, meaning it starts to consume more energy than it produces itself. A byproduct of this "decision" is then also the immortality of the cell. Tumors do not occur because your cells divide too quickly, but rather tumors occur because the old cells no longer die. Critics always maintain that these types of programs do not exist in our cells. But this is naturally not true because the program: "without oxygen", meaning the ability to generate necessary energy from fermentation is naturally in all of our cells, otherwise we could not have survived the first days after conception in our mother's womb.

There are two points in our body whose electricity we can measure with simple means (more precisely stated the ECG and the EEG) – our heart and our brain. Precisely at these points it is impossible for tumors to develop; or do you know someone with heart cancer? With heart cancer no, but perhaps you are thinking, with a brain tumor, yes. But in reality there are no brain tumors. It is known that our brain consists of nerve cells, and since nerve cells cannot divide, there cannot be any brain tumors. What there are, are tumors of the glia, which is a supporting tissue of the brain, whose cells can also multiply throughout life.

This supporting tissue with mesodermal origins comprises the major portion of our brain and consists of cells like glia cells, astrocytes, or oligodendrocytes, from which the names of brain tumors like glioblastoma, astrocytoma etc. are derived. Because nerve cells cannot multiply, naturally there are no brain tumors. With our heart whose cells multiply constantly it is a totally different picture. Our cell membranes have a voltage from -70 mV to -90 mV and as long as this voltage is maintained, it is not possible for a cell to ferment, thus they cannot become a cancer cell. Because our heart is known to be under slightly more current than other cell structures, it is not possible for the cells in our heart to degenerate. This fact alone indicates that the mitochondria theory is a much more suitable model to explain cancer, than is the mutation theory. Unfortunately for years this theory has simply been passed over and dismissed as if such "noticeable appearances", as our heart not developing tumors, or metastases occurring principally in the liver and lungs, do not exist.

The mitochondria approach to therapy:

Nutrition therapy, 3E program and orthomolecular medicine. The overarching concept could be termed protection or healing the mitochondria. For adherents of the mitochondria theory genes play only a conditional role.

Dr. Fryda's adrenalin theory

When I first heard that that a lack of adrenaline causes cancer I unjustifiably relegated the subject to a stack of unfinished work, for far too long. If I had known then that Dr. Waltraut Fryda is one of the few people who can maintain that she has successfully treated cancer patients for decades, and that she has developed a logical and easy to understand cancer theory, I would have put all the other literature aside.

How did she develop her theory? Years of research on the part of this holistic thinking physician revealed that there were no findings in medical literature relative to a lack of adrenaline. In hindsight this is even harder to comprehend, because there are known underfunctions and overfunctions for all other hormones. Adrenaline is produced by the so-called chromaffin system in the body and it is the great antagonist of insulin in our body. But what actually happens when a person is subjected to stress over a long period of time and the body is no longer capable of producing enough adrenalin? This is the question that Dr. Fryda researched, and she found, for instance, with cancer patients the adrenalin level is very very low, sometimes it is almost zero. Since now insulin is the winner, so to speak, in the insulin vs. adrenalin match (insulin = sugar into the cell and adrenalin = sugar out of the cell), a healthy cell is swamped with sugar. However since cells that are full of sugar can no longer perform their normal activities, at some point the body is forced to employ other "sugar breakdown measures". Parallel to this process, the body continues to produce another hormone, noradrenaline, in sufficient quantities, consequently the oxygen supply in the outlying blood vessels is limited.

At this point a survival mechanism kicks in. The cells must get by with less oxygen and burn more sugar. They do this primarily by switching over to fermentation. However fermentation is a primitive method for obtaining energy. Although it does indeed burn a lot of sugar, it only supplies a little energy to the body. In addition, there is the fact that now much too much lactic acid rotating to the left (L-lactic acid) occurs, which first, increases the cell division rate, and second, significantly disturbs the acid base balance in the body.

However the cells have achieved the most important thing for survival: Sugar combustion through a higher rate of cell division and through fermentation processes. Here again it is evident that evolution has supplied our body with extraordinary systems that enable it to survive even under extreme stress conditions. From this perspective, initially a tumor is naturally something very healthy that prevents greater damage. Just think of what would happen to the body if it did not develop any cancer cells under these circumstances? Sooner or later we would go blind, our kidneys would fail, our blood vessels would break with severe bleeding, or we would fall into a coma. And now the general question: What is better? All these illnesses that result in death within a short time, or a tumor?

Naturally in her statements, Dr. Fryda also satisfies scientists who want to know about the processes occur in precise detail. She precisely explains which inflammation processes are blocked, why the immune defense by lymphocytes is no longer adequate, why cancer patients usually are "healthy" for years before the tumor is discovered, etc. However the most important thing for a cancer patient to understand is that his cancer illness has something to do with physical stress and/or psychic stress and that equalizing the acid base balance via detoxification and nutrition is extremely important.

I am always astonished to learn how successful therapies such as the Dr. Fryda's are suppressed for decades, or are dismissed as quackery by physician's circles, but also by groups of patients. As early as 1988 she published a study with 48 cancer patients. Considering that almost all the patients were people who were not given much to hope for by other physicians, and that of these 48 patients, 33 were still alive 5 years later (and almost all of this number were still alive in 2003), it is astonishing that none of Dr. Fryda's colleagues ever studied her therapy in more detail.

It certainly had nothing to do with her personally, as Dr. Fryda is a very charming and intelligent woman, who has dedicated herself to the welfare of her patients for years. In the adrenaline theory I found confirmations for my own considerations, which are: Cancer is a stress and energy problem. Cancer must be countered with a therapy of nutrition, detoxification, and stress relief. Cancer can only occur with an alkaline blood value and acidic tissue pH etc.

Even my thoughts relative to the frequently discussed (negative) immune increase are not only confirmed here, she also explains this process in detail.

The adrenalin approach to therapy:

Nutrition therapy with a lot of right-rotating lactic acids, anti-stress therapies, Dr. H. Dyckerhoff's regeneresen (regeneresens consist entirely of biologically active ribonucleic acids (RNA) Dr. Fryda started instructing German and English doctors in her therapy in 2004.

The theory of the 2nd liver

Disregarding allopathy, for which cancer is simply a genetic pre-disposition, which cannot be countered anyway, many researchers around the world are considering whether there is a reason that our body produces a tumor. Primarily psychological theories often view the tumor as a sensible product. Dr. Hamer has described this in detail or there is a theory in which the tumor is viewed as a new intellectual challenge, in the sense of: Now I've got to change something. This would also explain the increased incidence of cancer in the elderly.

However there are also very interesting theories that are mainly based on bodily processes. I would like to introduce one of these theories, as it is very impressive to me, and with it I can explain a lot of things that were not clear to me previously. But before I explain this thesis to you I would like to ask you something. Imagine three groups of mice. The first group is the healthy comparison group. The second group consists of mice that are in a preliminary stage of cancer, and the third group has already developed tumors. And now two cardinal questions come to bear:

1. **Which compare group has the best immune system?**

2. **Into which group of mice can the most poison be injected before they die?**

I would like to deal with both of these questions in more detail, or more precisely stated, discuss how most proponents of allopathic medicine would answer these questions, and then cite the correct answers, which may surprise you.

1. Which compare group has the best immune system?

1a = the group of mice in the preliminary stage

This question can be answered both ways. You could say that the immune system/defense system of our body is more active or stronger because it has to defend itself against the toxin, i.e. the cancer illness. But you could also say that the immune system is weaker because it is already fighting against the cancer cells. Even among allopathic practitioners there are varying opinions.

1b = the group of mice with tumors

This question is clearly answered in allopathic medicine, but also by non-conventional doctors. Mice with tumors have a poorer immune system. Actually all doctors are unified here. Don't we read in many books that cancer is a problem of the immune system and that cancer patients must do everything possible to stabilize or improve their immune system?

2. Into which group of mice can one inject the most toxins before they die?

2a = Depending on 1a many would say that the mice in the preliminary cancer stage can bear more or less toxin.

2b = for the group of mice with tumors, everyone is in agreement. Logically this group can bear less poison because the immune system is already weakened by the tumor.

But what if a tumor actually occurs in our body because our old detoxification systems like liver, kidneys, lungs, and skin, either no longer function, or they have collected too many toxins? Then the mice with tumors would be able to bear a lot more toxins than healthy mice! And this is precisely what the nutrition scientist Dr. Catherine Cousmine published decades ago. In her work she demonstrated that mice in the preliminary cancer stage can be given only 34% of the total quantity of toxins that healthy mice can be bear.

On the other hand mice that have already developed tumors can be given 200% of the toxin quantity that can be given to healthy mice. Even mice with transplanted tumors were able to bear higher quantities of toxins. Not as well as with tumors that the mice had developed themselves, but all the same they were able to bear significantly more than the healthy mice.

If the tumors are cut out, then 1g of the tumor mass is even cable of neutralizing fifteen times(!) the quantity of toxin. With previous vaccinations, Dr. Cousmine was even able to increase this number by a factor of 90!

In the body only liver cells have a comparable capability of neutralizing toxins. From this viewpoint, a tumor functions, so to speak, as a second liver in our body. It can neutralize toxins in a manner similar to the liver and perhaps it is even capable of neutralizing certain substances more productively than the liver. However if we accept these incontrovertible facts, then we must also accept the conclusions that are derived from these facts:

1. No operation on the tumor, certainly not before an intensive detoxification therapy has been concluded. Removing the tumor would mean removing a portion of the necessary detoxification possibilities from the body. In this process we force the body to produce a new tumor. By the way this would also be the answer to the question: Why do most people always have metastases in the liver and the lungs? The body builds a supplemental detoxification organ precisely at those points where it is most urgently needed, in our liver and in our lungs. By the way most people are not aware that next to our liver, it is our lungs which perform the most detoxification work.

2. People with cancer do not need immune increase. The fact is that in the diagnosis most cancer patients do not have objective deficits in their blood relative to their immune system. And even if this were to be proven in the course of the illness then the question can still be asked whether external intervention with mistletoe, thyme, etc would not be effective.

3. The incredible detoxification capacities demonstrated by tumors explain why allopathic practitioners often are unsuccessful in destroying cancer cells, even using such strong toxins as carboplatin. Then there is still the issue of the intelligence of the cancer cells. If our body is capable of producing cells as intelligent as tumor cells, whose task is neutralization of toxins, then first, it is crazy to attack these cells with toxins, and second, we are forced to assume that the cells will develop a defense mechanism (resistance) should they not already have one.

4. Holistic practitioners have often experienced what "miracles" can be effected by intensive detoxification measures. These facts have not just been known since Pfarrer Kneipp (Bavarian priest and hydrotherapist 1821-1887), they have been part of the history of medicine for a long time. However with her experiments Dr. Cousmine has supplied a theoretical, and above-all, an easily-verified foundation.

Personal summary:
When I read Dr. Cousmine's work for the first time, I was very happy. Her work fits precisely into my picture of cancer, or it also explains a lot of what I and many other therapists have experienced. For example, patients who did not allow themselves to be operated on, and were healed. Therapists who, based on their years of experience with cancer patients, were mainly against operations (which previously I considered bad). Studies that showed that increased metastases occurs

after operations. Studies proving that tumors grow faster after the first chemotherapies (naturally because more cells are required for detoxification), and much, much more. But also the life and effectiveness of Dr. Cousmine have brought the correctness of her theories home to me because she helped many people who were seriously ill, and detoxification and nutrition where her principle therapies. Until her work and her total theoretical approach relative to tumors are disproved, we cannot ignore her research. If she is right, then the current therapies can no longer be maintained. How come no one researches in this direction? Don't we (meaning "alternative" doctors as well) need to rethink everything.

Therapy approach in accordance with Dr. Cousmine: Nutrition therapies and detoxification.

Dr. Hamer's New Medicine

These days, whoever writes about Dr. Hamer runs the risk of being thrown into the same pot with the "greatest quack in oncology"; particularly since Dr. Hamer was arrested again on the 9th of September 2004 in Spain and was extradited to France on the 20th of October. The official reason given by the French government for his arrest, as stated in the warrant, is: "Incitement against allopathy and instigation to new medicine, with the objective of practice".

Unofficially however, totally different things are involved, because if the same "legal charges" were brought against all people, then thousands of authors, including myself, and hundreds of therapists would also be immediately imprisoned. You can tell how important this issue is by the fact that not a single mass media (TV, print media, etc.) in all of Europe was brave enough to report it. In contrast to 1997 when Dr. Hamer was first incarcerated, that time in Germany, now there are thousands of healed patients, and more importantly, supporters of Dr. Hamer. Negative reports in the mass media would have resulted in the exact opposite This is why the "tactic of ignorance" is being used, as it has been used in many other cases. This is the same tactic that has functioned perfectly for decades in allopathic practice. Or can you think of any other reason why your family doctor has never heard of the successful cancer therapies that can be found in the world?

Without wanting to rank myself above Dr. Hamer, I must say that up to this point I have only met a few people who have really studied the theory of New Medicine intensively. (By the way since 2004 Dr. Hamer has called his therapy, German New Medicine, which I personally consider to be very unfortunate). Usually what is said is that Dr. Hamer is a crackpot, a dreamer, a fraud; however I never hear phrases

like: "His 3rd criterion of the iron rule is incorrect because…".
When I visited Dr. Ryke Geerd Hamer in his Spanish exile, I found that the man sitting across from me was certainly not a crackpot, rather he was a man who has intensively studied medicine, and oncology in particular. However what impressed me most was becoming acquainted with people who told me that they are still alive thanks to Dr. Hamer. Also impressive is the fact that Dr. Hamer is completely willing to prove his theories under university conditions at any time.

All that would be required to prove or disprove his theories is a university, a few professors, and a few patients, who would have to be interviewed. If all these proceedings were done publicly then we could very easily dismiss Dr. Hamer as a quack. Although Dr. Hamer had already made this offer many times, in recent years the "more convenient path" through the legal system was always pursued. What is it that all doctors are really so afraid of? Permit me to briefly explain Dr. Hamer's theory and then you will be able to answer the question for yourself.

In Dr. Hamer's view, cancer, and other disturbances as well, are caused by a biological conflict. The term biological conflict in this regard means a serious, acute, conflict-experience shock for which a person was not prepared. The problem in this regard is that, which may be a conflict for you may mean absolutely nothing to me, and vice versa. This conflict then has impact on the three levels of psyche, brain, and organ. Depending on how a person experiences the conflict, this conflict (the energy) manifests itself in the brain in the form of so-called Hamer Herds, which according to Dr. Hamer can be identified in the CT scan. And this is where the problem comes in. From this point on the organism switches over to permanent sympathicotonia, in English: Constant stress.

Dr. Hamer divides cancer types into groups that belong to the various blastodermic layers: thus ectoderm (external), mesoderm (middle) and entoderm (inner). Depending on the blastodermic layer to which an organ belongs, for example stomach and intestine belong to the entoderm layer, the conflicts cause different tumors or different growth.

There is also a significant difference depending on the phase of the illness in which the tumor is detected. According to Dr. Hamer app. 40% of all tumors are detected in an encapsulated form and should be left alone. A further distinction is whether the patient is a in stage before or after conflict resolution. If you would like to study the theory of New Medicine in detail I recommend the book: Legacy of a New Medicine, volumes 1 and 2 (only in German). Volume 1 is particularly important for those with cancer. You can also read about the theory in detail at the websites, www.newmedicine.ca.

By the way this is not first time that I have been massively attacked just for mentioning Dr. Hamer. However the data that he submits speak for him not against him. Several universities (Vienna, Trnava, Düsseldorf ...) have confirmed his work, and the question remains; why doesn't somebody publicly discredit him, if it so easy to do so? There are many "official sources" even in the alternative scene, that permanently attack Dr. Hamer, however up to this point no one has been successful in refuting the New Medicine.

On the contrary there are more and more allopathic studies that confirm Dr. Hamer's ideas, such as the work of Dr. Alexander Friedmann from the University Clinic for Psychiatry in Vienna, a man no one could accuse of being a friend of Dr. Hamer (published in the Medical Tribune No. 8, February 18th 2004). This work deals with the fact that the most serious psychic conflicts, we could also say energetic manifestations, leave visible changes in the brain. The fact that "psychic conflicts" can also been seen in the brain, is slowly but surely being confirmed around the world by more and more brain researchers thanks to functional MRT or dou-

ble spin echo proton spectroscopy (keyword: brain imaging) –
20 years after Dr. Hamer.

Psyche and body – Dr. Hamer's discovery?

Of course not; Dr. Hamer has never made this claim. All the
same more and more people understand the influence the psyche has on our body. As early as 1701 the English physician
Grendon published "Enquiries into nature, knowledge, and
cure of cancer", which dealt with the correlations between
psyche and cancer. This study as followed in 1846 by Dr.
Walsche in his, "The Nature and Treatment of Cancer" and at
the latest when Dr. Snow treated 250 women with cancer in
the London Cancer Hospital and described in his book Cancer
and the Cancer Process, that more than 200 of these women
had noticeable psychic stress, there should really have been
more research in this direction. Also the work of Dr.
Grossarth Maticek from Heidelberg relative to cancer and
psyche clearly shows such a connection.

What really disappoints me is that the turn of the century
ushered in the century of psychoanalysis in Europe. Today
there are hundreds of thousands of psychologists and psychoanalysts building on the work of Freud, Jung, Adler, Berne,
etc., who should be capable of better understanding the correlations between cancer and psyche.

But where are all these therapists? Why do we have to wait
for Americans like Le Shan, Siegel, Simonton, etc. to come
over and explain to us Europeans how important the psyche is
for cancer? In this book you can read a lot about energy and
psyche. The importance of this relationship cannot be overemphasized, and from this point of view I concur 100% with Dr.
Hamer.

If you carefully read the paragraph on the "because – in
spite of" theory, then you will also understand why Dr.
Hamer's New Medicine simply must help in many cases. Two

points are conspicuous in this regard. First, he does not injure any patients with his therapy, and thus he naturally supports the self-healing forces. The second and at least equally important point, particularly for cancer patients, is that Dr. Hamer takes the fear away from his patients. As you will yet learn in this book is that fear, or the diagnosis of cancer, often has a more destructive effect than does the tumor itself.

However Dr. Hamer explains their illnesses to his patients, how they can return to health, and what symptoms they will have during the self-healing process. When these symptoms then occur, even if these include new tumors or an ascites (water in the stomach), then his patients gain more and more confidence in their self-healing processes and thus become healthier.

However there are also points where I disagree with Dr. Hamer. One is certainly in the area of nutrition. Doubtless the self-healing processes are the most important, but when we have a tumor in the body, then concurrently we have purely bodily problems such as an increased lactic acid production, and a person with cancer must deal with this. When Dr. Hamer says that what a person eats is absolutely irrelevant, then I can understand this very well within his own explanation structure of the New Medicine. However for persons with cancer this can be very dangerous and a nutrition therapy will at least support the self-healing process, if not trigger it.

A second area where we do not agree concerns the explanation possibilities of the New Medicine. For example, in his book, Dr. Hamer describes that lung cancer has nothing to do with cigarettes. Although in this case as well I completely understand his manner of explanation, the whole contains a very dangerous component in the form of: "If everything is psychological, then from this point on I can immediately smoke, drink, and just eat fast food." This is certainly an extreme position, and most people would not react this way. However it is a fact that Dr. Hamer does not adequately deal with this point in his works, and this can lead to dangerous misunderstandings.

There is also a big difference in whether a "mortal conflict" encounters a healthy lung or an asbestos or tar lung. At the latest when the tumor is supposed to be decreasing in size, then it is "more than helpful" if well-functioning lung tissue exists Given this argument, which naturally applies to other organs as well, the New Medicine can be harmonized very well with detoxification and healthy nutrition.

Another thing that I cannot understand is why there are no studies of the many Dr. Hamer supporters and Dr. Hamer patients. I have absolutely no doubt that Dr. Hamer can present enough cases and with only 10 cases of healed ductal adenocarcinoma of the pancreas his adherents could take the wind out of the sails of all doubters.

Moreover I only know a few therapists who would be capable of diagnosing cancer based on a CT scan. Since according to their own statements Dr. Hamer or his students can do this, then it would be quite a simple matter to demonstrate this publicly. This would certainly also be legally feasible, and nobody can hide behind the words, "But I would be arrested". My hope is that something will finally move forward in this area, and I concur with Dr. Hamer's own statement that he will retract all his New Medicine theories, if just one person is successful in refuting him.

The New Medicine approach to therapy:

Conflict resolution and explanation of the development of the illness.

Additional information: In the meantime there are many other therapy directions that are based on Dr. Hamer, such as Meta-Medicine, biological decoding, Holo-Medicine etc.

The frequency theory

How do the trillions of cells in our body actually communicate? How does a cell know what kind of cell it actually is? A lot is being said these days about our genes, but one thing is certain: Normally we have the same genes in all of our cells, regardless of whether these cells are in our knee or in our eye. It is absolutely impossible that all of this information is stored in our genes. While morphogenetic fields are being researched in Russia and in China knowledge of meridians (energy paths) has been part of the traditional education of all doctors for millennia, in the modern west these "things" are still relegated to the "esoteric corner" as is cell-to-cell communication via photons (light).

Even if we still have not found any sure answers to these important questions in the 21st century, the statement can still be made that light or waves play a significant role. What Dr. Rife started in 1930, the physicist Schrödinger first expressed with his term of inner order, and what is continued in the modern photon and frequency research, in may quarters is referred to as the future of medicine.

Today we know that in the cell membrane there is a so-called potassium-sodium pump in almost of our cells that generates energy, and indeed that energy that we require for life. For energy practitioners, among which are frequency scientists, there are no illnesses in the medical sense of the word, but only two states, that cells can be in; energetically normal or energetically abnormal. According to American, Russian, and German researchers, thus abnormally functioning cells (e.g. cancer cells) withdraw up to 60 times the normal amount of energy without generating energy themselves. This is also the reason why a small tumor of consisting of only a few hundred cubic centimeters can cause so many difficulties for an adult. It is not the tumor alone that is responsible for the illness, but rather the abnormal energy withdrawal from the healthy cells.

This is precisely the point where the frequency theory comes in, its task is to bring this depolarization (change in the cell voltage) back into order. The cell membrane, consisting of a double layer of phospholipids (fats and phosphates), which is approximately 10 nanometers in thickness, forms the skin of the cell. Membrane proteins are integrated in this membrane. These "antenna" (see also Dr. Budwig's oil-protein diet) or receptors transfer sensor inputs to the cell, this means that the cell establishes contact with the "outside world" through these antenna, and determines what will come into the cell and what will leaves the cell. Consequently cell behavior is controlled via stimuli from the cell environment and not through the genes in the cell.

Each receptor is calibrated to receive only one type of signal from the environment, and to respond to that type of signal. Through this physical filter a cell is capable of ascertaining its environment and absorbing the necessary substances. The membrane, which is protected by fat, acts like an electric insulator which enables the cytoplasm (cell content) to accept a negative charge condition, as opposed to the layer that surrounds it.

Thus the cell acts like a battery with a minus pole and a plus pole. For the cell the change of its energy state is an electrical signal, which can activate or block specific genetic programs, for example. Cells recognize the surroundings by converting energies of the electromagnetic spectrum into biologically useful information. Different receptor proteins transform light, tones, x-rays, radio oscillations, microwaves, and extremely low frequencies (ELF), into cell combinations by activating effector proteins, which in turn can induce depolarization of the membrane, activation of the enzyme system of the cytoplasm, or a regulating of genetic processes.

The energy environment controls the behavior and well-being of cells and tissues in this manner. This energy regulation always takes priority over the regulation of cell activities through chemical influences.

The frequency approach to therapy:

According to frequency therapists every illness occurs through a reduction of energy production on the part of the potassium-sodium pump. In practical terms this means that if we succeed in supplying the body with the correct frequencies/waves, we can basically cure any illness. What today still sounds like a utopia can very quickly change the entire world of medicine.

Interesting in this regard is also the aspect that the mitochondria theory, the New Medicine theory, balance theory, and frequency theory, are not mutually exclusive – rather they are totally complementary. There is no reason why the disturbances of the potassium-sodium pump cannot occur through disturbances as they are explained in the other theories. It is just the approach to therapy that is different, since frequency therapists believe that it suffices to transfer the correct frequencies to the body so that it can heal itself.

Personally I concur with this opinion. Unfortunately we are not far enough along to understand which frequencies or which transmission possibilities are required for healings to occur. If all the research funding did not go into still more chemotherapy logs, then we would certainly be very close to really effective solutions.

The balance theory

This theory states that a tumor occurs because certain cells can no longer perform the tasks they are supposed to perform, and consequently they attempt to create a balance through over-production, (by the way, this is explained by others, including Dr. Hamer, in somewhat different terms).

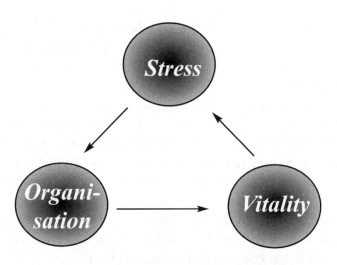

The trigger is always a stress situation, which can be of a bodily nature (poor nutrition, radiation exposure, toxins etc.) and/or a psychic nature. This stress situation prevents a cell from organizing itself in its usual manner (e.g. cell membrane voltage, mitochondrial activity, etc.) This lessens the vital cell functions and the cell tries to find its own ways out of this situation. Unfortunately this "attempt" leads to more stress and the cancer circuit cannot be stopped.

We recognize this problem with the fatty liver syndrome. With disturbances of the liver, e.g. excessive alcohol consumption, the liver cells are under permanent stress, which no longer allows the liver to organize itself. Consequently the liver can no longer perform its detoxification functions and produces more cells in the hope that these new cells can "help out".

In order to be sure, our liver does something very intelligent and produces many more cells than before and thus clearly increases in size. It is precisely this process that could also be taking place with cancer cells. Since certain cells are disturbed in their function, the body attempts, in spite of this disturbance, to perform the tasks that are intended for these cells, and produces "like crazy" to more and more of the same type cells. Unfortunately this excess production results in cells that are not 100% identical to the original cells, and which as a consequence can cause great damage to neighboring cell structures.

You can easily test this theory for yourself. Do not give your plants any water for a brief period, and you will note they grow faster then the "properly nourished plants". If you believe that conclusions cannot be drawn from plants that apply to people, then you are mistaken in this case. Do you know how scientists generate laboratory clones with today's genetic engineering? It is not by providing a sufficient supply of nutrient solution, rather precisely the opposite is the case. If you want human cells to divide faster then you let them starve. This is precisely what probably happens with a tumor. The cells are "hungry" because they are not getting enough of what they need. Applying this theory it is easy to see why nutrition and detoxification play such an important role with cancer.

The balance theory approach to therapy:

The most important thing is to exclude all stress factors. This naturally includes the bodily factors like teeth, intestines, skin, mesenchyme tissue, scars, etc., and the psychological factors. Considering allopathy treats cancer with toxins, and considering that psychological stress through the diagnosis and the lack of sensitivity of many doctors, then from the perspective of the balance theory one can only say that everything that could be done wrong is also being done wrong in allopathic practice.

The Reich theory

The famous doctor Wilhem Reich, who opposed his teacher Sigmund Freud and wrote a lot about freeing natural sexuality, was one of the first who considered cancer to be an energy deficit. He describes in detail how cancer cells have lost the relationship to the whole (body) and that their energy charge is no longer sufficient to handle the tasks intended for them.

Naturally, as a psychoanalyst, it was clear to Dr. Reich that such cell disorders are the result of great emotional blockage. What Reich only described in theory, Dr. Albert Popp was able to prove in the laboratory recently – namely the changed radiation of biophotons from cancer cells. Also Kirlian photography (photos that are made in a dark room, in a high-frequency field) brings more and more verifications for this theory to light.

We have Reich to thank that today we know that our immune system does not just produce antibodies, and that white blood cells eat up antigens, but that there is also a bioenergetic immune defense. This means that how strongly a cell is charged with energy is very important. His work with blood cells clearly showed that they are capable of withdrawing energy from pathogens and thus they are capable of killing them. If the blood cell is too weak then the energy flow towards the blood cell does not occur and the pathogen can continue to spread out. Interestingly enough this applies for pathogens from outside as well as from inside after a structural breakdown process.

Reich was able to determine that an immense number of T-bacilli (Reich's definition) are present in the blood of cancer patients, and that the few red blood cells quickly break apart. Since logically these T-bacilli withdraw a lot of energy, a cancer patient also becomes more cachectic (weaker), and dies due to this loss of energy (see the frequency theory in this regard). Every oncologist is aware of this problem, since most cancer patients do not die because of the size of the tumor, rather they die of this process.

Many unusual successes (also called spontaneous healings or miracles, by allopathy) can be explained scientifically with Reich's theory. I can also confirm this theory as I have personally shaken hands with many people who have returned to health through this "energy work".

The Reich theory approach to therapy:

Detoxification, nutrition, energy work with the orgone accumulator (a specially built box that a person can sit in).

The parasite theory

The word parasite comes from the Greek and means, one who eats at the table of another. Colloquially, freeloaders are also referred to as parasites, i.e. life forms that live at other's costs. Thus, for example, the Russian scientist, Tamara Lebedewa, has maintained for years that what which pathologists make out to be cancer cells under the microscope are really trichomonads. At first glance this seems to be absolute scientific nonsense, a second look however reveals that this is not so crazy at all, particularly in light of all of the research done by Ms. Lebedewa and her Russian colleagues.

The thought that parasites are responsible for cancer is not all that new. Karl Michael described this almost 200 years ago, and in 1893 Pfeiffer wrote that cancer was induced by the parasite amoeba sporidium. In the last century it was then Professor Koch in Germany, Newjadomskij in Russia, and Hulda Clark in America (see under cancer therapies: Clark), who again and again came back to a parasite theory,

Trichomonads are small flagellates that can exist in three different stages: in the amphitrichous stage, as a kind of amoeba, and in cyst form. Because this parasite reproduces asexually, each time a totally different organism occurs. With the aid of hyaluronidase (an enzyme) these parasites can wander around the entire body. Due to their various forms of appearance, naturally they also have various antigen characteristics. What is phenomenal is that they eliminate antigens on their surface which are absolutely identical to antigens of human origin. This naturally irritates the immune system and would explain why our immune system is so powerless against tumors.

According to Lebedewa's theory a tumor cell is a non-amphitrichous type of parasitic flagellate. Thus a tumor is nothing more than a collection of non-amphitrichous trichomonads and their daughter cells that separate. But why do trichomonads suddenly form large groups? There are also theories that explain this. First it may be the case that daughter cells do not cut themselves off, secondly there can be a fight for survival with the host (person), which is why as many new cells as possible must be formed, and third, naturally it makes sense that a group has better chances for survival then do lone warriors.

Based on the theory of evolution however we must ask ourselves three questions when parasites are involved:

1. Are parasites always our enemies, or do they perhaps assume important tasks in our body.

2. Which came first? The parasite or the cancer cell?

I have discussed parasites, mainly with Dr. Budwig, who as early as 1959 in what is probably most extensive book, <u>The Fat Syndrome,</u> reported in detail about the "wormlike life forms", as she called them, in the hemogram. She showed me microscope photos, how these life forms were increasingly degenerated, and then later were no longer to be found a few days after using the oil-protein-diet. However at the latest when Bavarian cell researchers at the Max-von-Pettenkofer-Institute discovered tiny protozoa and published their findings (Ärztliche Praxis: "Ungewöhnliche, korpuskuläre Elemente im Blut!", (Unusual, corpuscular elements in the blood!), and at the very latest when Dr. Alfons Weber published his research films, everyone should have understood that there is more in our blood than just the blood cells that are usually cited.

But just as the allopathic practitioners consider the tumor to be something malignant, now many non-conventional doctors make the mistake and vilify the parasites. Just consider for yourself. Can it be that all of these "little creatures" live inside us permanently and are only waiting to do us harm. Just as bacteria are not bad, neither are all parasites bad. Naturally bacteria or viruses can also harm us, but this depends more on the milieu than it does on the germ. Anyone can see this for himself under the microscope. "Damaging wormlike life forms" are suddenly no longer visible through a simple conversion of nutrition and/or detoxification therapies, or in other words: through a change of the milieu. Particularly the pH value of the blood plays a major role here and since everyone is talking about the deacidification of the body, I must tell you that parasites are happiest in the blood if the pH value is too high and not too low. This is precisely why acidification of the blood through d-lactic acid is very important.

Naturally the above does not exclude the fact that parasites can cause symptoms, particularly in large numbers, and that through short-term "antiparasitic measures" these symptoms can be also be fought effectively. But we must be careful to not draw the opposite conclusion, which is that we must kill the parasites. Milieu changes are much more important, they enable us to live in a healthy symbiosis with parasites. It is certainly utopian to believe that we can avoid parasites. First this is impossible and second it is absolutely unnecessary.

The parasite approach to therapy:

Detoxification, nutrition, anti-parasite medication.

Acid base theory

A lot has been written in recent years about the importance of the acid base balance, also with reference to cancer. However, when we finally have to explain why for cancer patients, the pH value of the blood increases while it decreases in the interstitial tissue, even the most basic logical explanation patterns are missing (the pH increases in the blood because the chlorine from NAC1 is intercellularly bound on proteins and the basis sodium forms alkaline salts).

I would like to introduce you to the work of Erich Rouka, who treated people who were ill with cancer for many years and theorized about the cause of cancer. In 1970 Rouka described how the increasing glycolysis (decomposition of sugar to lactic acid), for cells that were subjected to stress via an inflammation impulse, contributes to normal cells becoming cancer cells. He was able to demonstrate that it was precisely this major acid production that keeps cancer cells alive, and at the same time damages the healthy cells.

As opposed to a "healthy inflammation" where there is pus formation, the protein fragments decompose only into larger proteins, like albumoses, peptones, or peptides, which then serve as components for new cancer cells. Moreover new inflammation stimuli, and naturally pains, as well occur through enervation (nerve cell stimulation) of the adjacent tissue. Rouka bases his hypotheses on work from Borst or Warburg, who at the beginning of the last century determined that embryonic cells have a major anaerobic phase, and the surface of the cells shows acidification similar to cancer cells. This situation only changes by growing into the blood areas of the placenta. The infiltrative (growing into a different tissue) type of growth however was only possible though acidification of the cell surface. Naturally this knowledge also confirms statements of many researchers, who again and again point out that all of our cells have stored anaerobic survival systems in the genes.

With cancer the issue of cell division rates always plays a role. Today we know that the pH value in the serum increases with age and in a parallel manner the cell division rate decreases. In many studies researchers have been able to determine that with increased cell division, an increased glycolysis and a decreasing pH value are also present. Researchers only need to put cells in cultures under pH value 7.4 and the cells will quickly start to divide. From this we can conclude that the increased glycolysis and the decreasing pH value are a consequence and not the cause. Also instructive here is the fact that cancer cells do not have a greater cell increase in a familiar milieu. However if the cells are given a piece of muscle tissue, then the division rate increases massively and the cells infiltrate into the muscle tissue just as in the human body, because the muscle tissue supplies them with the necessary nutrients. By the way in this case growth runs parallel to lactic acid production.

However Rouka also brings the current mutation theory into harmony with the previously described facts. First he describes the fact that cells have an astonishing ability to adapt themselves to changed situations (in this regard see also the Cousmine theory). This is important because practitioners today refer to non-differentiated cells and under the microscope pathologists identify these cells as cancer. According to Rouka however these are nothing more than cells, which due to certain conditions, (toxins, radiation, parasites, pathogens, aging processes etc.) have adapted to the changed environment.

It is known that our DNA (Deoxyribonucleic acid) so-to-speak determines the type of cell via collaboration with messenger RNS (Ribonucleic acids), the recombinant RNA, and the ribosomes. But the DNA is by no means a rigid non-changing structure, rather it constantly obtains information via the recombinant mechanisms of the RNA. Thus adapted inherited material occurs via enzymatic processes, or in other words, the inherited material has adopted the increased acidification as a new characteristic of the cell. This in turn means that this mutation of the cell naturally also allows a new messenger RNA to occur. At the beginning of this process a new cell generation occurs with an ever-increasing acidification (e.g. as with leukemia cells) finally producing a cell with a significantly greater capacity for acidification = the cancer cell.

Naturally at this point a vicious cycle also occurs, since the cancer cells not only trigger an increased rate of division, but rather they also allow the connective tissue to become ever thicker, so that fewer and fewer oxygen molecules and vital substances penetrate. In addition, the body sends white blood cells to the occurrence location, these white blood cells also consume oxygen, where there was already an insufficient supply. Naturally from this perspective increasing the immune cells, regardless of the compounds through which this is accomplished, is extremely questionable. Today we must assume (as we can also see under the microscope) that with cancer cells adaptation processes have also taken place in the genes, as this is the only way to explain why cancer cells survive the extreme acidifications. Studies by the researcher Werth, who blocked the formation of cytochromoxidase-c with malachite green (cytochromoxidase-c is an enzyme that is important for oxygen utilization and which is referred to again and again by Dr. Budwig and Dr. Seeger in all their work) also speak for this. She was able to demonstrate that when laboratory animals were given malachite green over several generations, the inherited material took on a lessened production of cytochromoxidase-c as a new characteristic.

The researcher Strong has also made contributions in this area. He injected 1 mg of methylcholanthrenes into animals for 60 days, and he did it over 21 generations. Thereafter one group of offspring were separated and these were not given any more methylcholanthrene. Of 797 animals, 528 developed spontaneous tumors (in the control group the number was three animals). The reduced utilization of oxygen also resulted in many tumors, i.e. Strong was able to prove which mutations lead to cancer, and that such mutations are adaptations to changed situations, in this case, a toxin.

I find Roukas statements and also his conclusions (nutrition and detoxification) very coherent. Particularly as his theories are substantiated in daily work with cancer patients, and they explain much of what seems so incomprehensible to lay people. Also impressive is the combination of the mitochondria theory and the mutation theory, which are not mutually exclusive, according to Rouka.

Erich Rouka's approach to therapy:

Detoxification, extreme deacidiciation, nutrition.

Other theories

Naturally there are still many other theories, such as the anthroposophic theories of Rudolf Steiner, in which the astral body can no longer penetrate the physical body. Pischinger and Heine also have an enlightening theory with their description of the morphogenetic inductors or the breakdown of the matrix. I do not want to deal with all the theories of traditional Chinese medicine or the Ayurveda here as I believe they would exceed the scope of this book. It is important to me that you understand that the "mutation theory", which is accepted by almost all doctors as "scientific fact", is not nearly as scientific as it is presented to be, and that there are other theories that are far more enlightening.

As Erich Rouka describes very well, and as we all know today, naturally there are changes of the cell nucleus. However consequently to now go and act like all the other changes are only a "repercussion" of this DNA change, can only be called ignorance and arrogance in light of today's knowledge. Unfortunately we must experience every day just to what point denial of "genuine" science has brought us.

The next time you hear something about a "malignant" or "degenerated" cell, which is supposed to be responsible for cancer, then at least you will know that these statements at best reflect the knowledge of the person making them, and nothing more.

3

Diagnosis
Cancer

When is cancer actually cancer?

For many years we have been told that we can get a better handle on the "problem of cancer" thanks to new preventative examinations. But the only thing that one can get a better handle on are the significantly increased revenues for the industry that manufactures the X-ray devices, PAP tests, etc. An additional advantage for the industry is that the statistics look better. Since the introduction of mammography women with breast cancer survive much longer. The truth however is that the numbers naturally look better, because the tumor is detected earlier, and as a consequence logically there are more women that still live 5 years after detection of the tumor. In reality in spite of millions of tax dollars, not a single woman's life is saved. Quite the contrary. The high rate of wrong diagnoses contributes to the fact that women in particular are unnecessarily mutilated.

In British Columbia/Canada, in a state where a PAP smear test is made for all women, the death rate from cervical cancer is just as high as it is in all the other states. In 1988, another study showed that within 2 years almost 50% of all abnormal smears regressed to normal status. In the British Journal of Cancer Research the authors presented a study showing that up to 60% of the results were wrong. It really became embarrassing in 1987, when in England 45,000 smears were re-analyzed and it was determined that the diagnosis was wrong in 911 of them.

Please consider that serious measures, including total operations and chemotherapies are initiated based on such a test; measures which then cause cancer where previously there were healthy cells. The situation with mammography is similar. In 1994, even the National Cancer Institute in the USA retracted its previous recommendation that women under 50 years of age should have a mammogram. Realy the truth is that the National Cancer Institute had to do this, although its financial sponsors were certainly not happy, because various studies demonstrated the negative effects. If you do not find this convincing then you should read the article in the British Medical Journal in 1994 by Susan Ott, in which she reports how Swedish researchers observed more than 350 women, for whom a mammogram lead to an incorrect diagnosis. She reported that these women had to subject themselves to 1,112 doctor visits, 397 biopsies!, and 187 additional mammograms, just to finally be told that they were never sick. It becomes really unpleasant when you know that in 1994 the Canadian government determined in examining 50,000 women from 40-49 years of age, that in the group that received mammograms, 33% more women died than died in the compare group. Indeed more tumors were detected in the mammography group, however this did not turn out to be positive for the women in question, as the result clearly shows. In passing I would also like to mention that in the meantime this result has been confirmed by additional studies in Sweden and in the USA.

Doesn't everyone know that X-rays generate cancer? Is it not logical to assume that when sensitive tissue, such as the female breast is pressed with great pressure between two plates, that this can lead to minimal injuries? Doesn't every doctor know by now that through mammograms cancer cells possibly present in other tissue parts are pressed, and that this precisely causes what one wants to prevent? J.P. van Netten from the Royal Jubilee Hospital in London demonstrated this fact in a 1994 study, when he was able to prove that incidence of so-called ductal carcinoma in situ (DCIS: ductuales carcinoma in situ, in English: breast cancer in a very early stage in the milk duct) increased by 200% through the mammograms.

Many women still believe that preventative appointments are important. Regardless of whether you are one of these that so believe, this preventative care also creates fears, which as we know today, can generate cancer. Let me be more precise in listing the benefit of preventative treatment using the example of mammography. First there is the question of starting when and how often. This is evaluated very differently, and even reviewing the best statistics there are no advantages for women under 50 and over 70 years of age.

In the evaluation of the data it is happily "forgotten" that women who participate in the early detection measures, usually come from the higher social classes and for this reason have a higher life expectancy. In addition, women are not told that slow-growing tumors are more easily discovered than are fast-growing tumors, as these naturally remain longer in a stage in which they can be discovered. These tumors naturally also have a better prognosis even without early detection.

The advantage of mammography is often demonstrated with studies, which prove that women apparently have lived longer, if they were permanently examined. Let us take a closer look at this. One of these positive studies is by Dr. Nyström. In this study over a 10-year period 4 women out of 1000, who were not examined died. In the group of women who had mammograms, 3 out of 1000 died. Expressed in other words, 996 women were subjected to radioactive rays, so that one could survive. To a marketing manager for mammography devices these numbers have a totally different meaning. He would write: "Through mammograms 25% fewer women die (3 instead of 4)". Be careful reading statistics.

If we look at all the numbers of the study then we notice that of 100,000 non-examined women, 89,550 survived, and of the examined women 89,020 survived. To be mean we could say that in the group of women who were examined, 520 more died. To be fair one must say however, that these numbers are statistically insignificant and one can assume that in both groups the same number die whether they are pre-examined or not.

But your doctor will not tell you about another examination of 26,057 women (Kerlikowske). In total 25,858 women did not have breast cancer, but the mammography was negative in only 24,187 cases. This means that 1,671! women were told that they probably had cancer and even if many were not told, then I am sure that almost all of them thought so, or at least had to deal with strong fears. Interestingly the mammogram was also negative for 20 of 199 women although they did have breast cancer.

If we add the 179 women for whom it was later determined that they had breast cancer, then we get the number of 1850 women with a tumor finding. In total, however only 199 women had breast cancer, or in other words, only 1 in 10 women with a pathological finding really had breast cancer. The number of incorrect findings is alarmingly high for women under 50.

Have you ever read in a newspaper about the enormous damage that not only women have through these examinations? Or how often have you read about what women had to deal with due to an incorrect mammogram report? How many women would die with their tumor (and not because of their tumor) without ever having any greater problems (similar to prostate cancer), and who actually discusses the issue that for many women it is a major problem having to live the last years of their lives with the knowledge of having cancer, with all the associated bodily and psychological problems.

DCIS is another term that plays a major role in breast cancer. This is what is often discovered in mammograms. Even allopathic practitioners (see Silverstein, Brit. Med. J. 317: 1998, 734–739 in this regard) estimate today that only half of the DCIS develop into invasive breast cancer after 10-20 years. Even a lay person can understand now why the 5 year statistics for breast cancer look so good. Another problem associated with mammography is also happily kept quiet: The radiation stress through the examination. Discussion usually concerns the most modern devices and the fact that radiation exposure is less than that experienced on vacation in the mountains. However no one mentions that Dr. Mettler in 1996 published that one woman in 10,000 will die through the radiation stress. According to estimates by Jung (1998), the additional risk of getting breast cancer through regular mammography is between 0.015% to 0.045% - in other words this means 1.5-4-5 women per 10,000. In other words this means for you: if you are one of the 0.015%, then your risk of getting cancer through a mammogram is precisely 100%.

Nor is the following mentioned: Although my wife would never have a mammogram, my wife and I pay for this expensive examination every month with my insurance premiums. In 1995, the well-known Rand Corporation calculated that between 166,000 Euro and 1,480,000 Euro must be spent to discover a single incidence of breast cancer illness. Let's be honest how long do we really want to pay for all this nonsense?

And men?

Men as well are not protected from unauthorized attacks. A study published in 1994 in the British Medical Journal proved that PSA (Prostate Specific Antigen) test, preferred above all others, is not nearly as precise as is always and everywhere maintained. In this study 336 men developed prostate cancer with a normal PSA value, while only 47% of the men who already had prostate cancer showed a higher value. OK let's be honest, how do you feel when you learn that every 2nd PSA test in this study was wrong.

We should also look at prostate cancer from a different perspective. In 1995, the American Cancer Society described in their prostate cancer information that cancer cells were found in the prostate of 15% of all men examined. This number increased to 40% in 70 year olds and to 50% for 80-year olds. First we should consider how active these cancer cells really are, and the PSA test certainly does not tell us this. P.J. Scerret impressively describes in his work, "Screening for Prostate Cancer", that only 1% of these cancer cells form into a cancer tumor, and just 0.3% of these prostate tumors cause the death of the individual. And if this is not enough for you, then you really must read the books by Professor Julius Hackethal, who has confirmed all this data in his research.

The earlier the tumor is detected the better?

We are always told that the sooner the tumor is detected the better. The truth however is that the earlier the tumor is detected the sooner the women died. Naturally this does not have anything to do with early detection – that is always an advantage – but rather this is due to: The earlier the tumor is detected in women (and men), the greater the chance, that a therapy will be prescribed for them, through which they will die earlier. To be fair it must also be stated here that perhaps it is not the therapy, but rather also the knowledge of the disease. You have certainly heard the words "self-fulfilling prophecy" at some time or other. There is nothing more behind this than the famous placebo effect, which means that what we firmly believe always happens. As in the proverb: "Our faith moves mountains".

Just ask patients to list the words they associate with the word cancer. You will certainly hear words like: Death, pain, God, purpose of life, why...! Unfortunately these words plunge most people into a maelstrom, which leads to the illness and not to health. Of all people, doctors should know what the placebo effect can trigger; but when cancer is involved they are so careless with the diagnosis, that we would have to assume the words oncology and psychology should never be mentioned in the same room. Also the statements of Dr. Hamer (see under New Medicine) and many other therapists naturally fit into this category.

When do I have cancer?

The diagnosis of cancer is primarily associated with pathogens. Now you certainly assume that there is an absolutely failsafe structure that Doctors use to determine when a person has cancer and when not. Unfortunately I must disappoint you here as well. In 1992 a study in England determined that in some parts of the country, 20% of all tests for cervical cancer and breast cancer were positive, and in other parts of the country only 3% were positive.

In 1987 in Liverpool 45,000 tests were re-analyzed and a wrong diagnosis was determined in 911of these cases. In 1988, in Manchester it was 3,000 tests of which 60 were incorrect. At Yale University 10 experienced radiologists were given 150 good-quality mammograms for their analysis. In all of 50 cases the doctors were not unified. This needs serious consideration. One out of every 3 mammograms was not read in the same way by experienced radiologists. I certainly do not need to tell you in detail what this means.

These studies show once again how unscientifically things are done in the medical field. Another point is that pathologists do not commit themselves gladly. In the reports we read: "It is most likely in agreement with disease pattern XY", or "most likely it is a…, differential diagnostically it could also be a…". After you have read hundreds of pathology reports then you could write a book about "probably, most likely, perhaps, cannot be precisely determined, etc. Funny enough, the probabilities in almost all cases are taken at 100% by the doctors, there is no other way to explain the fact, that that which still appears somewhat uncertain in the pathology report is always described as 100% certain in the discharge summary.

Also, today the standards of the pathology text books are evaluated as certain, without anybody questioning the whole procedure. One example. Certain cells are viewed by pathologists as cancer cells with 100% certainty. Now however there are people who neither die with this diagnosis, even without therapy, nor does their tumor continue to grow.

An additional example is provided by the Basel Bone tumor Reference Center, where more than 9,000 bone tumor cases have been diagnosed. Of this number more than 5,000 cases were sent in for a second expert opinion. And now please read carefully: The diagnosis had to be changed in 2,289 cases out of the app. 5,500 cases sent in for a second opinion. In other words – almost every second diagnosis was incorrect with reference to the type of cancer, and in 492 cases the diagnosis was even 100% incorrect (the patients did not even have cancer). All previous diagnosis were sent in by "specialists in their field", professors, leaders of pathological institutes etc.

In this example we must not lose sight of the fact that the diagnoses involved are very serious indeed. Particularly with bone tumors the decision often involves "removing" entire members. By the way, in 236 cases this was the case, e.g. for 236 people, many of them young people, cancer was diagnosed where there was no cancer. Expressed statistically this means, that for at least every 20th patient a catastrophic therapy would have been initiated, if a doctor or the patient had not insisted that the first pathology report be rechecked. Now if we assume that this only occurs rarely, then you can imagine the kind of things that are going on today. And please do not forget: Every pathologist had maintained before the second examination that his diagnosis was correct.

Because I am quite aware of the "sensitivity" of this issue, I want to be very clear that pathologists in many cases most likely "are right", when one considers cancer from their point of view. Unfortunately many roads lead to Rome, and to be honest Mr. Pathologist, would you recommend an immediate mastectomy (removal of the breast) for your wife after the diagnosis of breast cancer? I do not want to go into more detail in this book about the problems associated with pathologists. For you as patient it simply means nothing more (but nothing less) than that you must absolutely ensure that the diagnosis is confirmed by additional examinations before you make more serious decisions.

The 1% hurdle

Doctors like to argue that tests are incorrect in 1% of all cases, maximum. At first this sounds good. Unfortunately many people understand very little of the mathematics involved, otherwise they would know that a test that is 1% incorrect, in truth is 99% incorrect when it is used to test millions of people. Let me explain all this with a computational example.

Let's assume that a lab uses a test that is 99% correct. Then let's consider an illness that only occurs in one out of 10,000 people, such as a certain type of skin cancer. And now calculate for yourself the result if one million people are tested with this test.

1. 100 people would be correctly diagnosed with cancer illness (1,000,000 : 10,000 = 100), since every 10,000th patient has this illness.

2. 9,999 would be incorrectly diagnosed with cancer (every 100th patient)

Now please count how many number people have been diagnosed with cancer and you get the number 10,099 (9,999 plus 100 = 10,099). Of the 10,099, cancer patients in reality only 100 are ill, which means that this test would be incorrect in 99% of all cases where cancer was diagnosed.

You can see that it is a very simple matter to deal with numbers when you present them the way you would like to have them. However the truth often looks quite different, and we must question every number. Patients tell me again and again that their doctor told them that if they would undergo this or that therapy, then they would obtain these or those better chances. I can only recommend that you please have these numbers confirmed in writing, or have your doctor write down the name of the book or the study where you can read about them. Why do I say this? It's simple! Unfortunately in recent years I have often experienced that therapists are not mathematicians, and apparently as a consequence they deal with numbers in a manner that would earn my son an F in grade school math if he did the same.

Please pay attention when your doctor tells you that your chances of survival will improve by ?? percent through therapy XY. Thoroughly review such numbers and if your doctor takes offence, which unfortunately quite often occurs, then I would pose this question to you: "Do you really want to be treated by a doctor who simply comes up with numbers as he needs them?"

Your life and the happiness of your family are involved here, not getting a prize for being the most agreeable patient. Good doctors have no problems with such questions – why should they be a problem for you?

Conventional examinations
for diagnosing tumors
or leukemia and lymphatic cancer

1. Blood examinations

In addition to the normal hemogram it is mainly the so-called tumor markers that are supposed to indicate that a cancer event is occurring in the body. Tumor markers are "tumor-associated signal substances", whose occurrence in human blood is supposed to be linked with the occurrence and growth of malignant tumors. Primarily doctors differentiate 2 groups:

1.a Non-specific substances which accompany tumor growth, such as plasma protein changes (BSG, acute-phase proteins), iron metabolism disorders (ferritin, transferin), enzyme and isoenzyme increases (LDH, AP).

1.b Specific substances that are produced by the cancer itself, such as the onco-fetal antigens (AFP, CEA), the onco-placental antigens (placental-HCG, HPLAP), the membrane antigens/hybridoma-defined tumor antigens (CA 19-9, CA 15-3, CA 125, SCC), as well as substances/hormones like (ACTH, PTH, STH, VIP (polypeptides).

With the exception of thyroglobulin (thyroid gland) and PSA (prostate) no tumor markers are organ-specific. Thus the CEA value can be increased with the intestinal, pancreatic, mammary, stomach and bronchial carcinoma. Often tests are combined, such as for breast cancer, CEA and CA 15-3, or for gamete tumors, AFP and HCG.

List of tumor markers and the associated tumors

CEA   Stomach -, Colon, Breast and Lungcancer

AFP   Germ cell tumors, Liver

CA 19-9   Pankreas -, stomach -, bile duct -, Ovarian CA

CA 12-5   Epithelial Ovarin CA

CA 15-3   Breast-, Ovarian -, Corpus CA

PSA   Prostate

NSE   Smallcell Lungcancer, Seminoma, Neuroblastoma

SCC   Squamos CA

CT   Thyroid CA (medullar, C-cell)

TG   Thyroid CA (papillary)

TPA   Surface activity marker

ß2-Mikro-globulin   Lymphomas, Plasmocytoma

M2PK   Colon CA

List of tumors and the associated tumor markers

Otorhinolaryngology	SCC, CEA, TPA
Thyroid CA (papillary)	TG, TPA
Thyroid CA (medullar, C-cell)	Calcitonin, NSE

Lung cancer
- squamos
- small cell
- adeno CA

CYFRA
SCC, CEA
NSE, CEA
CEA

Breast	CA 15-3, MCA, CEA
Pancreatic CA	CA 19-9, TPA
Stomach cancer	CA 19-9, CEA
Colon cancer	CEA, CA 19-9, M2PK

Liver CA
- hepatocellular
- cholangior
- metastatic

AFP
CA 19-9
CEA

Ovarian CA
- epithelial
- muzinous

CA 12-5, TPA
CA 19-9

Testicular cancer
- Seminom
- Non seminom

HCG, SCC
AFP, HCG

Prostate cancer	PSA-RIA
Bladder cancer	CEA, TPA
Plasmocytoma	ß2-Mikroglobulin
Lymphomas	TPA (Ferritin)

I do not dare evaluate how precisely tumor markers indicate a cancer event, and I particularly do not dare evaluate what an increase or lowering of the values really mean, because there are just as many different statements on this as there are tumor markers themselves. I know many patients whose tumor markers in part have drastically increased, and who shortly thereafter returned to health, and I know other patients who died after the increase. I have also documented many cases in which patients with completely normal tumor markers died, and other cases in which patients whose tumor marker levels have been increased for many years did not show symptoms. Interestingly enough tumor markers often increase before tumors become smaller. And precisely at this moment patients frequently come to the doctor and...

1.c. Immune status

Naturally for all blood tests it must be mentioned that for cancer the primary importance is what is happening in the cell; what is found in the blood is of lesser importance. Particularly this applies for that which doctors refer to as an immune status. In this regard special cell groups should be considered in more detail in a blood test. Primarily the following cell types are examined:

Cell types	Standard values
Leucocytes	4000–8000
Lymphocytes	20–50
T-Lymphocytes	60–75
B-Lymphocytes	5–20
T4-helper cells	30–50
T8-Suppressors	20–30
T8-Cytotoxic	3–16
NK-cells	10–14

These cell types can be subdivided even further, for example into LAK cells, etc. But here the question quickly arises as to why. On one hand these examinations, which unfortunately are very expensive, permit an assessment of the progress of the cancer. On the other hand, I experience again and again that patients and oncologists totally depend on these values in the sense of: "How are you doing Ms. Miller?" "Thank you Dr., my killer cells have already increased by 2.3%." Here as well the idea is that patients also die if the population of killer cells doubles. We know far too little about their significance. What is sold today in this area as "scientific" much more reminiscent of Wall Street than it is of a physician's practice.

Free yourself of blood tests. Please do not misunderstand. I am not against these tests, I just do not think that you should go to your doctor full of fear each time because you do not know which blood values you have. And when you have started listening to your inner self, you will not require most of these blood tests anyway.

2. Imaging processes

These include X-rays, ultra sound, CT, resonance, PET, etc. Please be aware that there is no small dose of X-rays. Be very careful and always keep copies of your X-rays at home to avoid unnecessary examinations.

3. Biopsies

Where diagnoses are involved no effort can be too high. As already cited with the mammography example, apparently for those of us in the western world no costs and no efforts are too high, when the objective is diagnosing an illness. Whether these diagnoses are harmful to the health or not, is not important. This certainly applies for all types of biopsies. A biopsy is a removal of tissue for purposes of examination under the microscope. In this regard there are various processes like fine-needle aspiration, core-needle biopsy, stereotactic biopsy processes, like vacuum assisted breast biopsy or ABBI etc. However, they all have one thing in common, they are very dangerous. Before you have one of these examinations, you should have read the following arguments very carefully:

1. Each biopsy releases millions of cancer cells into the bloodstream and in many processes they also get into a different tissue, because doctors often poke several times with the same needle. Thousands of professors at numerous universities around the world teach the theory of micrometastases and it is precisely these same doctors who distribute cancer cells throughout the body through biopsies.

2. In particular with fine-needle aspiration, the pathologist only gets a little cell material and this small amount of cell material is then often torn. Naturally this means for the pathologist that this material is much more difficult to evaluate.

3. With many biopsies bacteria or viruses get to a location where they do not belong, for instance with prostate aspiration biopsy hundreds of thousands colon bacteria can get into the prostate.

4. Each biopsy leaves a scar behind, and each scar is an interference field. However the last thing that I would want is an interference field which is close to a tumor.

5. Almost all surgeons still believe that every pathologist is capable of determining whether the tissue that the pathologist sees under the microscope is cancer or not, within a few seconds or minutes. You must know that these diagnoses must often be made very quickly, while patients are lying on the operating table under anesthesia. I am not sure whether I

would want to let a pathologist, who has just separated from his wife, and who since yesterday has a paternity suit hanging over him, make a decision in a few seconds about whether my tissue now has cancer or not.

6. We know today that there are encapsulated tumors that are not very aggressive and with which patients can perhaps live until their natural death, without having problems due to the tumor. We do not know what it means when we puncture this tumor with a needle and destroy the encapsulation.

7. The pathologist Professor Kemnitz in Essen, apparently made systematically incorrect diagnoses for years. More than 170 women sued the pathologist, who released himself from his responsibility through suicide. To this day we do not know why Professor Kemnitz did this. Was he a poor pathologist, was he angry at women, or …?

We will never be able to find out why, because he is dead. But we also do not know how many practitioners like Professor Kemnitz are in Germany or in other countries. Anyone who maintains that this is a unique case apparently does not know how Professor Kemnitz was actually found out. It was not the surgeons in the hospital, or the oncologists that were treating the patients who uncovered the scandal, rather it was a family doctor who noticed that many of his patients suddenly had breast cancer, and that all of them had been diagnosed by Professor Kemnitz.

This case, which is referred to as the Essen scandal, raises many questions that remain answered. Instead of questioning the entire system, all the responsibility is placed on Professor Kemnitz – because this means that everything can stay as it is.

Nothing, absolutely nothing has been undertaken by surgeons, hospitals, politicians, or health insurance companies, to ensure that such a scandal cannot occur again. For me this is the real scandal. This is tragic and it also indicates how completely patients are subjugated by a healthcare system – or should I say: to a sick system? In any event, the Kemnitz case demonstrated how uncertain doctors can be with the diagnosis of cancer, how dependant patients are on the statements of individual pathologists, and how quickly surgeons are prepared to cut parts out of you that are completely healthy. Please do not make the mistake and believe that there are no more Professor Kemnitzes on this planet.

Non-conventional examinations
for diagnosis of a tumor
or leukemia and lymphatic caner

Introduction:
What applies for conventional diagnosis also applies for non-conventional diagnosis. Until we know what cancer is, we are incapable of 100% sure diagnosis. However in contrast to the usual blood tests there are three serious differences:

1.   Fees for all of the following examinations will not be paid by any   health insurance company because they are not scientifically recognized. What this really means, we now know.

2.   The reputations of these examinations are much worse than those of the usual examinations, although there are many practitioners who   have often demonstrated with these examinations that   they can diagnose much more precisely.

3.   The principle of many examinations is different. They involve, detection of cancer or tumors before they occur. Because conventional oncologists can only detect cancer in a very advanced stage, (when a tumor is already larger than 6 mm), they naturally maintain, that all of these examinations are nonsense.

I always find it interesting that those therapists stating an opinion about a diagnostic process, are usually the ones who have never worked intensively with the process in question. At the same time in my opinion, they are using processes, when it has already been proven a thousand times over, just how wrong those processes can be. Please do not misunderstand me. This is no advertisement for non-conventional diagnostic processes, but I am simply upset when I hear from "experts" for the hundredth time, that dark-field diagnoses, or thethermography diagnoses are the same as a lottery, while the same therapists rely 100% on the statement of every pathologist or laboratory. I ask myself in this case who is the greater gambler.

Dark-field microscopy

In dark-field illumination special optics are used in which incoming light rays bypass the lens. Only when a preparation is brought into the path of the rays does the light, bent by the preparation, reach the lens and contribute to the image. The structures appear illuminated against a dark background. In this diagnostic process a blood is taken from a drop of blood from the ear and viewed under the dark-field microscope.

In the examination in addition to evaluating the acid base ratio, verification of differentiation of symbiotes is of particular importance. Symbiotes are the smallest life forms that get into the blood through the food we eat, and which are found in all bodily fluids. According to Professor Enderlein these symbiotes can develop abnormally and are an indication of how healthy a person is. Good diagnosticians believe with this microscope that they are able to determine the quality of the blood platelets (thrombocytes) and the white blood cells (leucocytes). In addition, the consistency and the bioaccumulation level of the blood, allergic and inflammatory reactions, a secondary oxygen deficiency etc. are also determined.

Many doctors are happy to equate dark-field microscopy with charlatanism, and I must say with good reason. Not because it is not a sufficiently meaningful technology, but because many hobby diagnosticians who have been to a one-day course in dark-field microscopy believe that they can make the most precise diagnoses with it. I have encountered this phenomenon many times and I also protect myself from this type of diagnosis. That being said, I have become acquainted with many practitioners who have been using dark-field microscopy daily for many years, and who are quite capable of using it draw exact conclusions.

HLB blood test (Heitan-LaGarde-Bradford)

The Heitan – LaGarde – Bradford blood test whose theory originates in the United States, was known as the H.L.B. blood test. The test was further developed and improved by the German doctor Heitan, who worked in Paris and died in 1977. Dr. LaGarde is a student of Dr. Heitan. In collaboration with many European doctors, Heitan and LaGarde attempted to detect cancer and graphically depict it. Dr. Bradford from the Bradford Research Institute is an American engineer, was the first to explain the biological reasons for the structural changes in coagulated blood with the test.

The two most important processes in this context are the different clot-forming processes and the pathological production of many kinds of bile salts that jointly anatomize the structure of the red blood cells, induce color changes, and destroy the fibrin network. The simple test can be performed in several minutes by a doctor or therapist. The test distinguishes between cancer and other benign or pathological conditions.

The test is not supposed to detect the initial stage of cancer in its earliest form, which is why a confusing the interpretations with other pathological circumstances is possible. In the test coagulated drops of the patient's blood are examined under a phase contrast microscope. The microscope shows multiple aspects of the drop of blood: the fibrin network, the characteristic transparent parts, and the color changes.

The blood of the cancer patient differs from normal blood in the following areas:

1. The fibrin network is partially or completely destroyed.

2. The cell membrane is eroded and looks jagged.

3. In the center of the drop of blood glue-like masses appear that are surrounded by transparent parts or "holes" of various sizes. Within these parts smaller bodies with other forms are recognizable.

Hormone stimulants and coagulants change the test results to an unknown, but always disadvantageous, degree. Likewise, all bodily trauma, such as operation, fractures, or heavy bleeding, also change the test results. The test is also age-dependent. With younger people the manifestations are less clear than they are with older people. In the blood of a cancer patient the open places are colored yellow or green, particularly around the edges of the transparent masses.

Erythrocyte examination developed by Sklenar

Dr. Sklenar was a contemporary of the well-known researcher and cancer specialist, Dr. Scheller, and he studied Dr. Scheller's methods of detecting cancer in the blood. For 12 years he worked with the Scheller method, and he gained a lot of experience with this method. After long, intensive research, he was able to bring the right dyes together for his blood examination method. He applied his method in practice for close to thirty years. The examination uses a light optical microscope with 1200-1500 times magnification. The erythrocytes are dyed with a special, modified, methylene blue solution. This method is based on the principle that healthy cells will not let any dye through. Only damaged cells are permeable, whereby the larger color molecules pass through the membrane and can dye abnormal structures.

The following stages can be differentiated in a cancer illness:

1. the preliminary phase of cancer, which according to professor Chiurco at the University of Rome is a conditio sine qua non (without other condition) for cancer.

2. the general cancer illness, with initial lactic acid fermentation in the cells, but still without visible carcinoma formation

3. the carcinoma

4. the distribution or metastases of the carcinoma.

During the preliminary phase of cancer, the erythrocytes change and granula occur in the erythrocytes. At the beginning of the lactic acid fermentation in the cells and with the carcinoma, smaller and larger blisters form that Scheller called lysomes. With healthy blood the dyed blood smear shows no changes in the erythrocytes, because the macromolecules of the dye cannot penetrate the fine pores of the healthy cell membrane.

Only a diseased cell membrane with enlarged pores can permit the large dye molecules to pass through, so that the structures within the cell become visible.

Chemotherapy sensitivity tests

In recent years more and more tests have appeared on the market, which are supposed to project how successful a certain chemotherapy will be for a certain patient. However all of these tests have the same problems:

* The question is no longer asked whether chemotherapy even makes sense, rather the question now becomes, which chemotherapy? Naturally this pleases all pharmaceutical manufacturers and a person must fundamentally question the "supposed" successes of this test.

* Various processes such as gene control, ATP measurements etc. are used. However the actual question is naturally: How meaningful is the result, in reality?

* Can laboratory conditions even be applied to people?

Also the various statements from within the allopathic community are also confusing. Hundreds of scientists write (and oncologists again and again cite what they write in their statements) that a chemotherapy is of no value at low p53 values, at the same time most therapies are administered without measuring a p53 gene value. For many years a p53 test or sensitivity test have been available. However most doctors do not use them. Why not? Is it because they themselves do not believe in their significance?. Are the costs too high, or is it because the health insurance companies do not want to pay for these tests because they are not "scientifically recognized?"

If you should want chemotherapy, particularly for epithelial tumors, then insist on a sensitivity test. What have you got to lose?

EVA (Ex Vivo Apoptotic Assay)

EVA is the designation that the American oncologist Dr. Nagourney has given to a laboratory test which stands for "Ex Vivo Apoptotic Assay". Apoptotic means "programmed cell death". In his examinations Dr. Nagourney tests a substance's capacity to cause the death of a cancer cell. The objective is to determine precisely which form of chemotherapy can really be used effectively for a certain cancer patient, i.e. which sensitivity or resistance occurs for various chemotherapy medications.

With his test the probable effectiveness of approximately 70 chemotherapy medications (that are either administered individually or in combination), and other substances, such as mistletoe are determined. More in this regard is available on the Internet at: www.rational-t.com.

ATP-TCA-Test

With the ATP test (adenosintriphosphate) fresh tumor material is removed after the operation, placed on test plates, and then mixed in various doses with the chemotherapy medications. These cultures are then incubated for 7 days and the ATP content of the cells is measured with a luminometer, and then we know to what degree a certain toxin can damage a cancer cell.

AMAS (Anti Malignin Antibody)

The AMAS test is a test for malignin, a polypeptide that occurs in most cancer cells. According to information from Oncolab USA, malignin is already present in the very early phases of a cancer illness, on the other hand, it is no longer verifiable in very advanced stages of the illness. In one study with over 8,000 patients the test has been proven to be more than 95% correct. The cost is approximately 150 USD plus the cost of transporting the blood to America. More information is available at: www.amascancertest. com.

CCR-Test

The Carcinochrome Reaction (CCR) developed by Gutschmidt is a photometric measurement of the red coloring formed in the urine after addition of a carcinochrome reaction for early detection of cancer illnesses. The test process assumes that increased polypeptides produced by a cancer cell can be measured in the urine. Many doctors use the CCR test particularly for early detection of a tumor event.

Hydroxylamine test by Professor Neunhoffer)

Professor Neunhoffer (†1998) was one of Germany's greatest cancer researchers and biochemists. His work on the proof of N-hydroxy-peptide groups in cancer cell protein was impressive for many people, and he developed a test which is capable of verifying the presence in the urine of hydroxylamine, which cancer cells increasingly excrete. For the significance of the test one must know that tumors do not permanently produce a lot of hydroxylamine, and consequently the test can also produce incorrect negative results. However if the test should prove positive then it strongly indicates a malignant event. The test can be performed in Germany for app. 80 Euro.

Scheidl thrombocyte test

In June 1996 the journal FOLIA CLINICA INTERNATION-ALIS in Barcelona carried the report of a cancer test which is the only test that satisfies World Health Organization (WHO) requirements for diagnosis certainty of 90% to 96%, for an ideal cancer test. This test demonstrated 95% reliability. The test is supposed to enable detection of tumor tendencies like sarcoma, carcinoma and leukemia illnesses even in the development stage – or even earlier – e.g. at a time when no symptoms can be identified with the other preventative examinations. In the Scheidl Test the thrombocytes (blood platelets) in the blood are measured. With the early detection test the thrombocytes are isolated, set to a certain pH value and incubated for 4 days. Then the preparation is examined in a darkfield microscope for certain criteria.

A trained medical specialist can analyze and evaluate the risk, or the occurrence, of a benign or malignant tumor illness based on the various growths, shapes and colorations. The most important aspect is determination whether a tumor tendency is present or not. However the localization of the tumor event cannot be predicted.

But the test can detect whether a carcinoma, sarcoma, or lymphoma, is involved. Also it is claimed that that a myeloic or lymphatic leukemia can also be detected. In addition a clinically existing tumor should also be clearly distinguished from a pure tumor tendency.

Regulation thermography

Regulation thermography developed by Schwamm/Rost involves heat measurement on the body surface (head, teeth, and chest) of the patient, with an electronic thermometer. In this process the temperatures are measured electronically at a total of 136 precisely defined measurement points of the body when it is at rest, and after a standardized cold stimulus. After the initial measurement the patient removes his clothes and remains seated for 10 minutes at room temperature (thermal impulse). The organism cools down. Then there is a second measurement in the same way, and the thermogram is created. A body that is healthy would show clearly defined normal regulation; even with a small regulation deviation, this is visible as disturbance on the evaluation sheet. Moreover this method is very well suited for therapy control and observation of the course of an illness. Also regulation thermography is often used to answer the question of an event focus.

Thermography

For decades the thermography has been a good method to detect tumors. However the process was displaced in the market after the invention of mammography. Naturally economic aspects play a major role here. This was wrong in my opinion, because the old formula still applies: Where there is a tumor, there is more blood, and where more blood is there is more heat. And precisely this heat can be made visible.

In this regard I quote Dr. Gautherie, former director of the Institute for Biomedical Thermology at the Louis Pasteur University in Straßburg. "In thermobiology studies there was a clear relationship between the specific heat generation of the cancerous tissue and the time necessary to double the tumor volume." In other words, the faster the tumor grows, the more heat it generates.

Philipp Strax M.D. at the Guttman Breast Institute in New York conducted 2 studies for breast cancer diagnosis using a brassiere with liquid crystals. 109 women from 16-70 years of age participated in the first examination. In 71% of the cases the diagnosis was excellent, in 19% it was good, and in 10% of the cases he was not satisfied with the examination results. Also Professor Tricoire at the Bobigny Clinic in Paris diagnosed breast cancer 1,046 times over a period of 30 months with only 1% false negatives and 4% false positives. These are better numbers than those for mammography, and in this case as well it is clear how money determines medicine. Or what other reason is there to subject so many women to the cancer-causing radiation of a mammogram. The manufacturer

Inframedic (www.inframedic.de) has developed a special thermography device, the so-called MammoVision, claimed capable of detecting tumors earlier than the mammogram can.

Radiothermometry

In this process the weak radiation of electromagnetic rays of the human body is measured in order to make a statement about temperatures inside the body. The radiated energy can be calculated in accordance with the Raleigh-Jeans formula. With the help of this technology it is possible to measure temperature differentials less than 1o degrees without subjecting patients to radiation.

Blood crystallization test

The principle of the copper chloride blood crystallization test consists of a copper chloride solution being added to the blood, and then being crystallized out in a chamber at constant temperature and humidity. This process usually takes app. 24 hours. In the process characteristic images form that can be evaluated by experienced diagnosticians. In Germany there are two experienced diagnosticians who have been doing this for years.

Decoder dermography

Decoder dermography is used to record electric signals inherent in the body, which are measured on predetermined skin zones and which are combined with non-detectable electrical stimulus sequences in the 10 Hz range. With this biolelectronic function analysis, which is similar to regulation thermography, disorders can be detected that serve as a very useful basis for an additional diagnostic explanation. Electric skin measurement involves three pairs of electrodes that are respectively connected to the forehead, hand, and foot.

EAV

EAV stands for Electro Acupuncture by Voll, which was developed over 40 years ago by Dr. Voll. Today EAV is a much-used diagnostic and therapy process. It is concerned with biological processes, as well as with control and regulating processes in the human body and their disorders. Consequently EAV is used to determine causes of acute illnesses, and particularly chronic illnesses. EAV is mainly designed to determine important disorder factors like residual infection, environmental toxins, herd/interference field stresses etc. However EAV has also proven itself in verifying incompatibility of dental substances such as amalgam, or for testing nutritional intolerances For the test electrophysical measurements are taken at anatomically defined and electrically significant skin points (acupuncture points).

Regulation diagnosis device
developed by Professor Popp

Professor Fritz -Albert Popp has an international reputation as a biophoton researcher. However up to this point only a few patients are familiar with his diagnostic method, which is a practical implementation of medical biophotonics. According to Professor Poll the order of an ideal healthy organism leads to ideal measurable skin resistance values. However if the order for a person is more and more deficient, then certain values in the skin resistance measurement also change. The breakdown in the regulation results in pure random distribution of the measured values. In the test process several hundred measured values are taken with an electrode at different points on the skin within a few minutes. This process attempts to determine the following diagnostic criteria:

* The measure for the control capacity of the test person
* The measure for the deviation of complete regulation incapacity.
* The measure for complete regulation incapacity relative to the remaining regulation capacity.
* The measure for the energy that the test person can supply, in order to regulate at all.
* The measure for the limited remaining reserves for ideal regulation and
  * The measure for the limited remaining reserves for the regulation itself for ideal regulation.

The interesting thing with Professor Popp's diagnosis is that it does not try to determine the presence of a tumor, rather it attempts to determine how well the regulation mechanisms of a body still react. From this data then the PC program analyzes the status quo. From a holistic perspective I consider this approach worthy of high recommendation and hope that many doctors in the future will collect enough data to better evaluate this principle.

The optic erythrocyte test from Professor Link

The invention of this test is due to professor Arno Linke, who died in 1992. It is based on the electric negative surface charge of the erythrocytes (red blood cells) which effects an enrichment of the higher molecular weight proteins in the peripheral zone of the erythrocytes. These are viewed under a microscope through fixing and dying processes and are classified in various levels. In this process two measurement numbers (PW and EVI) determine whether the person has cancer or not, according to Professor Linke.

Preventative care and aftercare

The concepts of preventative care and after care also part of the subject of diagnosis. Is it really clear to you that these two terms include the word "Care" (as in worry)? This is precisely what is involved here because a lot of people earn a lot of money when you are worried. The term preventative care, and in particular the preventative care examinations themselves, are acknowledged to be in the interest of early detection of cancer. But the term early detection certainly does not earn its name, because as a rule a tumor must divide thirty times before it is discovered. If one assumes a rate of division of 130 days with breast cancer, the tumor is already 10 years old when it is detected through magnetic resonance imaging processes. If a person would suggest this kind of early detection for any other illness then that person would be ridiculed immediately. This is not the case with cancer.

Under the false pretence that we can better treat breast cancer allopathically if it is detected earlier, women get more and more prescriptions for mammograms, although we have known long before Tschernobyl that precisely such radiation generates cancer. Yes the word is generate – even according to allopathic opinion. Aren't medical students around the world taught that DNA changes are responsible for the occurrence of cancer, and is it not a physical fact that mammogram devices generate precisely these DNA changes. While doctors still talk about "low doses" and safe radiation, this is only because they have never read Dr. Golfmans book: <u>Preventing Breast Cancer</u>, or they have not continued their education in physics and biochemistry. Otherwise they would know that there is neither safe radiation when the destruction of DNA in individual cells is involved, nor is there a low dose, as even hits of the smallest quantities can induce major damages.

Aftercare

After the destruction or removal of a tumor many patients want to know from their doctors which examinations they should take in order to determine whether the tumor has returned. On first glance this is an understandable question in light of the fact that almost all tumors return, sooner or later. The question presupposes faith that their doctors knows more about how they are doing than they do themselves. Let's take a look at why this is so.

1. Faith in the hemogram

In most cases your doctor checks your hemogram and attempts, based on so-called tumor markers or lymphocyte values, to assess whether a tumor has returned, or to determine the status of your immune system. However what would you say if I told you that there are cancer patients who have had increased tumor markers for decades, and with most cancer patients their immune system is not particularly bad. Ask a cancer patient sometime shortly after his diagnosis, how his liver values are or about his immune status. In almost all cases he will tell you that his doctor could not find anything. Other than the tumor or increased antibody antigen reactions (increased tumor markers) there are no "symptoms".

In March of 2000, in the Russian Institute for Basic Research (IISP) I met with Professor Fudin and Professor Glazachev, and we spoke about the work of what is most likely the most famous Moscow Academy which can count figures like Tolstoy, Bechterev, or Pavlov among its alumni. By the way Pavlov's grandson, Professor Sudakov is the head of the university today. Among the many studies one is particularly worth mentioning, namely the one involving the Nentsi people. These Russians live in the northernmost part of the Union and they have been observed and studied for many years, because Nentsis do not know any cancer or other chronic illnesses (with the exception of lung illnesses) and almost without exception they live to be very old. For my work what seemed most important to me was that the immune system of the Nentsis is so poor that a western doctor would immediately prescribe immune strengthening medication. Please think about this point for a moment. Although (or because) the Nentsis have a miserable immune system, they stay healthy and in the process, they live to be very old. While oncologists around the world learn the fundamentals of immune stimulation, in Russia the discussion is whether with cancer the immune system should be increased at all, in any way. Strengthening the immune system is absolute standard practice in today's oncological clinics (mistletoe, thyme, oxygen, ozone, cell therapies, etc.).

If we assume that nature or evolution is always right, then we must assume that there is a very important reason why our body changes the production (increase or decrease) of certain cells in the event of chronic illness. Could it perhaps be possible that it is easier for our bone marrow to produce 3,000 healthy leukocytes, than to produce 6,000 leukocytes that do not work so well together? Is it perhaps possible that energy is pulled out of the bone marrow because it is urgently needed somewhere else or...? Questions and questions to which he have no answer today. However whoever knows something about cancer therapies will quickly note similar thoughts in the work of Dr. Hamer, or Dr. Budwig, who have always consistently maintained that we should not destroy our self-healing system, and that tumors are nothing more than a portion of this process. Also my experience with People Against Cancer confirms these thoughts as we have come to know many patients who have returned to healthy primarily because they did not subject themselves to the tortures of conventional (and often also alternative) therapies.

In order to avoid any misunderstanding. I am certainly not against tumor markers or checking the hemograms, as long as they are used as supplements, and if the patient needs them, as a part of the diagnosis. unfortunately however many patients still come to their doctor and he says: "Dear Ms. Miller I am sorry but I must tell you that your tumor marker XY has increased from 12.3 to 14.5". Unfortunately what the doctor does not say is that this increase can be very positive, as tumor markers often increase before a tumor becomes smaller. When we consider this antibody- antigen reaction chemically then this is also logical and should first be viewed as a good reaction on the part of the immune system. In addition the values are subject in part to greater fluctuations and one also forgets unfortunately that there may be times when the devices in the laboratory do not always measure the same, or that human error can occur.

But at this moment the patient only hears: "Oh no I have a relapse. No, anything but that". The whole energy flow of the body collapses and the immune system is so strongly suppressed that whether the words of the doctor are correct or not is no longer significant at all. It also does not help when the doctor says one should not attach too much importance to this now, and that we (why we) must now wait to see whether the values get worse or not. Yes Mr. Doctor, what do you believe will happen when you, through your careless words have caused the collapse of your patient's immune system for days, if not for months. Naturally these values will worsen.

At this point I would like make an appeal for much more careful handling of diagnosis, because it is not just me, but a lot of doctors around the world must experience again and again that patients get very poor, very quickly, after a diagnosis. An additional point should also be considered by doctors. That which doctors say and that which patients hear is not always the same. A small example:
Doctor: "Well, Ms. Miller on the whole I am very happy with your hemogram."
However the patient thinks: "On the whole. He is certainly not

telling me the whole truth."

Doctor: "But in order to be completely sure we should take another CT scan".

However the patient thinks: "Why do yet another CT scan? They probably cannot help me anyway."

Doctor: "At this time there is nothing else to do by wait."

However the patient thinks: "He is not even offering me another therapy. Nothing to do except wait is only a nice way of saying: Go home and try to have a few more nice days. What nonsense. How can I have a few more nice days when I only have a few more weeks to live"?

The misunderstanding is naturally not always so extreme as presented in this example, and many doctors have a very good feeling for their patients. However even the most sensitive doctors cannot realize what the patient construes out of his words, and this is where the great question can be asked; as to whether the only possibility of avoiding this misunderstanding would not simply by dispensing with this type of aftercare.

2. Faith in the importance of the tumor size
Try to evaluate the following situation as a patient. You have completed the third cycle of chemotherapy and you have an appointment with the head physician. Together with other doctors the head physician enters your room and says to you: "Dear Ms. Smith. I have good news for you. Yesterday's CT scan shows that your tumor has become somewhat smaller, this means that the chemotherapy is working very well for you." In my experience most patients understand this news as an indication that they will thus live longer. However the truth is that in most cases a decrease in tumor size does not mean

an extension of life, as countless studies demonstrate.

In this regard I will cite Dr. Blumenschein, author of several books about cancer and a walking encyclopedia of non-conventional cancer therapies: "If doctors would only understand that with cancer the tumor is not that important, and would finally start treating cancer and not tumors, then we could save the lives of thousands of cancer patients – I would no longer have to treat patients whose bone marrow has almost always been destroyed through therapies and which unfortunately renders a sensible therapy nearly impossible.

My own experiences with doctors on all continents confirm Dr. Blumenschein's view. The size of the tumor is a secondary consideration if not even a tertiary consideration in a cancer therapy. This does not mean that the objective of a cancer therapy should not include disappearance of the tumor or a reduction in its size, however all of us, doctors and patients, should finally come to an understanding that this cannot be the primary goal of a cancer therapy.

If you have not studied the illness of cancer intensively then this may sound somewhat odd to you, certainly many people have most likely told you that with every cancer therapy the tumor must first be destroyed if the patient is to survive. However this view is still part of the totally outdated perspective that cancer is a local illness and when the tumor is gone, then cancer is also conquered. The fact that this is not the way it is, is proven daily by thousands of cancer patients, who must die, even though their first tumor disappeared after a therapy.

3. The belief that a tumor will return
The reason for aftercare is to check whether the tumor or cell changes have returned. Naturally the prerequisite here is that we also believe that the tumor can return. But what would happen if we were 100% sure that the tumor will not return. Doesn't the Bible teach us that our faith can move mountains?

Do not leaders of all religions in the world teach that we must create our future ourselves through prayer, meditation, and our thoughts in general? Don't the best motivational trainers and psychotherapists prove to us daily that our visualization and affirmation capacities make the difference between personal happiness and unhappiness? Do not spiritual leaders on all continents teach that we can only harvest that which we have previously sown (thought)?

We now naturally assume that all the wise people of this world are wrong, and that only doctors know how to prevent a relapse. You should only assume this if you are totally certain that your psyche or your soul has nothing to do with your health or illness. If you should have the slightest notion that you psyche or your soul may have something to do with your status quo, then you should start thinking intensively about how you can create your own future, today. Programs such as MindStore (www.mindstore.com) can help you to design your future systematically. In recent years I have shaken the hands of many people who have survived their cancer in spite of an incurable prognosis. There was not one of these patients for whom words like visualization, purpose of life, or God were unfamiliar terms. Every single one of them told me in their own way of the changes in his life or paradigm shifts (more about this in the chapter: Mental Energy).

Even if you consider this to be nonsense or exaggerated, you cannot get around the fact that I know many healed cancer patients, who told me that they were or are 100% certain that their tumors will not come back. This includes the story of Karl, a young man who was sent home to spend his last days with his family. While everything pointed to his immanent death, he signed a contract with his tumor, (see tumor contract) and although the tumors continued to grow, he calmed his attending doctor by telling him, "Don't worry. I know that my tumors will hold to the contract and that I am now healthy. I am 100% sure of it." When I had dinner with him, he told me that he was 100 certain that he would become healthy and would stay healthy.

My question to you: Do you think that it would be good for Karl if he went in for an aftercare examination every 6 months? (Info: Karl has been healthy since 1994 and has dispensed with all aftercare appointments).

4. The belief that my doctor knows how I am doing – even better than I do myself!

Frank Wiewel, president of People Against Cancer in the USA, certainly the man in the USA where non-conventional cancer therapies are involved, often tells the story of an old woman, who he visited in an American cancer clinic. Right at the beginning of his visit he asked her how she was doing and she answered: "My doctor is very happy with me, he says that I am doing well." You must understand however that the lady sat hunched over in a wheel chair, a yellow/pale face and she hardly had the strength to speak, as she had already completed several chemotherapies. I have also received many similar responses. When I ask how someone is doing, I get answers like: "My hemogram looks better", "the tumor is still growing", or "they say that I will soon be released to go home."

All of these answers have one thing in common. They are bound to the answers of third-persons, as if we are no longer capable of answering the question about our own well-being ourselves. When we want to know how we are doing, we have 2 powerful "tools" , which however are no longer used by most doctors and patients. The first is the mirror, and the second is "going inside".

A mirror shows us not only the condition of our skin and our body relative to shape, but it also reflects our state of being. Here you must take a few minutes to look at yourself in the mirror and then write down everything that goes through your mind. If you have not yet tried this exercise then now is the right time to do it.

Another exercise is to look into your own eyes for 5-10 minutes. If you have never tried this exercise then you will be amazed at the things that happen when you do this regularly. What earlier was totally normal, namely looking at the patient carefully and then making a diagnosis from precise observation, is rarely practiced by doctors today. We have forgotten to go inside just as we have forgotten how to look into the mirror. Many people in our hectic world have lost the feeling for their own well-being.

Klaus Pertl, MindStore motivation trainer, asks his clients in his seminars, what they do when they are hungry, and the answer naturally is "eat something". But what do the same people do when they have stress? Have they learned to relax and to go inside to find out why they are stressed and at the same time to dissipate the stress? Usually the answer is no. It is precisely the same for cancer patients. They have also learned or forgotten to listen inside themselves, in order to find out how they are doing, why they are stressed, what their goals are, and what makes them happy today, etc.

Why do so many people believe that doctors are more capable knowing how they are doing, then they are themselves? What does an Hb (hemoglobin) value of under 10 really mean for my life? Who is to say that it is fundamentally something bad to be sick? It is not recent news that illness can be an important self-healing process. Buddhism teaches its adherents that there is Yin and Yang, good and bad and that these form a whole.

As you see with these questions, we are the only ones who can answer the question about our well-being. In the future do not leave the answer to this question to third-persons.

4

Chemotherapy and radiation

Chemotherapy!
A curse or the last resort?

To address the subject of chemotherapy without getting into an emotional discussion is probably no longer possible in the 21st century; and the reason for this is relatively simple. Nobody really knows precisely for which people chemotherapy will prove helpful in destroying a tumor, nor does anybody really know precisely if it would be better not to undergo the chemotherapy. To this day there is no medical measuring instrument that shows us whether a chemotherapy will help this person or that person. I emphasize the word people here because we are even less certain about whether a chemotherapy will help this or that type of cancer.

If you have not studied the subject of chemotherapy intensively then perhaps you will think: "But surely the doctors must know whether a chemotherapy can help me before they prescribe one for me." Unfortunately I must disappoint you. If you study chemotherapy scientifically and intensively then you will quickly determine that we are really just beginning to understand, (or that we have stopped understanding) the real effects of chemotherapy. What is certain is that in 1944 the physician Peter Alexander described that bone marrow is seriously damaged and that sooner or later people die due to an "exhaustion of the white hemogram". By the way this fact had already been described in a magazine in 1919! Dr. Alexander examined the sailors who came into contact with mustard gas through the accident in the Italian harbor Bari, in December 1943. Afterwards the victory march of this preparation, which was actually designed to kill enemy soldiers, was unstoppable, and today "modern" oncology is unimaginable without this toxin and all of its relatives. Now we could assume that we have made enormous progress in the new millennium, and that we can no longer compare present day chemotherapies with the mustard gas used in the Second World War.

But let's take a closer look at the status quo. As you will remember from the biology class in school, our cells divide over and over with some few exceptions. Every second millions of cells in our body renew themselves. Cell division occurs in specific phases. Biologists designate these as prophase, metaphase, anaphase, and telophase.

Many new cells must still reach maturity. The entire process of cell division and cell maturity is called cell cycle and this complete cycle is divided into G0 phase (rest phase), G1 phase (RNA and protein synthesis), S phase (DNA duplication), G2 phase (DNA repair phase) and finally the M-phase, the actual cell division. This is important for cancer patients to know, so that they better understand how a chemotherapy works, because different preparations influence different phases of cell division. Cells are more vulnerable during the cell division process. Cytostatic agents now attempt to exploit this lowered immunity of the cells, by disturbing certain metabolic processes of the cell. In this regard the desired result is the death of the cell. I would like to emphasize this point, the desired effect is the death of the cell, and not transformation of the cell into a healthy cell.

Since many tumor cells divide very rapidly, they are naturally more sensitive to such toxins and are destroyed in increased number. If you read the last sentences carefully then you will certainly recognize the problem posed by these cell toxins. If tumor cells do not divide more rapidly then other cells in the body, what then? And how do these toxins actually identify tumor cells?

You can certainly answer the first question yourself, and you already know at least part of answer to the second question. Cytostatic agents do not detect tumor cells at all. They simply destroy everthing that grows faster (and a lot more). This is the reason for the known side effects of all body systems whose cells usually divide more rapidly:

* our epithelial cells, e.g. in the mouth, stomach, or intestinal tract.

* our lymphatic system, e.g. destruction of the lymphocytes.

* our gonads, consequently the temporary or often permanent sterility after a chemotherapy

* our bone marrow, e.g. destruction of the leucocytes, the erythrocytes and the thrombocytes.

* skin, hair, and also nails.

If you are aware of these main effects, not side effects as they are always called, then it is not hard to understand why everyone must reconsider three times over whether he should undergo a chemotherapy. The influences on bone marrow and on the lymphatic system particularly are so devastating that many people justifiably wonder if this is not precisely the opposite what they need when tumors are present in the body. We all know that we urgently need our immune system when we have a tumor in the body, and yet in spite of this we believe that we can continue to destroy our immune system for many months when we have cancer.

This is precisely the dilemma associated with chemotherapy preparations. Their entire objective is targeted on the destruction of cells, it is targeted on communicating to cell structures, so-to-speak, how they should divide correctly. An additional problem is the resistance to these preparations. It is not just the fact that these preparations do not even recognize cells that divide slowly, or that do not divide at all, there is also the factor of resistance, which is even more serious. Many tumors ignore certain substances from the very outset. Consequently "cocktails" of different substances are usually given in the hope that one of these substances will help. The fact that multiple substances also have greater side-effects goes without saying. Perhaps you would also be interested in the results of multiple surveys (Makillop/Hansen/ Moore/Tannock ...) wherein oncologists responded to the question as to whether they would undergo chemotherapy, with no (what kind of world is this where doctors prescribe therapies that they themselves would never use).

However these cocktails do have one advantage. Huge costs can be billed for each patient, which is extremely gratifying to every manufacturer. This sentence may seem exaggerated, ironic, or even insolent to you. But it does not change the following fact, which is happily forgotten. If you are not resistant to a certain substance, then your chance to very quickly become resistant to this substance increases very quickly, from infusion to infusion, and indeed much more quickly than you are accustomed to with antibiotics. The reason for this is that our body has astoundingly intelligent capabilities for protecting itself against toxins. For example one of these capabilities is changing the permeability of the cell wall.

In addition the chance of metastasis is increased, as various studies have demonstrated. Studies indicate that the larger the tumor the greater the number of resistant cells. It has also been determined that over time, tumor cells learn to defend themselves against every type of cytostatic agent. This also explains why changing to a different combination of cytostatic agents so often results in failure.

Many are also pleased to forget that cells become more malign (aggressive) after a chemotherapy, as was determined by Wenzel-Seifert and Lentzen and others years ago. Such cells also have an increased "potential for metastasis"?, which means nothing more that the chemotherapy can trigger the feared metastasis.

The more toxic a substance is, the more your body will undertake to ensure that this substance does not cause as much damage the next time it is encountered. Thus resistance to medication is nothing more than part of an ingenious defense system called man, which brings us right back to our subject: Evolution is right.

A short list of the most commonly used chemotherapy preparations and their areas of application is provided below:

Alkylates
This is a group, which at least in theory, reacts at multiple points with the DNA at the same time, and networks the DNA (cross-link). In other words this means that alkylates change our genetic code which consequently can no longer be read. An old term that is also used for this is radiomimetic agents A nice word for something quite diabolical, namely the fact that cells divide as if they had been exposed to strong radioactive radiation. The consequences of this are most likely familiar to everyone.

Yperite also belongs to this group. Yperite is the substance which was still called mustard gas in the First World War, and which killed thousands of soldiers. Today's yperite is a nitrogen yperite, with an effect however that is not much reduced. It still destroys bone marrow and other tissue structures. Additional known compounds are chlorambucil (Leukeran) and melphalan (Alkeran).

A subgroup of nitrogen yperite includes representatives of the oxazaphosphorines like cyclophosphamide, whose most famous representative is probably Endoxan. However ifosfamide (holoxan) and trofosfamide (Ixoten) are used just as

158

often. "Relatives" of nitrogen yperite are also used for brain tumors, since in theory these overcome the blood brain barrier. In these cases primarily nimustine (ACNU), fotemustine (Muphoran), carmustine (BCNU), bendamustine (Ribomustin) and Lomustine (CCNU) are used.

Another group of cross linkers are the so-called platinum combinations like Cisplatin (Platinex) or Carboplatin (Carboplat), which are feared by patients because of their strong side effects. As you can see, the possibilites of subgroupings and additional derivatives are almost infinite. But I do not want to bore you any longer with additional subgroups like hydrazine derivatives or mitomycins. Instead let's look at the next group of cell killers, the

Antimetabolites
The theory of how this group works assumes that if certain combinations that are similar to the DNA bases are introduced in the metabolism of the cell, then these false bases will be integrated into the DNS strand, which cause the stand to break, i.e the death of the cell. This form of therapy becomes quite reminiscent of Dr. Frankenstein when we go one step further and prevent certain bases from being built-up through so-called folic acid antagonists. To prevent the patient from dying too quickly through this treatment, the patient then is given high doses of a medication like 5FU and then shortly thereafter folic acid (e.g. Leucovorin).

I have noticed something very interesting in this regard. For more than 20 years, this combination is established itself in Germany as the standard treatment for advanced intestinal cancer, although it was never been approved by Germany's highest authority for the approval of medication, the Federal Institute for Drugs and Medical Devices BfArM (see facsimile of letter dated March 26th 1999 on the next page), because it has been demonstrated that this combination was responsible for "Fatalities due to therapy". The fact that the German

159

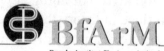

BfArM

Bundesinstitut für Arzneimittel
und Medizinprodukte

MENSCHEN GEGEN KREBS E.V.
Postfach 12 05

71386 Kernen

Hauptsitz und Postanschrift:
Seestraße 10
D-13353 Berlin
Telefon: (030) 45 48 - 30
Telefax: (030) 45 48 - 32 07

Ihre Zeichen und Nachricht vom	Gesch.-Z.: Bitte bei Antwort angeben	Telefon: (030) 45 48 - 30	Berlin 2 6. März 1999
16.03.1999	1-A21014-18978/99	4548 3324	

Kombination 5FU / Calziumfolinat

Sehr geehrte Damen und Herren,

zu Ihrer Anfrage können wir Ihnen mitteilen, daß gegenwärtig
kein Calziumfolinat enthaltendes Arzneimittel für die Kombination mit 5-Fluoruracil bei fortgeschrittenen colorektalen Karzino-
men als Indikation zugelassen ist.

Mit freundlichen Grüßen
Im Auftag

gez.

Dr. Mohrbutter
Dir. u. Prof.

beglaubigt:

*Short Translation: „We hereby confirm, that 5-FU in com-
bination with any calcium acid has not been approved in
Germany."*

government knew this is proven by a letter dated August 30th 1999.

Also most German doctors knew what was published in issue 31/32 of the Deutsche Ärzteblatt on August 8th 1994. I quote: "The Federal Institute for Drugs and Medical Devices notifies medical circles that the treatment of advanced colorectal carcinoma with the combination of 5-FU and CF (calcium folinate as Leucovorin, author's comment) has not been approved, rather it represents an experimental therapy. The serious risks of the combination treatment are pointed out because it has already been widely used in the past."

In a letter I received from Dr. Manfred Hoffmann of the BfArM, Dr. Hoffman writes that the combination of 5-FU and CF has been approved since November 1999. It is interesting in this regard to note that in a letter dated February 23rd, 2000, i.e. 3 months AFTER the apparent approval, Mr. Ulrich Heier from the BfArM writes: "An application for approval of 5-FU for combination treatment with folic acid/folinate has been submitted. The evaluation has not yet been concluded". In this letter Mr. Heier again points out that: „.... "...use outside of the approved indication and under the special conditions of a clinical test is approved. The prescribing doctor bears the possible criminal law and civil law responsibility". Question: was the combination not yet approved in March 2000, or is Mr. Heier telling a lie? And if the answer is yes, then why?

In response to months of persistent inquiry on my part to learn which studies served as the basis on which the combination had now been approved, on the 6th of December 2004 I received a letter from Dr. Hoffmann and a list of studies based on which the combination of 5-FU and CF has been approved. In this list studies are cited e.g. that motivated the BFArM in 1994 to warn: "Our analysis of the data revealed that more patients died in conjunction with the combination treatment 5Fu/CF, (2.3%) than died with a treatment of 5-FU alone

(0.5%). At the end of 2004, these same data are now provided to me as proof (among other things) as to why 5-FU/CF is supposed to be so successful. In other words: "It is not just the cancer patients who are really being hoodwinked in this case". Just how stupid do the employees of the BfArM think we really are? Which group of people gave final approval for the medication? Has it really been approved, and why are there such drastic lies associated with this medication?

I do not have any certain answers to all of these questions, other than coming back to the conclusion that cancer is a huge industry, and that it is not always easy for thinking people to accept these lies. Fundamentally this issue involves people's lives, and yet in many of the 5FU studies that I have reviewed carefully the statement still occurs again and again: "drug-related death occurred in each regimen".

One can only imagine how small the famous tip of the iceberg really is here. Here an explanation in this case is urgently necessary in the interest of so many cancer patients. But how will this happen? The only solutions that I can come up with would be either too expensive or much too dangerous. On the other hand this "little 5-FU/CF example" shows how risky it is to blindly place trust in others when one submits to a therapy, which can lead to death, or to be more precise, has often resulted in death. Let's be honest. If doctors would explain the advantages and disadvantages of 5-FU and Leucovorin in detail, how many patients would then undergo these therapies?

And something else is quite clear. Theoretic constructs are much further removed from practice than they appear to be on paper or in the lab. Additional representatives of this group are: Cladribine (Leustatin), Pentostatin (Nipent), fludaribine phosphate (Fludara), Cytarabine (Alexan), Fluorouracil, 5FU (Efudix) and gemcitabine (Gemzar).

Likewise Gemzar is an interesting preparation that has "secretly" established itself as standard preparation for pancreatic carcinomas. If we disregard pleural mesotheliom (pleura / lung cancer, mainly caused by asbestos), then statistically pancreatic cancer has the worst prognosis of all types of cancer. This year app. 12,000 people will die of this illness in Germany alone. In recent years as far as allopathic treatment is concerned either resignation, or the chemotherapy preparation Gemzar (Gemcitabin) are the norm when dealing with this diagnosis. Gemzar is a medication that disturbs the DNA synthesis, or to be more precise, influences cytosine.

Even with our own intensive research we could only find a few cases of healings or long-term survivors of pancreatic carcinomas (which by the way were almost exclusively possible due to intensive nutrition therapies like Budwig's oil protein diet, NutriTherapy, Gerson's diet or Dr. Gonzales' therapy). The literature primarily cites studies that compare Gemzar with 5FU. Once again these are studies in which two or more chemotherapeutics are compared, so that in the end at least one of them can be evaluated as positive. In the most frequently cited study involving 126 patients, half of the patients were given Gemzar, and the other half were given 5FU. Pharmaceutical companies and doctors cite this study again and again and tell their patients that the patients who received Gemzar clearly lived longer.

But what does "clearly longer" mean for people whose vocabulary is enriched with an abundance of Latin expressions? In this study patients who were given 5FU lived 4.2 months on average. Patients who were given Gemzar lived 5.7 months. To this day this difference is called "a small breakthrough in the therapy of pancreatic carcinomas". Again it was "forgotten" to include a group in the study, which either did nothing, or which pursued biological therapies.

Would you as patient really undergo a Gemzar therapy, if instead of saying to you that you would clearly live longer with Gemzar, your doctor said: "Dear Mr. Miller, statistically you will live a maximum of 6 more months. I know of no therapy that can heal you. However what I could offer you would be a chemotherapy with all of its side effects. However your survival chances increase with this measure by 6 weeks compared to a different chemotherapy that I could naturally offer you as well. I cannot tell you whether your life will be any longer or shorter through using this chemotherapy than it would be if you did absolutely nothing, because there are not any studies about this." Now ask yourself: "Would you still undergo a therapy with Gemzar if the doctor told you the truth in these words?

Gemzar is a good example of how medications can develop themselves into a gold standard, without the prescribing doctor having a single proof that his patient will live one day longer through its use. If this were a homeopathic medication without side effects you could still say: "OK, why not"

Gemzar however is a chemotherapy that is given to people in the last weeks of their life and which clearly lowers their quality of life. Not to mention the costs borne by the general public. Doctors of all people should be much more open with their patients when dealing with the diagnosis of pancreatic carcinoma, and if doctors are not familiar with therapies provided by Gerson or Kelley, who have demonstrably provided therapy to patients who are long-term survivors of pancreatic carcinoma, then they should perhaps consider in more detail how a person would like to spend the last weeks of his life.

Intercalants
The first antinomycin was extracted during the First World War. This substance, which is extracted from bacteria, belongs to the group of intercalants. An intercalation is nothing more than a molecule inserting itself between 2 base pairs. The more important intercalants however are the anthracyclines or in other words; antibiotics – extracted from streptomycin. These cell killers work primarily in the S-phase of cell division, and consequently they are used for leukemias and lym-

phomas. Although this treatment can cause permanent damage to the heart muscle, there is a whole group of these preparations like adriamycin, doxorubicin (adriblastin), and the familiar epirubicin (farmorubicin).

Taxanes

The taxanes are a group that was only approved in the 90s, and which are produced from the bark of the yew tree. Paclitaxel (Taxol) and Docetaxel (Taxotere) are the best known. Although revenue figures for both medications have now reached dizzying heights, to this date there are no hard facts. For breast cancer the best study gave an extension of survival time from 14 months to 15 months. This is a purely statistical deviation possibility and it does not necessarily have anything to do with the medication. All the same 87% of all patients had additional complaints with its use (J Clin. Oncol. 1996; 14:58-65).

Also its use with lung cancer (non-small cell lung cancer) is recommended by the manufacturers in glossy brochures due to the "significant advantages". But where are these significant advantages? In a study of the M.D. Anderson Clinic, still the largest cancer clinic in the world, there was no difference between the placebo group and the two other groups, who were given Taxotere in a higher or in a lower dose (J Clin. Oncol. 2000; 18:2354-62). Is this just another numbers game at the patients' expense?

And now?

If you start reading a book about cytostatic agents and their effects on cells or cell division, then you will most likely require 2-3 new dictionaries. However what is really impressive is reading how much the scientists know about cell division, DNA, and genes in general. The things you can read about hybridized and co-hybridized cells, plasmids, nucleotide sequences and primary clones, are really fantastic.

But at some point a thinking person cannot escape the question: And now? How does all this knowledge really help me? If these scientists know so much, and given the prerequisite that what I have read is really true, then why don't all of these substances work they way the studies say they work? Is there any scientific field where theory and practice are so far removed from each other as oncology.

The more I study the theory of cancer and the more people I become acquainted with who are ill with cancer, the more I distance myself from a satisfying answer to all these questions. It is a fact that chemotherapy, as it is used today, has reached a total dead-end. The wall at the end of the dead-end street, is made of large heavy stones, on which unsatisfactory or wrong answers to frequently asked questions are written. You have certainly read at some time how successful chemotherapies are for cancer. These cancer types are primarily testicular cancer, leukemias, and lymphatic cancer types. A closer look at medicine reveals that cancer types like leukemias have been described by many doctors for centuries, but these "cancer types" have only been included in the big group of "Cancer" for a few decades. When it was determined that mustard gas destroys bone marrow, which in turn is responsible for the increased cells in these types of cancer, the thinking was that a magic remedy had been found for these types of cancers. However apparently only a few doctors question whether leukemia has anything in common with a tumor in the pancreas. Is "cancer" of the lymphatic system really the same as lung cancer? And even more important, is a disturbance in the formation of erythrocytes (leukemia) of a child who is still growing, really the same thing as prostate cancer in an adult?

You will now say certainly not. However at the same time you accept the concept that both illnesses should be treatable with the same medication. We cannot close our eyes to the history of chemotherapy, and this history shows us that there were successes in the treatment of bone marrow disorders, and as a consequence governments and approval authorities around the world were convinced to approve these preparations for treatment of other types of cancer as well. There are still those today who consider this a chess move that brought in billions.

In my daily conversations with cancer patients and with oncologists I experience (with the exception of certain leukemia and testicular cancer illnesses in young people) only that a chemotherapy (and to a much worse degree radiation) indeed can often stop tumors from growing, but it never heals cancer. The few critical statistics that have managed to see the light of day have show the same conclusion. In this regard the public learns even less about how many people die due to these treatments. I often think of a member of People Against Cancer, who died after his first dose of chemotherapy, although he was quite healthy except for a tumor that was still very small. Or the case of a 35-year old mother with two small children who died in a clinic in southern Germany, because she was told that, with her breast cancer, it would be better for her if she took a high dose chemotherapy. What was not given her to read were the studies showing that there is absolutely no advantage in undergoing high dose chemotherapy for breast cancer.

I do not know how you feel but when I see a report on the television about cancer, usually the report involves leukemia and more often than not it concerns children and cancer. This is most likely due to the fact that it is easier to get donations with the emotions thus generated, and because there is something positive that can be said about chemotherapies. The fact that these illnesses do not even account for 0.6% of all cancer illnesses in Germany is usually not mentioned.

Imagine that you are at the airport and there are 20 airplanes outside that will take you from Munich to Hamburg. You know in advance that 19 of these will crash, nevertheless a pilot tries to convince you to fly. Let's be honest, would you board one of these airplanes, or would you rather look around for an alternative means of transport to your destination?

Certainly you would not board any of the airplanes, yet nevertheless similar situations occur almost every day in German clinics. According to the best statistics you have a 5% chance of surviving a chemotherapy, yet in spite of this the majority of epithelial types of cancer are still being treated with chemotherapies. However the big question of why remains unanswered by allopathy. Please consider this again. Although even the best statistics for the major cancer illnesses like breast cancer, lung cancer, intestinal cancer, or prostate cancer, clearly show that the use of chemotherapies offers very little or nothing, nevertheless thousands of cancer patients are treated with chemotherapies on a daily basis. Apparently no allopathic practitioner has hit on the idea of questioning the whole procedure, regardless of how many books Dr. Ulrich Abel will still write (Dr. Abel is author of the book: Chemotherapie fortgeschrittener Karzinome (Chemotherapy of advanced carcinomas), in which he as an employee of the German Cancer Research Center examines most of the chemotherapy studies in detail, and in the process has determined, that there are virtually no studies that prove that chemotherapies contribute to patients with epithelial cancer living longer.

The cancer business is a billion dollar industry

In the meantime the number of people who earn their living from cancer patients, is greater than the number of cancer patients themselves. It is easy enough to imagine that companies that annually earn hundreds of millions of dollars in cancer medications, mammography devices, laboratory examinations, and radiation devices, will do everything they can to satisfy their shareholders. What this struggle looks like we experience again and again. Have you ever wondered that a government minister of health supports cigarette advertising (Germany) or why it is illegal to sell a vitamin C tablet containing more than 250 mg of vitamin C in a supermarket, even though 80% proof alcohol is for sale next to the cigarettes. An even greater problem is caused by a few criminals who are responsible for the fact that thousands must not only suffer, they also must die. I would like to cite the example of Professor Herrmann to show the dimensions of this problem.

In 1997, at 47 years of age Professor Herrmann was still considered to be the shooting star of German cancer research, at least that is how he was described by the news magazine Focus. As student of the "leading" German gene authority Professor Mertelsmann, he received cancer research projects from German Cancer Aid, the Thyssen Foundation, or the German Research Foundation. He won seven research prizes, he was an authority, a member in many scholarly associations and spokesman of German gene therapists.

But in the middle of March 1997, the image of this professor of the medical faculty in Ulm started to crumble. Professor Hofschneider from the Max Planck Institute for Biochemistry in Munich, and Mr. Bertram from the Institute for Human Genetic Engineering at the University of Heidelberg, indicated in a letter to the medical faculty, that Professor Herrman and his assistant and companion Prof. Brach had falsified cancer research.

To make a long story short – it was revealed that Professor Herrmann and Professor Brach had falsified at least 50 research results. Interestingly enough 28 of these were in Freiburg where Professor Mertelsmann was active, and seven other "scientists" from Freiburg were co-authors of 32 of the studies. In other words, most of the major cancer research studies in Germany had been falsified. I am writing this in detail so that you really understand how "scientifically" things are approached in conventional oncology.

Now one would assume that Professor Herrmann and Professor Brach have been incarcerated, and in addition that they must repay millions in research funding. Not be a long shot. Neither of them even lost their appointment (position), and neither has spent a single day in prison. Cancer medications are approved based on such research; and these medications are then administered to thousands of cancer patients. Have you ever seen a list citing which medications have been tested and which approvals have been withdrawn? I have not!

While tax evaders are immediately incarcerated on suspicion, falsifiers never see the inside of a prison. You can see with this example, that the chance that you will be given a medication that has been approved on the basis of false research results, is much greater than is frequently assumed. Even if your doctor means well, how does he really know, that the statistics have not been produced by such criminals? And have you ever wondered why Professor Herrmann never went to prison – isn't he responsible for the death of many cancer patients? How was it possible that no one caught on to Professor Herrmann for years. Who was responsible within the German Cancer Aid organization for seeing how the funds were used? The original text of the Task Force F.H. that was responsible for the investigations stated. "In the publications flawed by falsification, listed here and in concrete publications suspected of falsification, the funding institutes cited are the German Research Foundation in 41 instances, the German

Cancer Aid/Dr. Mildred Scheel Foundation in 43 instances, and the Federal Ministry of Education and Research in 12 instances. Additional funding institutions are also listed. In total 14 of the works listed here have already been withdrawn (as of January 3rd 2000). In the case of 5 publications some of the authors withdrew their own names from the publication (as of Jan 3rd 2000)."

I find it extremely interesting that of all organizations German Cancer Aid was the one that most frequently financed the studies of Professor Herrmann. Naturally any thinking person would now immediately ask the following questions: Did German Cancer Aid cover for Professor Herrmann for years, because his study results were counter to the German Cancer Aid strategy, or did German Cancer Aid pay many people's charitable contributions to Prof. Herrmann for years, without ever examining the results of the studies in more detail? Honestly at this point I do not know which of these alternatives would be worse.

If you survey the German Cancer Aid's official membership list you will find an abundance of professorial titles and political names. However for years not one of these professors or politicians noticed (officially) what was going on here. I do not want to say anymore about the role of the German Cancer Aid in this book. However you can order their "blue booklets" free of charge at: Deutsche Krebshilfe, Thomas-Mann-Str. 40, 53111 Bonn, Germany – and then determine for yourself whether the content of these books will help you along your path.

Certainly Professor Herrman and Professor Brach were not the only people that were indicted by the Task Force F.H., for manipulating research results. Thus you can read in the concluding report: "The Task Force investigated 170 joint publications (publications in journals and book articles) by Professors Mertelsamnn and Herrmann. Of these, 58 studies showed indications of data manipulation, where Mr.

Mertelsmann took the position of last author in 15 of these publications, which normally indicates special responsibility for the publication. In our opinion it contradicts every aspect of reality to assume that a person whose professional activity over a long period was so closely associated with that of another person, did not notice that this procedure or that procedure was incorrect." In December 2001 Professor Mertelsmann (University of Freiburg) was pronounced innocent by the court. I have no comment on this.

However other professors were mentioned, for instance Professor Lindemann: "Professor Herrmann co-authored 53 of the 129 journal publications. Of these 53 publications 27 are on the list of the incriminated publications, 6 of them with his first authorship. Also of 25 book contributions 4 are on this list. In addition, several falsified illustrations were found in the professorial dissertation (see Appendix 18). These accusations resulted in the retraction of the professorial dissertation. .... In our view it remains for the record that Mr. Lindemann disqualified himself as scientist. ..... Even for his professorial dissertation Mr. Lindemann did not want to assume any sustainable responsibility; rather he attempted to withdraw the work after revelation of the apparent data manipulation contained therein, and to submit a new cumulative work, which referred exclusively to "Herrmann-independent" work. To this day this appears to us as an unusual process, when after the accusations are made known a new, "cleaner" work is submitted and it is submitted in a simultaneous exchange for the work flawed by falsification. Mr. Lindemann did not consider it necessary to lay down his position as professor due to these revelations, which he apparently obtained with work that was flawed with falsification.

On the following pages I could list more professors from the oncology field whose manipulations have been "uncovered". However my primary objective is to demonstrate to you how high the probability is that you will be prescribed chemotherapies or other conventional cancer therapies, that are only prescribed because money-hungry, egocentric, and power-hungry doctors, simply stated are walking over corpses. But the biggest scandal for me is how the German judicial system (and not only the German judicial system) deals with these results. Not a single doctor went to prison after this scandal.

If you still believe that your chemotherapy or cyto injection is only prescribed because it has helped so many people in recent years – then you will not be helped if you keep reading this book.

An exception?
More than one fourth of scientists surveyed by the American Association the Advancement of Science admitted that they have personally come into contact with at least 2 cases of research where they suspected falsification or plagiarism in the last decade. In this regard I think of Dr. Poisson from St. Luc Hospital in Montreal/Canada, who falsified the data about the tumor size of his patients.

Or think of the scandal involving Professor Hübener from the University Hospital Eppendorf (UKE) in Hamburg. Hundreds of patients were radiated with a dose, which the courts later said patients died of through the irradiation. The expert report for patients with intestinal cancer said: "A total of 51 patients suffered severe side effects from EORTC/RTOG level >= 3 (51/83 = 81%). An actuarial analysis according to Kaplan-Meier projected a side effect rate of 85% after 5 years and 93% after 10 years. In total at the time of the analysis 20 patients were living (20/63=32%). 43 patients are dead, 23 primarily to tumor ailments, 11 primarily due to long-term effects, and 9 due to the causes/illnesses." Later the 11% was projected as 20%. Now let's take a good look at what has never been discussed in public to this day. Here is the comment of Professor Trott, University of London, in the expert report dated July 7th 1993 concerning patient S. who was irradiated according to the Hübener sandwich method: "In conclusion I have determined that according to the present state of radiology-biological knowledge in 1987 the combination of pre-operative irradiation with 4 times 5 Gy, and post-operative irradiation with 15 times 2 Gy (2.4 Gy), lead to a non-tolerated overdose in the target volumes, which resulted an unjustfiably high risk of chronic radiation sequelae for the pelvic organs."

In total the Professor Hübener's patients received a total dose of 50-55 Gy. This however is an absolutely normal quantity, which is actually at the lower end of the scale in today's cancer therapies, where standard irradiations are often 30-35 times 2 Gy. Because this point was unassailable the 4 x 5 Gy was taken up and was considered to be the culprit for the dilemma (plus the questionable sandwich therapy, i.e. irradiation prior to, and after the operation).

This tactic was used to avoid a larger discussion, namely a discussion of how effective irradiation really is for certain types of cancer. I really have no interest in relieving Professor Hübener of his guilt, but in the numerous expert reports many "colleagues" go easy on themselves by placing all the blame on Professor Hübener's sandwich therapy. On any given day these same colleagues often prescribe a much higher dose than did Professor Hübener and feel that they are justified in so doing as long as the individual dose remains under 2.5 Gy. But we have known for a long time that exposure doses accumulate and do not solely dependent on an increased individual dose.

Don't these doctors ever ask themselves whether many patients die of the therapy and where to draw the limit. Is it 50 Gy, 70 Gy, or 100 Gy? And regardless of the number that is cited here, the next logical question is: "How do you know that this number is correct?"

Response rate and survival time

Chemotherapy also involves an additional issue: Response rate and survival time. You must learn to separate these terms because doctors unfortunately do not always separate them. If a doctor says to you that there are breast cancer studies for example by Henderson and Canello, by Schwartsmann and Pinedo, or by Plosker and Faulds, which prove that chemotherapies like Doxorubicin or Epirubicin in high doses have acheived reponse rates up to 70%, then this is absolutely true. Usually the doctor does not elaborate and "forgets" to tell you that even response rates of 70% in the best studies did not achieve a 25% remission (disappearance of the tumor). However the most important thing is that understand that neither a 70% response rate, nor a 25% remission rate, have any effect on your survival time. Should you still doubt that the tumor, or the tumor size is not as important as it is always made out to be with cancer – all these studies prove it.

Now should I undergo chemotherapy or not?
In my opinion, sooner or later the use of chemotherapy as first strategy will certainly go down in history as medical malpractice, and it is certainly a medical error today to use it as the sole means of treating cancer types like breast cancer, intestinal cancer, prostate cancer, pancreatic cancer, kidney cancer, or lung cancer, – and the legal grounds in support of such use are slowly but surely becoming more difficult to defend.

The fundamentals concerning irradiation

Since you do not feel it,
you will hunt it down in the future

Dr. Seeger

In my opinion irradiation is still considered far more harmless than it really is, and I cannot believe the nonsense that is printed in books or cited in presentations. Many professors maintain publicly that irradiation only damages diseased cells. In response I can only say, "Are there any limits to how much nonsense can be stated publicly?"

Naturally I know that many doctors only say such things to assuage their patients' fear of irradiation or because they want to exert more pressure on the patient so that he really does undergo radiation therapy. I could also say at this point that many doctors consciously lie because they (should) know better due to their education. And this returns us to the old issue which is; How can a patient make an objective decision for a therapie if he only gets one-sided information. And if there is one thing of which I am 100% certain, it is that irradiation with 30 x 1.8 Gy most certainly and most sustainably destroys healthy cells, influences, and in many cases is the direct or sole initiator, for new tumors.

In the literature there are hundreds of findings that prove the hazard of irradiation therapy, as you will read later in this book. The big question however is why is iradation therapy so popular? Several influences come together here. First naturally irradiation can destroy cells, tumors too, completely – it depends on the amount of radiation. Since all of oncology rests on the long outdated statement: tumor gone = cancer gone, it is naturally a logical process to implement destructive therapies for all types of tumors. However the financial aspect is at least as significant. Irradiation therapy is real big business and the magnitude of the revenues for the machines and the therapies is astronomical. Naturally people don't talk about this, because certainly a doctor would not prescribe a radiation therapy for financial reasons – and certainly not a chemotherapy, and certainly not a bone marrow transplant for which a university clinic bills a "laughable" ≠ 190,498.07. Yes, you have read the number correctly. A single therapy costs more than 190,000 Euros, plus additional charges.

In addition, radiation therapy can be simply executed, requires relatively little "doctor time" for the therapy, and it makes sense for the patient, because the patient usually believes that the cancer illness will be gone when the tumor is destroyed. Here as well radiation therapy works extraordinarily well in conjunction with the explanation of the destruction of the micrometastases. There are not many patients who think of asking a doctor whether he has ever seen a micrometastasis under a microscope. These micrometastasis apparently are going to be destroyed with the radiation. In studies, irradiation therapies are only compared with other conventional therapies, so that one of them naturally comes out on top in the contest.

The greatest advantage and disadvantage of iradiation is that irradiation cannot be seen and at first they it does not hurt. Frequently the side effects only kick in often after months, and if things go wrong the primary response is: "The cancer was stronger". All of these reasons together have made it possible for radiation therapy to attain a position in today's oncology, that is totally unexplainable based on the statistical data. The statistics that see the light of day in most cases are not earth shaking, a thinking person is almost afraid to ask how many studies have never been published. However in spite of all, this or precisely because of all this (depending on the individual perspective) there is a reason why radiation therapies are still considered to be the first standard therapy, and many people who worry more about the stockholders than the people who are ill, will also ensure that nothing changes in this regard.

I am absolutely certain that neither this book, nor any other measure can stop the "daily oncological insanity of irradiation". To avoid misunderstanding. I am not always fundamentally against irradiation, but from what I have been able to learn, I am of the opinion that 99% of all irradiation therapies do not benefit the patient. When you consider that doctors irradiate a tissue after an operation just because they **believe** (not know!!!) that cancer cells could still be present there, although the surgeon maintains he has cut "in healthy tissue", then you can see how far removed modern oncology is from scientific medicine.

All of oncology is built on theoretic constructs and radiation therapies happen to fit very well within these theoretic constructs. I know that this sounds like heresy, but believe me, nobody would be happier than me to learn all of these theories are true. What is true however, is that patients get cancer again, precisely at those points where they were radiated. What is true is that all "safe radiation quantities" are only theoretical constructs and it is also true – whether radiologists like it or not – that precisely these irradiations generate cancer.

I do not want to put radiologists or doctors in general in a bad light. But where irradiation is involved, apparently entire groups of professions can no longer distinguish between truth and fiction. I have to say this with such hard words because we are just starting to understand the significant influence of even low frequency waves like transmitted by antennae, and we are very far away from knowing what a radiation quantity of 60 Gy can effect in our bodies. Any doctor who maintains that he knows better in this regard should nominate himself for the Nobel Prize, because he would be the only one in the world. First I find it irresponsible, and second I find it legally unsound for a radiologist to tell his patient that the recommended radiation therapy does not damage healthy cells, or causes little damage to healthy cells. The fact is namely that the radiologist hopes this is the way it is, knowledge is something else. Apparently many medical specialists do not read the literature about X rays; otherwise they would know the following:

As early as 1960 Dr. Zabel described that a tumor only bears the brunt of 0.5-4.0% of the total radiation, the remaining tissue absorbs at least 95% of the amount of the radiation. However because there is a fight around the tunor involving various immune system cells, and it is precisely these immune system cells that are attacked or destroyed by the irradiation. Every person who as undergone irradiation can confirm this due to the increased vulnerability to infection during and after the irradiation. This is a paradoxical situation because the body is then robbed of its defensive function against the rest of the cancer cells.

The famous Otto Warburg described the increased H_2O_2 production of cells caused by irradiation. Since today we know that cancer cells likewise have an increased H_2O_2 production, this can be responsible for an increased cancerization. I am not the only one who has had to experience this "phenomen" many times; namely that a tumor undergoes explosive growth during or shortly after a radition. Allopathic practitioners basically assume that an increased H_2O_2 production leads to the death of cancer cells, but closer examination also leads to the opposite conclusion.

In 1959, Dr. Astaldi published his explanation of how X rays block oxygen consumption, in a parallel relationship with the dose. This is is an important indication, since leukemia cells, for instance, can bear a lot more than healthy leucocytes. In the same year Noyes and Smith published their findings that X rays with 0.2 Gy destroy mitochondria, and that nitrogen content is increased in the mitochondria. On the average patients are radiated with 1.8-2 Gy per session, often this is done 30 times. Thus per session the patient receives 10 times the quantity required for irrevocable destruction of possibly millions of mitochondria! The patient is unfortunately unaware that destroyed mitochondria do not regrow, and thus energy production is impaired for the rest of his life.

These are two arguments that speak strongly against any type of X-rays. In my opinion, whoever denies the importance of mitchondria relative to cancer is beyond help. Mitochondria are vital, not just for cancer, but for our health, and whoever denies this does not really understand anything about biochemistry. However the second part as well, the increased nitrogen content of the mitochonrdia, plays a major role (see mitochondria theory under nitrous oxide).

In 1961 the work of Wohlfarth, Bottermann, and Schneider confirmed that mitochondria under X-rays completely crumble just 15 minutes after the iradiation, fatty acid oxidation is destroyed, and changes are visible in the cytoplasm. We must also thank the researcher Kuhl for his contribution relative to cancer and irradiation. In 1966 he brought the following research together, which Dr. Seeger published in his best German book: Krebs – Weg ohne Ausweg (Cancer – Path with no Return):

1. In 1903 the Berlin Professor Dr. G. Schwartz was able to demonstrate that X rays, radioactive radiation, etc. destroy the cell phosphatides; this means the lecithins in the the the cell membranes and erythrocyte membranes. Thus these rays invoke the same effect SEEGER was able to demonstrate histochemically in 1937/38 as initial phase of the cancer genesis. Because the phosphatide-containing (i.e. lecithin containing) base structure of the mitochondria is also destroyed, as a consequence of the associated disengagement and destruction of the structure-bound oxidation ferments, especially the cytochromoxydase (SEEGER 1938), succinodehydrase and cytochromes (von EULER 1939), an oxygen utilization disorder occurs in the cell, and thus resulting in an electron accumulation of increased negativity, i.e. cancerization of the cell. J. THOMAS (1959) confirmed through oxidation blocking caused by radiation exposure as a consequence of ferment inactivation at concurrent increase of glycolysis.

2. The consequence of oxygen utilization disorder (SEEGER 1938/51) is the fact determined as early as 1925 by C. and F. CORI at the Berliner Charité clinic, (who later won the Nobel Prize), that the blood from a revulsive vein of a leg tumor has a greater oxygen content than blood from the vein of the healthy leg. J. THOMAS (1959) likewise confirmed a significant oxygen increase in the venous blood of cancer patients as a result of blocking or damaging the oxidation fements. Thus the experimental findings of SEEGER (1937/38) and the results derived in 1951 from these findings afford a brilliant confirmation.

3. Through the ionizing radiation therapy, the lipoprotein membranes of the lyosoms in the cell plasma, (these are cell organelles that are 0.4μ in size), are destroyed and hydrolytic proteolytic ferments are freed, which SEEGER as early as 1938 was able to demonstrate with the aid of ABDER-

HALDEN ninhydrin reaction. Their optimum effect is in the acid area which initially is provided by the left-hand lactic acid, occuring through the glycolysis, although this is quickly eliminated.

4. Through ionizing irradiation the lymphocyte defense wall (compare the work of SEEGER: Über die Wirkung von Mistelextrakten (On the Effect of Misteltoe Extracts), Erf. Heilk. 1965) is destroyed and the cancer cells can swarm out; the entire lymphatic system is damaged and thus the body's own defence against cancer cells is destroyed. Even after low doses of 25-50 r an increased decline of lymphocytes takes place through pyknosis and cell disintegration. Spleen, thymus and lymph nodes shrink and degenerate to 50% of their normal weight (A. MARQUARDT and G. SCHUBERT).

5. The mitochondria of the normal cells in the tumor environment, in which only the ferments of the oxydation are membrane-bound contained (SEEGER 1937/38) are damaged and decimated. Reduction of the mitochondrial ferment depot on one hand and inactivation and destruction of the respiration ferments in the still existing mitochondria on the other hand, causes transformation of these normal cells to cancer cells through the ionizing irradiation.

6. The ionizing irradiation resuts in an abrubt cell disintegration. The cancer patient's entire body, which is already overloaded with the toxins of cancer cells like malignolipin, toxohomone (polypeptides), mucopolysaccharides etc. that it cannot handle, is suddenly explosively flooded with cell detritus of the melted down tumor masses D(-)= left-handed pathological amino acids (KÖGL und ERXLEBEN), pathogenic left-hand lactic acids (WARBURG), hydrogen peroxide etc. and the condition of the cancer patient becomes cachetic and life threatening. The cancer patient does not die from his tumor, rather the patient dies from the toxins that are released from the tumor. The toxic effect of ionizing iradiation is best shown in the effect that a dog, which is parabiotically associated with a radiated dog, suffers a fatal poisoning.

7. According to J.SEGAL (1963) ionizing irradiation leads to a shift of the isoelectric point of the serumglobulins to the acid side, the H-bridges in the protein molecule break, a "Faltentrommel" model of polypeptide chains occurs and this leads to an increased occurrence of irreversible denatured proteins in the cell, which SEEGER was able to demonstrate histochemcially with several methods in 1938.

8. The X-ray irradiation results, according to the target theory (concentrated energy shoots through the room like a bullet SEGAL 1960) in a healthy cell mutating into a cancer cell, in addition to production of substances, which are nonphysiological, chemically very active, and that have a highly toxic effect. Peroxides and chemically very active free radicals occur, which secondarily reach and damage the "target molecule" at great distances. According to WITTE (Expert report 1960) there is no real tolerance dose; even the smallest possible x-ray dose, the photon, is capable of generating distinct damages, because it is so rich in energy that it can destroy a large number of the living body's organic molecules.

According to a finding of the well-known physicist B. RAJEWSKI (1960) any influence of X-ray radiation exerted on living tissue results in damage of its structural and functional elements (as already demonstrated in Berlin in 1903 by Professor SCHWARZ) of the units hit by rays. This also applies for any small dose of radiation. BENDER (1910) found that chromosome restructuring mutations or chromosomal breaks, (which have a lethal effect on the cell), occur in 3 of 1000 cells, even with 1 r of irradiation Even the skin dose of a serial x-ray examination of 0.2 r generates an average of

400 ionizations and app. 800 electron stimulations in each cell with a diameter of approximately 10μ. In total, 30 million cells are damaged through chromosome mutations, many fatally, this means through 1-2g of bodily substance are destroyed through a serial X-ray examination.

9. According to E. HECKER (1969) through physical carcinogins like X-ray radiatoin, ultraviolet radiation, or high-energy electron radiation, the bases guanine and thymin in the DNA are irreversibly damaged, in vitro as well as in vivo, in which the six-membered ring of the thymin with loss of 3 carbon atoms is decomposed to urea, and the 5-membered ring of the guanine is transferred in a formamide derivate, whereby the information content of the affected nucleac acids is changed and a somatic mutation or a lethal mutation is caused due to modification of the base sequence of the polynucleotide strand of the DNA and RNA.

I am always surprised that "experts" act today as if all of these facts do not exist. Granted, not all doctors have as much time as I have to go through all the literature and acquire the necessary knowledge about irradiation. But isn't this what a patient could legitimately expect from a radiologist, who, in the final analysis is the person who decides whether the patient will get a radiation therapy or not.

Older studies are often disregarded just because they are old. But the radiation of 1960 is still the same as it is in the 21st century and 60 Gy are still 60 Gy. Also our mitochondria are still structured the same and today are even more severely damaged than they were 40 years ago. If radiation therapies today are trivialized, then this is certainly not because radiation is so harmless for our healthy cells.

5

Conventional
therapies

Conventional therapies

Below I would like to provide you with a list of what the gold standard of allopathy (standard treatment) is for certain types of cancer. Perhaps you are thinking, "But there are certainly conventional text books for this". Yes that is correct, but they do not include my critical comments. And from my years of experience I know that it is often the little things that make the difference as to why patients decide for this treatment, or for that treatment. Does the patient like the doctor, do the doctor's statements come across well, is the clinic conveniently located often are more important decision-making factors than all the statistics in the world.

On the followint pages I have put together a list that is compressed as possible, of those therapies that conventionally thinking doctor will offer you for your type of cancer. Space limitations prevent me from listing all possible therapies, or all that are known to me. However I am sure that I have listed the main theories and I offer my point of view.

Many a doctor would naturally clap his hands to his head and say: "It's just not right. The author can't keep patients away from such "vital" therapies as chemotherapy and radiation. But my response is that I am not keeping any patients away from anything.

If I permit myself to evaluate significant studies in a somewhat different manner than does your oncologist, then I am certainly not trying to confuse you, rather I would like to show you the other side of the coin. The fact that many doctors cannot take this much criticism is just something that I will have to live with and take their responses in stride.

But dear Dr. there is one thing that you should never forget in this regard. We share the same goal, and just as I accept your view of things, I also expect that in the interest of thousands of cancer patients you will accept the fact that there are other points of view. This is the only way that we can jointly be there for all the people who urgently need help. For those that maintain that their way is the right way, I can only recommend that rereading the Gospel of John (most importantly chapter 8, verse 7).

Let's be honest. Isn't it incredibly arrogant to maintain relative to cancer patients, that this or that is cancer and that it can only be treated with three or four therapies. I wouldn't say anyting if objective progress had been made in recent years, particularly with epithelial types of cancer. But this is not the case; it's not even close. All the statistics in the world clearly speak a different language. And as long as there are no proofs for a new beginning, I will permit myself to question therapies, again, again, and again.

Nor should we forget the studies that the Journal of the American Medical Association (Vol. 284, July 26th 2000) published, namely that the allopathy has now become the third largest factor relative to fatality (after heart disease and cancer illlnesses). According to these studies approximately 225,000 people die in the USA due to doctors alone. Just imagine how many people die due to therapies. We should all tread a little more carefully when we maintain that we know how to treat cancer.

Now regarding treatment. Scientists at the McGill Cancer Center in the USA sent a questionaire to 118 oncologists and asked them which of the 6 usual therapies they would use on themselves. 79 doctors responded and of these, 64 said that they never would undergo a therapy with Cisplatin – quite a normal chemotherapy, with annual sales over 100 million Euros. Much worse however was the response of 58 of the 79 doctors, who said that they would never undergo chemotherapy because in the first place it is ineffective and secondly it is much too toxic. When I read this for the first time I only thought: "It is nothing new that doctors treat themselves or their wives differently." But after I thought about all this and considered what it really means that app. 75% of the doctors written to prescribe therapies that they cannot stand behind, then I only had sympathy and anger. Sympathy for the patients who are sacrified. Sympathy for the doctors who daily must subject themselves to the schizophrenia of oncology, and a lot of anger directed toward all those who represent such a system as permenantly positive to the rest of the world.

Frequently I am caught in the contradiction of oncology when allopathic practitioners condescend to ask a non-doctor like me for advice, when they themselves or their families have cancer. On one hand such contacts confirm my work, on the other hand it is not always easy for me to deal with people who have fought against me for years. But I always think of a specific sentence in such situations: "Only dumb people never change their opinion and then I welcome every doctor who uses his intelligence positively. In addition it helps me to remember what I would have done if I had had cancer.

When your doctor says to you that only the therapy that he prescribes is successful and that a, "Mr. Hirneise, who is not even a doctor, doesn't know anything about oncology in Germany", then at least you know that this is not right.

What is the gold standard of conventional oncology?

In the following pages I will show you as briefly as possible and in as much detail as is required

*   The allopathic definition of your type of cancer

*   The incidence of this type of cancer

*   The subdivisions

*   The stages of the illness

Attention:
The TNMG system is employed worldwide to evaluate the tumor stage. This means:

$T =$ *Tumor stage. Stages 1-4.*

$N =$ *Nodes (Latin nodus). Stages 0-3.*
                       For anal cancer:
                       N0 = No lymph node metastases
                       N1 = Perirectal lymph node metastases
                       N2 = Inguinal lymph node metastases (in the groin) and on the internal iliac artery on one side.
                       N3 = Inguinal lymph node metastases (in the groin) and on the internal iliac artery on both sides.

$M =$ *Metastasis. Stages 0 (none) – 1.*

G =   *Degree of cellular degeneration. Stages 1-4.*
             Practitioners call this differentiation.
G1   *means that the cell is well-differentiated, i.e.*
             quite similar to a normal cell.
G4   *means a poorly differentiated cell, i.e. a cell,*
             that is significantly different from a normal
             cell.

* How it is diagnosed by allopathic practitioners

* The allopathic therapy concepts,
  usually organized in:
  - Operation
  - Chemotherapy
  - Radiation
  - Additional therapies like hormones, interferone,
    antibodies etc.

The data come from medical textbooks and from published statistics. Perhaps you know the joke about statistics: What is the progression of a lie? Answer: "One lie, two lies, a statistic."

Moreover you must know that statistics are flexible, they can be "bent" in all directions. I maintain that if you tell me the result that you want to substantiate in advance, then I will make each study appear to be right in my consideration through an appropriate study design, a "bent" evaluation, or by posing the "right" questions. This is why we must be very careful with the specified numbers.

There is something else that is often not taken into account. If a medication helps 99% of all patients, but triggers the most serious side effects for one percent, then initially this sounds quite positive. However if you belong to the 1% then this medication represents a 100% failure for you. If you are told about a particularly positive or negative study, then first ask:

* Who paid for the study?

* Who is served by the result of the study?

* What advantage is there for the person who is telling you about this study?

You should only include the study in your considerations if all three questions can be answered to your satisfaction. I know from my own experience that this requires a lot of effort and often can only be accomplished with difficulty or with a significant time commitment – but what is the alternative? The alternative is clear: Faith instead of knowledge. Unfortunately in today's medicine, the complete treatment of chronic illness (not emergency treatment) is built on this framework. And unfortunately we know how successful it is.

Acute lymphatic leukemia (ALL)

1. The allopathic definition:
Malignant degeneration and dysmaturity of white blood cells. Here the body produces immature white blood corpuscles (lymphocytes), the so-called blasts.

2. How frequently does ALL occur (incidence rate) in Germany (USA appr. x 3)?
Currently one per 100,000 people.

3. Subdivisions:
L-1, l-2, and l-3 blasts are differentiated morphologically. L-1 blasts are small and have a homogenous nucleus. Approximately 20% of all blasts have a large nucleus with indentations and in general they are heterogeneous (different types). L-3 blasts are all large and homogenous (same type).

4. How is ALL diagnosed by allopathic practitioners?
Fatigue, fever, subcutaneous bleeding (ecchymosis), paleness, bone pain, general neurological symptoms, joint pain. Bone marrow punction, (blast count higher than 25%), blood tests (leucocytes, Hb, thrombocytes, measuring the size of the liver and spleen, testicular examination, ultrasound, CT. Basically every physician should make a precise differential diagnosis of rheumatic disease or of an osteomyelitis (bone marrow infection). In detail such a diagnosis should also be made of neuroblastomas, rhabdomysarcomas, and naturally lymphomas. Cytogenetic changes of individual chromosomes are evident for approximately 50% of the patients. The translocation of the cABL protooncogene (paternal chromosome 9q34) designated as "Philadelphia chromosome" and the BCR

(Breakdown Cluster Region/maternal chromosome 22q11) is present in 4% of the incidences of childhood ALL, and 20% of the incidences of adult ALL.

Stages:

As opposed to solid tumors, there is no stage subdivision for acute lymphatic leukemia. The type of treatment depends on the age of the patient, the patient's hemogram, and whether the patient is undergoing the first, second, or third therapy. Otherwise the groups are divided the same way they are divided for AML, in induction therapy, consolidation phase, maintenance therapy, and recrudescence therapies (see AML for more detailed information).

What are the allopathic therapy concepts?

Chemotherapy
In general the treatment protocol for ALL prescribes that chemotherapy will be administered in different blocks in as high a dose as possible over a 6-month period, followed by an additional two years of lower-dose chemotherapy. Usually the following toxins are used: Ara-C, daunorubicin, cyclophosphamide, asparaginase, vincristin, prednison, mercaptopurine and methotrexate.

There is no doubt that there are studies that seem to speak for a chemotherapy. Careful reading however reveals that almost all studies compare old chemotherapy protocols with those that are more recent. Again we do not know what these protocols would look like in comparison with holistic therapies.

Bone marrow therapies (BMT)

In recent years bone marrow substitution therapies in particular have become more and more of a standard; for instance:

A. Allogenic bone marrow transplant / stem cell transplant:

Here the patient receives stem cells from a donor. First high doses of chemotherapy are administered with or without supplemental radiation, in order to destroy all the bone marrow in the body. Then healthy bone marrow is taken from a different donor. The donor's healthy bone marrow is then injected into the patient, and this is supposed to replace the patient's destroyed bone marrow.

B. Autologic bone marrow transplant / stem cell transplant:

In this therapy bone marrow / stem cells are removed from the patient, then the bone marrow is treated with medication to kill all cancer cells, and after high-dose chemotherapy it is returned to the patient. The bone marrow is frozen for storage. The patient then receives a high-dose chemotherapy with or without supplemental radiation therapy to destroy all the remaining bone marrow. The stored, frozen bone marrow is thawed and then injected back into the patient.

Naturally one should not forget that bone marrow transplant involves a high risk of the patient dying due to the therapy. Neither of these therapies is undisputed, even among allopathic practitioners.

Irradtion
Radiation therapy, usually with 24-26 Gy, is recommended for patients, particularly in the case of mediastinal tumors.

Additional therapies like hormones, antibodies, etc.

Although there are approaches with interferon, other therapies like cytokine therapies or monoclonal antibodies, are not used for ALL, because next to testicular cancer and AML, ALL is considered to be the stronghold of chemotherapies.

General

Please read the additional information listed under AML. Even if the individual protocols are different, the therapy approach for AML and ALL are identical.

Acute Myeloic Leukemia (AML)

1. The allopathic definition:
Malignant degeneration and dysmaturity of the blood-forming stem cells. In this regard the word acute means that leukemia cells occur morphologically as blasts and a major portion of blasts are present in the bone marrow (25%-30%).

2. How frequently does AML occur (incidence rate) in Germany (USA appr. x 3)?
The current incidence rate is 2.5 per 100,000 people. On average the patients are over 60 years old. Primarily patients who were subjected to multiple incidences of radiation exposure (tumor therapy, radiation therapy, etc.) are affected. But also patients are affected after a chemotherapy.

3. Subdivisions:
M0 - M7

4. How is this type of cancer diagnosed by allopathic practitioners?
Fatigue, fever, subcutaneous bleeding (ecchymosis), paleness, bone pain, general neurological symptoms, joint pain.

Bone marrow punction (blast count greater than 25%) blood tests, (LDH, leucocytes, Hb, thrombocytes, GOT, GPT, quick, PTT, PTZ, fibronogen, lysozyme, etc.), measurement of the liver and spleen size, testicular examination, ultrasound, CT. Bear in mind here that with hemograms can return values that are too high and too low. Many physicians also use the lactate dehydrogenase value (LDH) as a measurement value of the disease.

General

AML therapy means = chemotherapy. Here there are also statistics showing that patients who received chemotherapy survived the five-year threshold. Naturally what many patients do not know is that there are only a very few patients who have not been treated allopathically with this therapy, naturally again giving rise to the question; "do patients survive because of, or in spite of, the therapy?"

Another point is also "forgotten" when allopathic therapy is recommended. After treatment with such an intensive chemotherapy that is used for AML, which as we know, is carcinogenic itself, there is no possibility of going back to a holistic therapy, because the damages caused by this therapy combination cannot be restored by any holistic therapy. In practical terms this means that the patient must decide for one direction or the other. The option of, "let's test this first, and if it fails then we will pursue a different path", is not possible in 99% of the cases.

Chemotherapy

In most therapeutic centers reference is made to the 4 steps of an AML treatment. These are:

1. In the first phase, the induction phase, a lot of chemotherapy is used to bring the cancer illness into a remission. Here, naturally a CR (Complete Remission) is the objective. According to the allopathic view this is achieved when the medulla blast count is a maximum of 5%, the peripheral thrombocyte count is less than 100,000, and the peripheral granulocyte count exceeds 1,500. In this regard cytosinarabinoside (Ara-C), anthracyclines (such as daunorubicin or idarubicin), thioguanin and VP16 are primarily used. In many clinics the standard has become the TAD therapy (thioguanin, Ara-C, daunorubicin) followed by the HAM therapy (Ara-C, mitoxantrone).

The "M3 patients" are an exception in this case. M3 patients are patients with a promyelocyte leukemia. Patients with this clinical picture initially receive all-trans-retinoic-acid, because apparently studies have shown that the promyelocytic blasts "normalize" and then divide normally again. Unfortunately the side effects of this therapy are very dangerous (embolisms), so that usually this therapy is only used for a short time.

Patients who do not respond to the above-named therapies, are referred to as Non-Responders by practitioners. I find this word very disrespectful; apparently no one has considered that it is not the patients, but rather the therapy that has failed. When referring to the patient as an NR, the underlying assumption is that the therapy was basically correct. What a fatal mistake for many patients.

2. In the second phase, the so-called consolidation phase, the theory is to reduce the recurrence risk with significantly more chemotherapy. This understanding of therapy in my opinion, should be challenged because patients are given no time to recover from the induction therapy and it is believed/hoped that the patient is then healthy enough that he will survive further chemotherapies. Unfortunately many times I have had to experience that this is not the case.

It is also interesting to note that oncologists are not at all unified as to what a successful consolidation phase must look like. To take a heretical stance I could say: Since oncologists have no idea at all of which therapies can help their patients, they simply "to at it and therapise". While many patients get allogenic or autologic stem cell transplants, others in turn are given high-dose chemotherapies with Ara-C or also another "normal" dose with Ara-C.

3. In the third treatment phase, the so-called maintenance therapy, chemotherapies are usually administered in lower doses.

I consider this approach to be questionable, since the chance of an immune/resistance relative to the previously higher, administered toxins is quite probable, and the question must really be asked in this case as to whether maintenance therapies are really anything more than unnecessary toxifications of the body.

4. For relapses, usually so-called "second-line" therapies are offered. Collectively these can be referred to as: Yet more chemotherapies in all variations. In my opinion the helplessness of many oncologists is manifest here. In any field other than oncology, other strategies would be used if the old strategies have failed. But this is not the case in oncology. Here more is administered of what did not work previously. The only answer here is logic, logic, logic.

Bone marrow therapies (BMT)

A. Allogenic bone marrow transplant / stem cell transplant: Here the patient receives stem cells from a donor. First high doses of chemotherapy are administered with or without supplemental radiation, in order to destroy all the bone marrow in the body. Then healthy bone marrow is taken from a different donor. The healthy bone marrow of the donor is then injected into the patient, and this then replaces the destroyed bone marrow of the patient. Unfortunately whether this really occurs is all to rarely investigated. I am not aware of precise test procedures that prove that new bone marrow is really just the bone marrow of the donor, and not partly new bone marrow produced by the patient himself. But as long as over 250,000 EURO are earned for each bone marrow patient, who is interested in answering this question?

B. Autologic bone marrow transplant / stem cell transplant: In this therapy, bone marrow/stem cells are removed from the patient and re-administered to the patient after high-dose chemotherapy. This means that bone marrow is removed from the patient and treated with medication to kill all cancer cells. The bone marrow is frozen for storage. The patient then receives a high-dose chemotherapy with or without supplemental radiation, to destroy all the remaining bone marrow. The stored, frozen bone marrow is thawed and then injected back into the patient.

Naturally one should not forget that bone marrow transplant involves a high risk of the patient dying due to the therapy. Neither of these therapies is undisputed, even among allopathic practitioners.

Radiation and operations
Radiation or operations are not used for AML. If you are offered radiation, then immediately demand to know the reason why, three times.
Additional therapies like hormones, antibodies, etc.

Monoclonal antibodies
There were studies and there are studies with antibodies e.g. CD3 (MAK). Here however it must clearly be stated that while these studies have not shown any significant advantages, they have shown many disadvantages.

Furthermore, in June 2000, one manufacturer of monoclonal antibodies, (Genentech), was compelled to send a warning letter to all physicians in the USA, warning of serious side effects, because 15 women died (within 24 hours of the infusion) through therapies with monoclonal antibodies.

Other approaches
Other medications like arsenic-trioxide, gene therapies etc. are currently being discussed and investigated. However again the question arises: Where are the convincing results?

Anal carcinoma

1. The allopathic definition

Malignant epithelial tumor of the anal region.

2. How frequently does this type of cancer occur (incidence rate) in Germany (USA appr. x 3)?

Currently 2-5% of all interstinal cancer illnesses. There are tests which indicate that a connection exists between anal cancer and homosexuality, chlamydias, herpes, and papilloma viruses. However these studies can be called into question as frequently in this case data is interpreted in ways would not stand up to strict scientific examination.

3. Subdivisions:

App. 90% of all colon carcinomas are plate epithelial and cloacogenic carcinomas (cloacae= end of the hindgut). In addition there are basaloid (from the basal cells) and mucoepidermoid (glandular-cystic structures) carcinomas.

4. How is this type of cancer diagnosed by allopathic practitioners?

Stool examination for blood, bleeding, sigmoidoscopy (endoscopy of the intestine), pain, pencil-thin stool, coloscopy, X-ray (with barium swallow) ultrasound, laboratory with increased CEA and LDH.

What are the stages of the disease?

The TNMG system is employed worldwide to evaluate the tumor stage. This means:

T =	Tumor stage. Stages 1-4.
N =	Nodes (Latin nodus). Stages 0-3. For anal cancer: N0 = No lymph node metastases N1 = Perirectal lymph node metastases N2 = Inguinal lymph node metastases (in the groin) and on the internal iliac artery on one side. N3 = Inguinal lymph node metastases (in the groin) and on the internal iliac artery on both sides.
M =	Metastasis. Stages 0 (none) – 1.
G =	Degree of cellular degeneration. Stages 1-4. Practitioners call this differentiation.
G1	means that the cell is well-differentiated, i.e. quite similar to a normal cell.
G4	means a poorly differentiated cell, i.e. a cell, that is significantly different from a normal cell.

Stages:

TX: Primary tumor cannot be assessed

T0: No evidence of primary tumor

Tis: Carcinoma in situ

T1: Tumor 2 cm or less in greatest dimension

T2: Tumor more than 2 cm but not more than 5 cm in greatest dimension

T3: Tumor more than 5 cm in greatest dimension

T4: Tumor of any size that invades adjacent organ(s), e.g., vagina, urethra, bladder

What are the allopathic therapy concepts?

Operation
Is employed in all stages and is certainly the first option. Unfortunately anal carcinomas infiltrate the musculature of the sphincter quite early so that an operation saving the sphincter is usually not possible. Moreover many men are impotent after anal operations.

For the reasons cited above you should always look for a physician, who is knowledgeable in the area cryosurgery. In this process the tumors are "frozen" and often this can prevent more extensive operations. Often laser therapies are also used.

Anus praeter
Anus praeter is the medical term for an artificial intestinal exit (usually on the colon transversum). Here the distinction is made primarily between a temporary anus praeter or a permanent anus praeter. This intervention also demonstrates the significant impact an intestinal operation has on the remaining quality of life and why this impact must always be carefully considered. Particularly where sexuality is concerned a permanent anus praeter plays a drastically negative role for many people. Basically in this case it must be said that there are studies that confirm life extension through an operation.

Particularly when removal of a large tumor is possible without anus praeter, then the operation should be taken into account when considering therapy.

If you must be operated on, then you should also consider a lectin blockade in the form of a D-galactose infusion for prevention of metastases (see also chapter: supporting substances).

Chemotherapy
For anal cancer usually chemotherapy is combined with radiation (RCT - Simultaneous Radio Chemotherapy) . Medications of choice are mitomycin C and 5-FU. Studies are cited again and again, (Allal 1993, Cummings 1991, Grabenbauser 1993, Panzer 1993), which maintain that you would live longer through these combination therapies, but a closer look again reveals only studies with different toxins have been compared, so that logically there must be a "winner" in the various categories. See Colon cancer for more information.

Irradtion
Radiation is used primarily for smaller tumors, in the hope that the operation can be kept to a minimum. Unfortunately the high quantity of radiation often destroys too much tissue, so that afterwards the operation is necessary anyway. For this reason many oncologists prefer internal irradiation with iridium, because here there are better study results showing that the complication rate is not so high.

Additional therapies like hormones, antibodies, etc.
Are listed under Colon cancer.

Astrocytoma

1. The allopathic definition
Brain tumors that consist of astrocytes, the so-called sheath cells of the CNS (Central Nervous System).

2. How frequently does this type of cancer occur (incidence rate) in Germany (USA appr. x 3)?
In Germany 1-2 people out of 100,000 get astrocytoma annually.

3. Subdivisions:
Astrocytomas belong to the subgroup of so-called astrocytic brain tumors, and here the distinction is made between: pilocytic tumors, (level 1), astrocytoma with low-level malignancy (level 2) , anaplastic astrocytoma (malignancy level 3) and then the glioblastoma (malignancy level 4).

4. How is this type of cancer diagnosed by allopathic practitioners?
In addition to the neurological examinations, imaging processes are used, primarily due to the many differential diagnoses: Electroencephalogram (EEG), evoked potentials (acoustically evoked potentials AEP, visually evoked potentials or VEP, sensory evoked potentials SEP), computertomogram (CT), blood tests (e.g. tumor markers), magnetic resonance tomography (MRT), angiography, positron emission tomography (PET), and naturally biopsies.

Stages:
The WHO grading of CNS tumors establishes a malignancy scale based on histologic features of the tumor. The histologic grades are as follows:

WHO grade I includes lesions with low proliferative potential, a frequently discrete nature, and the possibility of cure following surgical resection alone.

WHO grade II includes lesions that are generally infiltrating and low in mitotic activity but recur. Some tumor types tend to progress to higher grades of malignancy.

WHO grade III includes lesions with histologic evidence of malignancy, generally in the form of mitotic activity, clearly expressed infiltrative capabilities, and anaplasia.

WHO grade IV includes lesions that are mitotically active, necrosis-prone, and generally associated with a rapid preoperative and postoperative evolution of disease

What are the allopathic therapy concepts?

Surgery
Here very clear distinctions must be made relative to the individual levels. For anaplastic astrocytomas the attempt is made to remove the tumor, if its location permits. With pilocytic astrocytomas, an operation is often even curatively (healingly) applied without additional therapy. However if the tumors are near the eyes or on the hypothalamus, then complete removal is usually not possible, i.e. complete removal is too risky for the patient.

Allopathy usually assumes fundamentally that the tumor mass should be reduced, if at all possible from the operation/technical view. I fundamentally disagree with this argument, because my personal experiences with patients who have conquered their tumor without operation, offer compelling reasons to the contrary. In addition the high relapse rate after operations should not be forgotten.

Chemotherapy

Also for anaplastic astrocytomas the value of a chemotherapy is very much disputed among allopathic practitioners, as the tumors of younger people, in particular, are resistant to most of the toxins. There have been and there are attempts with cisplatin, vincristin, doxorubicin, taxol, 5-FU, cyclophosphamide, carmustine, cytarabine und etoposide, but unfortunately the results to this point have not been promising, and basically the question arises here, as to whether chemotherapy is really the right approach for anaplastic astrocytomas.

For pilocytic astrocytomas, chemotherapy does not play as significant a role as it does for anaplastic astrocytomas. Nevertheless here as well polychemotherapies are often recommended if there is tumor infiltration in neighboring regions of the brain.

Irradiation

For an anaplastic astrocytoma usually there is percutaneous (through the skin) radiation after the operation. Today electron accelerating devices (teletherapy) are used almost exclusively. In the meantime cyclical accelerators (betratron) have been displaced by linear accelerators. The fundamental distinction is between total brain radiation and radiation of the tumor alone. You must realize that with total brain irradiation these rays primarily destroy cells that are well supplied with oxygen (healthy cells). However as we know (see cancer theories) this is not the case for cancer cells and consequently the side effects (like strong edema formation) are never foreseeable. Interestingly enough accelerated tumor growth is one of these side effects. I emphasize this point because unfortunately physicians often do not tell their patients this.

In the meantime there are a wide variety of irradiation techniques like stereotactic irradiation, "internal" irradiation with radionuclides like radium 226, iridium 192, cesium 137, cobalt 60, gold 198 or iodine 125. Catheters are operatively implanted in the tumor via bore holes in the skull (overloading process) and in seed implantation radionuclides (seeds) are "worked into the tumor tissue" as small pellets or rods. For pilocytic astrocytomas, usually 125 iodine seeds are used.

But regardless of the type of irradiation used you must clearly understand that the rays pass through your head and thus always destroy more healthy cells than changed cells. Ask any physician who maintains the contrary, to please explain to you how anything else could be possible. Since Hiroshima, Nagasaki, and Tschernobyl, we also know that this radiation in particular generates cancer many years later, yet nevertheless the standard today is still irradiation with up to 70 Gy.

General

The prognosis for pilocytic astrocytoma is very good and in this case, it certainly cannot be said that an extremely aggressive tumor is involved. Consequently you must treat even the "positive statistics" with extreme caution, as many patients also survive without therapy, or they survive "just" with an operation. I refuse to ascribe these successes, particularly for this type of tumor, to irradiation and chemotherapy, although most of the literature does ascribe these successes to these treatments. The fact is, that to this date no one knows how a chemotherapy actually functions in the brain, because biological rules apply for the brain that are different than those that apply for other organs (e.g. blood-brain barrier).

Caution

Since allopathy offers few promising therapies for advanced brain tumors, this is a major field for "experts", and naturally for pharmaceutical companies. For example, currently lenti viruses and herpes viruses that have been altered through genetic engineering are being extensively researched, and it is only a matter of time until new trials will also be made here;

perhaps with you as a test case. Thus be on guard if you are told: "In animal experiments...! Frequently we hear about wonder drugs alike hypericin, SU101, thermal neutrons etc. but here we must deal firmly on the basis of facts, and patients should also be told that these therapies are nothing more than trials, on or with sick people, which have not produced any significant results to this date.

Hyperthermia
For example in the Charité Clinic in Berlin, tests are made with an interstitial thermal therapy (hyperthermia) using liquid magnets. In this process a magnetizable liquid is injected into the tumor and via an externally-applied magnetic alternating field the magnetic liquid, and thus the tumor, can be heated. To this date there are no significantly positive results with people.

Antibodies
Scientists at the Duke Medical Center in Durham have attempted to achieve successes against the tumor antigen tenascin using a radioactive monoclonal antibody. In this process radioactive iodine 131 (coupled antibodies 81C6) is introduced into a intracerebral cavity, which was previously created in an operation of the tumor.

This technique however has already been used by employees of the Duke Comprehensive Cancer Center without success, even if they did not use any iodine 131. To this point mention has only be made of "partial successes". This could be also be termed as stockholder satisfaction.

Gene therapies
After more than 300 glioblastoma patients in 45 clinics in Europe and North America (study 117) were treated with a gene therapy starting in 1996, the study had to be broken off in 1999 because all patients died. Other than earning money

209

the official idea was to sluice "suicide genes" into the tumor using certain viruses. The external hereditary information first results in formation of the protein thymidin kinase. Then the patients received an infusion with ganciclovir, which is transformed in the tumor into a strong cell toxin by the thymidin kinase.

In animal tests it was an outstanding success, however artificially generated tumors in rats are a little different than human glia cells, a group which also includes astrocytomas.

Cortisone and Boswellia acids
The prevention of edemas plays an important role with astrocytomas. Usually this is accomplished through cortisone (e.g. dexamethasone). However Boswellia acid (incense) is used more and more frequently. In studies at the universities of Gießen and Bochum, the best results occurred with a dose of 3 x 1,200 mg / day (DÄ, 94; 18, 2.5.97, A-1197).

Mistletoe therapy
Often mistletoe (s.c. or i.v.) or other immune-stimulating medications are used to reduce the side effects of the cortisone, in particular, but also for recurring prophylaxis. Here however I cannot deny that some holistically thinking therapists refuse the use of mistletoe particularly for astrocytomas, because, according to their experience, it is counterproductive (faster tumor growth).

Basalioma

1. The allopathic definition:

For basalioma (also referred to as basal cell cancer, basal cell carcinomas, or basocellular epitheliomas) the discussion involves malignant cell formation of the basal cell layer of the epidermis (outer skin).

2. How frequently does this type of cancer occur (incidence rate) in Germany (USA appr. x 3)?

Incidence rate: 50-100 per 100,000 annually. This makes basalioma the most frequently occurring epithelial skin cancer.

3. Subdivisions:

The diagnosis can only be ensured through biopsy (cell removal). Polarized light microscopy can be used for differential diagnosis of pigmented basal cell carcinomas. In addition CT or MRT scans can be used. Basically it can be said that basaliomas grow very slowly, often over years, and that they are only "noticeable" at a late stage.

Appearance: First an often unnoticed knot or a hardening of the skin is formed at the affected site. Fine red veins (telangiectasia) on the edge of the tumor are typical. Over months or even years, a glassy or spherical tumor forms with accumulated edge. An additional form appears more like a scar. The moniliform edge (like a string of pearls) is characteristic. The real size of the tumor can extend beyond the visible skin changes.

Stages:

TX: Primary tumor cannot be assessed

TO: No evidence of primary tumor

Tis: Carcinoma in situ

T1:   Tumor =2 cm in greatest dimension

T2:   Tumor >2 cm but =5 cm in greatest dimension

T3:   Tumor >5 cm in greatest dimension

T4:   Tumor invades deep extradermal structures
        (e.g., cartilage, skeletal muscle, or bone)

4. How is this type of cancer diagnosed by allopathic practitioners?

Surgery
An operation is the absolute first choice for therapy and is performed under the aspect of a healing. In the initial stage this is usually an out-patient operation performed under local anesthetic.

In the advanced stage the tumor is usually operated on twice. In the first operation the tumor is surgically removed but the operation incision is not closed. The incision is only closed depending on the biopsy results for the tissue that has been removed. If the examination shows that the tissue removed was not healthy, then another, more extensive operation follows. If the tumor tissues cut out were removed in healthy tissue, then the second operation closes the still-open incision.

Caution
Because particularly in the initial stages of the basilioma, surgical measures are the "easiest" for the patient/doctor, and the 5-year statistics look good for basaliomas, the assumption is

frequently made that an operation would be sufficient therapy. However the good statistics look good, first because basiliomas are often detected at an early stage, and second they grow very slowly. Even for the malignant melanoma (black skin cancer), which usually grows much more aggressively, the Chipsa Clinic in Mexico published a study in which 100% of the patients with T1 stage 5 survived for 5-years (mainly through the Gerson therapy).

As patient you cannot let yourself be lulled into thinking that with removal of the tumor, the cancerous event has also been operated out, just because the cancer is a type that grows very slowly.

Chemotherapy

For basiliomas there is a distinction between local and systemic chemotherapy. With local chemotherapy the medication of choice is the cytostatic agent, 5-fluorouracil (5-FU). Mostly it is used for 4-6 weeks (1-5% in cream or salve). There are no statistically relevant data to indicate that this therapy holds out any more promise than does an operation.

Although there are repeated trials with systemic chemotherapies for metastized basiliomas, particularly with 5-FU (fluorouracil) in combination with cisplatin, all therapy approaches have failed and they could not contribute to a significant extension of life. If your doctor suggests a systemic chemotherapy, then this should not be regarded as anything other than an act of despair.

I am aware that what I say may be hard to take. However I cannot support a situation wherein patients who have been given up on by the treating doctor, (hence the systemic chemotherapy), are then used as study objects.

Irradiation

Today the allopathic view is that radiation offers prospects for healing that are comparable to those offered by conventional surgical treatment (Silvermann et. Al. 1991a, Rowe et al. 1989c; Rowe et al. 1989b; Dubin, Kopf, 1983; Silverman et al. 1992b; Smith, Grande, 1991, Lovett et al. 1990, Grieb et al. 1995). This is why patients over 70-years in age with basiliomas in the nose, corner of the eye, ear, or mouth area, are advised that radiation is preferable over an operation.

In my opinion this gross error is based on the assumption that radiation destroys the tumor just as effectively as does an operation. What is totally forgotten in the process is that this therapy is carcinogenic and comes at a cost of side effects and risks which are a thousand times greater, because therapists are employing a radiation dose of 15-25 Gy weekly over several weeks.

Additional therapies like hormones, antibodies, etc.w

Photodynamic therapy

Photodynamic (PTD) therapy is recommended to patients, particularly for larger basiliomas. Here a special agent (e.g. HPD) is applied on the tumor mass, and then after 24 hours it is exposed to red or blue-green light, which is supposed to kill the tumor cells.

This therapy could represent an alternative to an operation in areas where operating is difficult. Unfortunately I could not find any meaningful data.

Interferon

There are studies with type I interferon (a, b) in which I.E. was given 3 x a week over a three-week period. Here as well there are no meaningful data that would indicate an advantage over the other therapies, as far as extension of life is concerned.

Imiquimod Aldara® cream (3M Medica)

Imiquimod is a so-called imidazochinoline derivative, which has really been approved for treatment of extra-genital warts (condylomata acuminata) that are caused by human papilloma viruses.

Imiquimod in this case is supposed to induce an immune-modulating effect. In scientific terms this means that it is assumed that imiquimod docks on the surface receptors of the cells of the immune system like monocytes, and macrophages, and stimulates the phosphorylation of the transcription factors NF kappa B (kappa gene enhancer binding protein) and of factors for the transcription of the tyrosine kinase and the protein kinase C. Synthesis of IFN, TNF, IL-1, IL-6 and IL-8 is induced in this manner. In English this means that the immune system is stimulated.

In a double-blind study performed in a Californian skin clinic with 24 patients, for 15 patients who rubbed in imiquimod 3 x a week, after 6 weeks the tumor could no longer be found. However there were strong skin reactions that compelled many patients to stop the therapy.

Cyrotherapy

Cyrotherapy with liquid nitrogen at -196° C in the contact process or spray process is a technique that achieves results that are comparable to those attained with conventional surgery, if appropriate safety distances are maintained. [Hall et.al 1986: Tuppurainen, 1995; Rowe et al. 1989c; Rowe et al. 1989b]. It can represent an alternative to an operation for well-delimited, surface tumors that are not too large, particularly for those patients who are advanced in age.

Fever therapy

The use of fever therapies (endogens through bacteria) has been proven positive, in my opinion, for all skin tumors, and should be taken into consideration in any case.

Breast cancer

in women (mamma carcinoma)

1. The allopathic definition:
Breast cancer is a disease of the female mammary gland.

2. How frequently does this type of cancer occur (incidence rate) in Germany (USA appr. x 3)?
The current incident rate is 75 per 100,000 women.

3. Subdivisions:
The majority of the tumors originate in the ductal (milk duct) epithelial and the remainder from the lobuli.

Stages:

TX: Primary tumor cannot be assessed

T0: No evidence of primary tumor

Tis: Intraductal carcinoma, lobular carcinoma in situ, or Paget's disease of the nipple with no associated invasion of normal breast tissue

Tis (DCIS): Ductal carcinoma in situ

Tis (LCIS): Lobular carcinoma in situ

Tis (Paget's): Paget's disease of the nipple with no tumor. Paget's disease associated with a tumor is classified according to the size of the tumor.

T1:   Tumor =2.0 cm in greatest dimension
T1mic: Microinvasion =0.1 cm in greatest dimension
T1a: Tumor >0.1 cm but =0.5 cm in greatest dimension
T1b: Tumor >0.5 cm but =1.0 cm in greatest dimension
T1c: Tumor >1.0 cm but =2.0 cm in greatest dimension

T2:   Tumor >2.0 cm but =5.0 cm in greatest dimension

T3:   Tumor >5.0 cm in greatest dimension

T4:   Tumor of any size with direct extension to (a) chest
        wall or (b) skin, only as described below
T4a: Extension to chest wall, not including pectoralis
        muscle

T4b: Edema (including peau d'orange) or ulceration of the
        skin of the breast, or satellite skin nodules confined to
        the same breast

T4c: Both T4a and T4b

T4d: Inflammatory carcinoma

4. How is this type of cancer diagnosed by allopathic practitioners?
Palpation of the breast, scanning processes like CT, mammography, ultra-sound etc. Definitive determination of the malignancy through pathology after previous biopsy.

What are the allopathic therapy concepts?

Surgery
Is employed in all stages and is always the first allopathic

therapy. Here there is a distinction between breast-saving operations and radical operations (mastectomies).

Comments: There are several studies, which show that radical operations do not provide any advantage for survival (e.g. L94; 334:1496-7). Even the removal of lymph nodes can result in unnecessary long-term damages. In the meantime there is the allopathic possibility of dying the so-called "first lymph node" and thus avoiding unnecessary removal of the lymph nodes.

Chemotherapy
Usually the approach involving CMF (cyclophosphamide/ methotrexate /fluorouracil) or similar combinations (CAF/VAC) is used. More and more physicians are also using taxol, taxotere, etoposide, idarubicin and even gemcitabine. Chemotherapy is also used more and more frequently prior to an operation, in order to reduce the size of the tumor.

Studies by Henderson and Canello, by Schwartsmann and Pinedo, or by Plosker and Faulds prove that chemotherapies like doxorubicin or epirubicin in high doses can achieve response rates up to 70 %. Unfortunately this has no effect whatsoever on your survival time, as the major studies demonstrate (Antman 1992, Walters 1991, Marschner 1994, Becher 1990, Focan 1990, etc.). These numbers are very significant, as they prove that destruction of tumors, or reduction of tumors really has no effect, and that it is much more important to fight the causes and not the tumor.

Comments
1. For you it is very important to know that to this date there are no sure tests that indicate that you will live significantly longer through any combination or single application of chemotherapy medication. Combinations do not produce survival times that are any longer (Baker 1974).

2. Even the NCI (National Cancer Institute) in America published that before the adjuvant chemotherapy was implemented throughout the country starting in the mid 80's, 91% of all women with localized breast cancer lived for more than 4-years, regardless of age (NCI/Bethesda 1994). This means nothing more than that the survival rate has declined since the introduction of the various chemo combinations.

3. High-dose chemotherapy plus bone marrow transplant.
If this therapy is suggested in your case then you should certainly first read the studies that demonstrate that this therapy has never left the experimental stages, due to the poor results (Lancet 1998, Rodenhuis, Eichel). As of this writing nobody has discussed how many women had to die through this therapy.

4. In October 2004 an article from Jörg Blech that appeared in the German news magazine Spiegel (again) shocked the oncology world, relative to breast cancer. The article published the latest data from Professor Dieter Hölzel from the Großhadern Clinic in Munich. Professor Hoelzel and his team have collected data on several thousand cancer patients since 1978, and in the process they found out something astounding (for lay people). Thus the survival time for women with metastasized breast cancer in the period from 1978 – 1986 was precisely 24 months. In the period from 1987 – 1993 it was 23 months and in the period from 1994 – 2002 it was only 22 months. This fact alone was and is shocking. If, in this regard, we also consider that the sales figures for chemotherapies increased from 5.93 billion USD to 16.11 billion USD, just in the 1996 – 2004 period alone, then we would must finally dismiss the whole pack of lies associated with the "new and better chemotherapies".

Since the 1970's women with breast cancer have been persuaded (or should I say forced?) to undergo chemotherapies and radiation with all types of lies. Some studies are cited, numbers are juggled, and finally the simple outcome is, that if you follow the counsel of your expert in white, you must die sooner. But not just that, this counsel costs billions of Euros, women go through the anxiety of a chemotherapy, and in many cases it has even cost women their lives, because they died directly or indirectly as a result of the chemotherapy.

Now I am enough of a realist to know that even this article in Spiegel magazine will not change anything. Insurance companies will continue to pay for almost any chemotherapy, governments will continue to approve almost any chemotherapy, and patients will continue to allow chemotherapy to be prescribed for them. I cannot prevent all of this. But I can ask you, dear reader, to you thoughtfully consider what you have read. Or in other words: Ask yourself the question; "Do I need any more evidence in order to understand that chemotherapy for breast cancer cannot contribute to my living any significantly longer, but rather it can possibly contribute to earlier death!

Irradiation
Although to this date there are no hard facts confirming that irradiation contributes to women living significantly longer, this therapy is still considered part of the standard program. The recommendations are usually that the entire breast should be irradiated with 50-60 Gy. Here in turn you must know why this is the case, because interestingly enough even leading oncologists say that the survival time is not significantly increased through this measure. This is why the studies usually refer to prevention of local recurrence of up to 40%", similar to the studies of chemotherapies.

In English this means that indeed tumors do not occur as often, however this fact does not mean that you will live a single day longer. Here again the assumptions are based on the micrometastases theory. A prospective randomized therapy from Dr. Wilhelm Friedl (Surgical Clinic Heidelberg University) for breast cancer showed that after 10 years, approximately 37% of the women were still living, regardless of whether they had undergone irradiation or not (MT, No. 6/82). The study by Dr. B. Fisher/ USA involving 2,000 women over a 9-year period showed no difference (NEJM 89; 320: 822).

Dr. Ian MacKenzie's study proved that for the 781 women he examined, the chance of getting breast cancer was 24.5 times (!) higher for women who had had irradiation, than it was for non-irradiated patients (1/510 und 13/271).

Additional therapies like hormones, antibodies, etc.

Monoclonal antibodies
In Germany primarily Herceptin (trastuzumab) is used. This is due to an American study. In this study one group was given chemotherapy and the other group was given chemotherapy and herceptin. After one year 67% of the chemo group were still living, and 78% of the other group were still alive. This study, which lasted precisely one year, and even though its differences can be explained by statistics alone, was enough to market Herceptin as the "new wonder drug" against breast cancer. In June of 2000 the manufacturer Genentech had to send a letter to all physicians warning of serious side effects, because 15 women died due to the therapy (within 24 hours of the infusion). The utmost caution is urged, particularly for patients with lung and heart diseases.

Hormonal therapies
If your estrogen or progesterone receptors react positively then usually a hormonal therapy is prescribed, such as tamoxifen. The idea behind all anti-estrogen medications is to sup-

press estradiol-specific cell metabolism stimulation. In theory this leads to stimulation of growth-inhibiting factors (TGF-ß) and it is supposed to inhibit growth promoting factors (FGF alpha and IGF).

To this day tamoxifen is a very controversial medication. On one hand there are "official studies", which are supposed to prove the effectiveness of this medication, on the other hand do not forget that the leader of the major tamoxifen study, Dr. Fisher had to rescind his study because he falsified important data (including the fact that there were 4 fatalities through tamoxifen, and that cervical cancer occurred more frequently). The most recent data from 2000 confirm the danger of tamoxifen. In Holland, 309 women who had developed cervical cancer after breast cancer illness were examined. These women were compared with 860 women who "only" developed breast cancer, and the result was that women who had been taking tamoxifen for a maximum of two years had a 50% greater risk. Women who had taken tamoxifen for two to five-years had a 100% greater risk of developing cervical cancer, and women who had taken tamoxifen for more than five years had a 690% greater risk of developing cervical cancer (Lancet 2000, 356). Moreover the cervical cancer was more difficult to treat for these women, than it was for the women who had never taken tamoxifen.

The national cancer Institute in the USA and the Sloan Kettering Cancer Center also reported that tamoxifen can induce mutations at the p53 gene, which naturally can be quite disadvantageous for cancer patients.

There is an another problem which also has not be investigated adequately. It is known that tamoxifen docks on receptors. However because tamoxifen does not fit into the receptors 100%, the receptor changes slightly. However this could result in the receptors becoming immune to their own hormones. This phenomenon has been observed for a long time in other medications. An alternative in this case could be perhaps Indole-3 Carbinol (see chapter: supporting substances). Professor Dr. Julius Hackethal has been pursuing an independent way of hormone blockade since 1985, by daily injecting buserelin (profact) a so-called hormone blocker (GnRh), in high doses (20-40x higher than recommended). Usually Buserelin was given for 6-24 weeks and thereafter for 3-6 months with pauses.

The 2001 and 2003 data, published in the WHI study, as well as the data provided by Dr. Chlebowski, Dr. Gann, and Dr Morrow, clearly demonstrate that women who have been taking hormones (estrogen and progesterone) for several years, develop breast cancer significantly more frequently, and that this cancer is even more advanced when it is detected. This is due primarily to the higher radiation resistance of the breast tissue of the women. In addition there is also the aggravation that mammograms often have a noticeable appearance and consequently lead to incorrect diagnoses. For decades doctors have warned of the dangers of the birth-control pill and against taking hormones in the menopausal years. The present recommendation can only still be: Stay away from hormones!

Aromatase inhibitors
In women after menopause estrogens are primarily produced in increased amounts in fat cells. Aromatase inhibitors can prevent this production, and consequently are often prescribed for older women. Aminoglutehemide, along with anastrozole and letrozole (Arimidex/Femara) belong to a new generation of aromatase blockers.

In the 2002 ATAC study involving 9366 women, (Arimidex, Tamoxifen alone or in combination were compared – again only toxins were compared), it was shown that Arimidex had significantly fewer side effects than did tamoxifen, however no significant advantages were shown relative to survival time. Personally I consider this international, much-discussed, study to be a joke, since the study was executed and evaluated by the manufacturer of both medications, AstraZeneca. I wonder if all the doctors who prescribe this medication or that medication on the basis of such a study, know who is behind the study?

Brassiere

With breast cancer there is a risk, which unfortunately is not mentioned in the media for various reasons. It is discussed in the study by the anthropologists Sydney Ross Singer and Soma Grismaijer. Both investigated a total of 4,700 women and they found that the chance of getting breast cancer is 125 times greater for women who wear a brassiere 24 hours a day, than it is for women who do not wear a brassiere. At 12 hours a day the chance is still 21 times greater. The reason for this is not known. Probably the fact that brassieres permanently block lymphatic vessels plays a significant role. Also the changes of the magnetic field through the mostly artificial fibers of the brassier could be responsible for this. Today we still do not know why brassieres have such negative effects, but after this study every woman should reconsider whether she wants to wear a brassiere in the future, or what kind she would like to wear.

There is something else that I have noticed in this regard. Japan has the lowest incidence of breast cancer in the world, and upbringing, nutrition, and many other influences are discussed internationally in an effort to determine why this is so. However the fact is that Japanese women wear fewer brassieres due to smaller breast size, this is at least one reason of perhaps many, but it could also be the main reason for the lower incidence of breast cancer in Japan.

Cervical cancer
(cervical carcinoma)

1. The allopathic definition:
With cervical carcinoma cancer cells are found in the cervical tissue.

2. How frequently does this type of cancer occur (incidence rate) in Germany (USA appr. x 3)?
Currently app. 7,000 women annually. There are statistics that are supposed to indicate that women who have not given birth, who became sexually active early in life, or who had infections with herpes or papilloma viruses, get cervical cancer more frequently. However these data are very difficult to evaluate and consequently must be considered carefully.

3. Subdivisions:
The distinctions are mainly based on tissue types. Most (app. 80%) are squamous epithelial carcinomas, followed by the adenocarcinomas (app. 10-15%). The rest are mixed tumors.

Stages:

TX: Primary tumor cannot be assessed

T0: No evidence of primary tumor

Tis: Carcinoma in situ

T1/I: Cervical carcinoma confined to uterus (extension to corpus should be disregarded)

T1a/IA: Invasive carcinoma diagnosed only by microscopy. All macroscopically visible lesions--even with superficial invasion--are T1b/IB. Stromal invasion with a maximal depth of 5 mm measured from the base of the epithelium and a horizontal spread of 7 mm or less. Vascular space involvement, venous or lymphatic, does not affect classification

T1a1/Ia1: Measured stromal invasion 3 mm or less in depth and 7 mm or less in horizontal spread

T1a2/IA2: Measured stromal invasion more than 3 mm and not more than 5 mm with a horizontal spread 7 mm or less

T1b/IB: Clinically visible lesion confined to the cervix or microscopic lesion greater than T1a2/IA2

T1b1/IB1: Clinically visible lesion 4 cm or less in greatest dimension

T1b2/IB2: Clinically visible lesion more than 4 cm in greatest dimension

T2/II: Cervical carcinoma invades beyond uterus but not to pelvic wall or to the lower third of the vagina

T2a/IIa: Tumor without parametrial involvement

T2b/IIb: Tumor with parametrial involvement

T3/III: Tumor extends to the pelvic wall and/or involves the lower third of the vagina, and/or causes hydronephrosis or nonfunctioning kidney

T3a/IIIA: Tumor involves lower third of the vagina, no extension to pelvic wall

T3b/IIIB: Tumor extends to pelvic wall and/or causes hydronephrosis or nonfunctioning kidney

T4/IVA: Tumor invades mucosa of the bladder or rectum, and/or extends beyond true pelvis (bullous edema is not sufficient to classify a tumor as T4)

M1/IVB: Distant metastasis

4. How is this type of cancer diagnosed by allopathic practitioners?
Unusual bleeding, abdominal pains, enlarged uterus, ultrasound, CT, magnetic resonance tomography, hysteroscopy (endoscopy of the cervix), curetting.

The PAP test is still performed frequently. Although many studies (for instance see the book: What Doctors don`t tell you, page 91-100) or the unnecessary expense involved, confirm the unreliability of this test, it is still part of the standard program of many gynecologists.

What are the allopathic therapy concepts?

Surgery
There are no studies confirming that radical operations, i.e. with removal of the cervix and/or fallopian tubes, produce better results, as Connors and Norris demonstrated in their 1990 study. Unfortunately this operation is still frequently performed. In this process the cervix as well as the lymph nodes in the pelvis are also removed. Usually the entire cervix, both fallopian tubes, both ovaries, the pelvic lymph nodes, and parts of the abdominal viscera (tissue covering within the stomach area) are removed (Wertheim-Meigs-operation). Usually the upper third of the vagina is also removed.

Cleaning out of lymph nodes is even disputed among allopathic practitioners, as there are no studies that prove that patients live any longer through this measure (Hannigan et. al.; 1992, as well as Leibsohn). Considering that the side effects however are clearly greater, then this option should be discussed with the surgeon in any event.

In later studies parts of the colon, the rectum, or the entire bladder are also removed (exenteration). Thereafter you usually require a new vagina, which must be surgically created.

Chemotherapy
There are many studies with chemotherapies, usually in combination with irradiation. Most studies have shown that chemotherapies plus irradiation in comparison with irradiation only, decrease the chances of survival (Souhami et al., 1991, Cardenas et al., 1992, Kumar et al., 1994, Tattersall et al., 1995).

In recent years primarily cisplatin as established itself as "Gold standard". What is interesting in this regard however (Malfetano et al., 1993 , Souhami et al., 1993, Runowicz et al., 1989, Potish et al., 1986), is that in all the studies only the response rates are cited (which naturally are quite high for cisplatin) and that the entire observation time amounts to a maximum of 44 months. In addition the groups examined were quite small, sometimes with 29 patients (Potish). However the most important thing here is that in the study, again there was comparison with a biological therapy, not to mention that the results were not all that exciting anyway (4-year survival 81% with cisplatin against 71% without it).

Another point is that with cisplatin, you are possibly giving up a chance for healing, as you damage your bone marrow so strongly, that you do not recover from the damage, or you die because of the therapy. This point is happily "forgotten" although countless people die through chemotherapy each year.

Irradiation

In 1992, Dr. Hannigan published a study in which he was able to prove that over 30% of all women with cervical cancer had been irradiated in the pelvic area due to other illnesses. This fact was immediately swept under the rug and the reason was given that these women had a predisposition to cancer anyway. From the conventional medical view, this is naturally understandable otherwise a radiologist would have to ask himself whether he had generated the cancer of these women! And it could even get worse. Someone could get the idea to likewise subject other types of cancer to an intensive examination. In this case it is certainly a lot better to certify "bad genes" for all women.

Irradiation plays a major role with cervical cancer. It used alone mainly for very advanced tumors and in the early stage, it is used instead of an operation. For local irradiation, a radiation probe is advanced through the vagina to the tumor region. This type if irradiation is referred to as afterloading. This measure is supposed to protect the tissue that is not affected by the tumor, such as the bladder or the intestine. Otherwise most women are offered a radio-chemotherapy combination, usually with a cisplatin supplement.

Additional therapies like hormones, antibodies, etc.

Hormonal therapies

Hormonal therapies are not used in treating cervical cancer, other than to trigger cancer. In this regard the medication tamoxifen plays a major role here.

Data published in 2000 confirm the danger of tamoxifen. In Holland 309 women who had developed cervical cancer after breast cancer illness were examined. These women were compared with 860 women who "only" developed breast cancer, with the result that women who took tamoxifen for a maximum of two years had a 50% greater risk; women who took tamoxifen for two to 5-years had a 100% greater risk, and women who took tamoxifen for more than five years had a 690% greater risk of developing cervical cancer (Lancet 2000, 356). Moreover the cervical cancer was more difficult to treat than it was for the women who had never taken tamoxifen.

Chronic Myeloic Leukemia (CML)

1. The allopathic definition:
Malignant degeneration and dysmaturity of the blood-forming stem cells. As opposed to acute myeloic leukemia, there is an increase of all three cell series in the initial stage in all maturation levels.

2. How frequently does this type of cancer occur (incidence rate) in Germany (USA appr. x 3)?
Current incidence rate: one per 100,000 people.

3. Subdivisions:
CML is usually divided into three stages.

1. Chronic stable phase
The main symptoms here are fatigue, loss of efficiency, and nocturnal sweating. There is an increase of leukocytes (leukocytosis) in the blood, and you can find an enlargement of the spleen (splenomegalia) that can also cause a feeling in pressure in the upper left area of the stomach. In addition there is throbbing or pressing pain in the breast bone.

2. Acceleration phase
In this phase there is increased leukocytosis, anemia (red blood cell deficiency) and thrombocytopeny (blood platelet deficiency). In addition there is tumor fever, bone pain, and possibly weight loss. Splenomegalia also increases.

3. Blast crisis
In this stage the bone marrow produces immature preliminary stages of blood cells (blasts) and gives them off into the blood.

The number of blasts increases to over 30% of all blood cells.

4. How is this type of cancer diagnosed by allopathic practitioners?
See the divisions cited above, and it is diagnosed by the presence of the so-called Philadelphia chromosome (possible for app. 90% of all patients). A more precise blood test must be performed (Brc/Abl etc.) for patients that are Philadelphia-negative.

What are the allopathic therapy concepts?

Surgery
Often it is necessary to remove the spleen. But otherwise naturally operations do not play a role with CML.

Chemotherapy
In contrast to acute myeloic leukemeia, chemotherapy does not play a major role, since chemotherapies do not result in healing. However they have been "tested" for years in all forms, indeed without success. Nevertheless, chemotherapies, usually hydroxycarbamide, are used in order to better control the number of cells and the size of the spleen. Prednisone, vincristin, or mitoxantrone are also used.

Allogenic bone marrow transplant / stem cell transplant:
Here the patient receives stem cells from a donor. First, high doses of chemotherapy are administered to destroy all the bone marrow in the body. Then healthy bone marrow is taken from a different donor. The healthy bone marrow of the donor is then injected into the patient, and this then replaces the destroyed bone marrow of the patient. According to allopathic opinion, this is the only therapy of CML that can result in healings. Unfortunately in this case you need an HLA-identical donor (HLA=human leukocyte antigen). Alternatively

HL-compatible donors are also accepted, but not with the same prognosis of success.

Irradiation

Radiation is not used, except for the rare exception of radiation of the spleen.

Additional therapies like hormones, antibodies, etc.

Interferon

Interferon-alpha is used for early treatment in a very high dose of app. 5 million units / m2 per day. In approximately half of the patients this should result in at least temporary normalization of the blood, and to a reduction in size of the enlarged spleen. But disappearance of the malignant cells with the Philadelphia chromosome only occurs in one patient out of ten. In addition there are some serious side effects, and as soon as the medication is not taken the illness returns.

STI 571 / Glivec / Imatinib

Since May 2001, the enzyme inhibitor, imatinib, has been approved as Glivec for patients with CML. With Glivec the idea is to inhibit the Bcr-Abl-protein which shows a certain enzyme activity (so-called tyrosine kinase activity), without the leukemia cells cannot survive. Glivec was highly praised in the press (once again) as *the* medication for CML, and in the meantime it has even been approved for other types of cancer, like stomach cancer. But the same applies here as well: "Let's wait and see", because the initial euphoria has long since faded after the medication did not even come close to achieving the projected successes.

This does not mean that Glivec perhaps could not be an important medication in the treatment of CML, but in the meantime, even among allopathic practitioners, there are some voices warning against viewing Glivec as a wonder drug. I can only agree, and say that my few experiences with Glivec have not been exactly overwhelming. In advanced cases (and there are a lot of these!) Glivec appears to be unable to prevent relapses, as reported by the journal "Science" in June 2001, and secondly it even promotes the growth of the cancer.

While many patients indeed get a remission, this condition does not last long. For approximately 80% the hopeful phase lasts for a maximum of one year, then a special gene again produces too much kinase protein, thus activating the growth of cancer cells. In California a team headed by Charles Sawyers claims to know why. His team discovered a point mutation in the Bcr-Abl-gene in patients, which changed the corresponding protein in such a manner that Glivec was ineffective. At the same time it maintained its activating effect with the consequence that tumor growth started up again.

With other patients the gene was present in extra copies and thus flooded the cells with the kinase. These investigations again show how intelligent our cells are and that destruction of cells can never be the solution to the cancer problem.

Colon cancer
(colon carcinoma)

1. The allopathic definition:
Malignant epithelial tumor of the colon (main part of the large intestine).

2. How frequently does this type of cancer occur (incidence rate) in Germany (USA appr. x 3)?
Current incidence rate: app. 18 men and 25 women per 100,000 people.

3. Subdivisions:
Approximately 90% of all colon carcinomas are adenocarcinomas (carcinomas that form glandular or duct-like structures).

Stages:

TX: Primary tumor cannot be assessed

T0: No evidence of primary tumor

Tis: Carcinoma in situ: intraepithelial or invasion of the lamina propria*

T1: Tumor invades submucosa

T2: Tumor invades muscularis propria

T3: Tumor invades through the muscularis propria into the

subserosa, or into nonperitonealized pericolic or perirectal tissues

T4: Tumor directly invades other organs or structures, and/or perforates visceral peritoneum

4. How is this type of cancer diagnosed by allopathic practitioners?
Stool examination for blood, sigmoidoscopy (endoscopy of the intestine), pain, pencil-thin stool, coloscopy, X-ray (with barium swallow) ultrasound, laboratory with increased CEA and LDH.

What are the allopathic therapy concepts?

Surgery
Is employed in all stages and is certainly the first option. Here a distinction is made between various operations:

A: Non-radical operations
In this process only the tumor is removed without cleaning out the lymph nodes. This operation is usually suggested for very old people or people with a high operation risk.

B: Radical operations
In this process the tumor and the lymph nodes are removed.

C: Anus praeter
Anus praeter is the medical term for an artificial anus (usually on the colon transversum). Here the distinction is made primarily between a temporary anus praeter or a permanent anus praeter. This intervention also shows what a significant impact an intestinal operation has on the quality of life and why this

must always be well considered. Particularly where sexuality is concerned a permanent anus praeter plays a drastic negative role for many people.

Basically in this case it must be said that there are studies that confirm life extension through an operation. Particularly when removal of a large tumor is possible without anus praeter, then the operation should always be taken into account in therapy considerations.

For the reasons cited above you should always look for a physician, who is knowledgeable in the field of cryosurgery. In this process the tumors are "frozen" and often this can prevent more extensive operations. Often laser therapies are also used. If you must be operated on, then you should also consider a lectin blockade in the form of a D-galactose infusion for prevention of metastases (see also chapter: Supporting substances).

Chemotherapy
Usually chemotherapy is recommended for patients with colon cancer, usually with 5-FU (fluorouracil), together with leucoverin or levamisol (a de-worming medication e.g. for sheep). One study from 1990 is cited over and over again. In this study patients with Duke C lived up to 33% longer through the administration of 5-FU and levamisol (Moertel 1990). However in a study previously made with levamisol only, it was determined that levamisol clearly shortened the life of patients (almost twice as many survived in the control group; 68% instead of 38%. This study confirmed previous studies in which levamisol also contributed to patients with lung cancer, for instance, dying earlier (Davis 1981).

Interestingly enough this study only showed an advantage for patients with colon cancer in stage 3. There were no advantages in stages 2 and 4, but rather only disadvantages. No one appears to have pursued the question as to why a combination of 5-FU, which on its own does not provide any survival advantage, and a medication like levamisol, which demonstrably contributes to patients dying earlier, suddenly when administered in combination should have significant advantages.

In recent years many physicians, also in Germany, have been prescribing a combination of 5-FU and leucoverin. There are two studies in which there were 20 therapy-caused fatalities (Petrelli, N. et al., J.Clin. Oncol. 7, 1989 1419-1426 and Laufmann, L. R. et al., J. Clin. Oncol. 11, 1993, 1888-1893), and yet this therapy is quite frequently prescribed! Ask yourself: Why is this medication prescribed daily in spite of such information, why do health insurance companies still pay for it, even though it has maybe never been approved in Germany?

This is a frightening example of the extent to which doctors get tangled up in systems. Several studies have demonstrated that the majority of physicians do not even know that this combination has only been approved for very strict trial conditions, and only if the patient consents to this therapy.

Another medication doctors prescribe for colon cancer with increasing frequency is campto (irinotecan – CPT-11). Like topotecan it comes from the group of so-called topoisomerease-I inhibitors. This anti-cancer medication's job is to break a DNA strand, in the hope that thus cancer cells are killed. I am familiar with this theory from many other cancer medications and I also know why it is basically a theory, and why it will remain a theory.

In the meantime many oncologists think that more is better and give their patients 5-FU, leucoverin, and campto. They present arguments to their patients that a study made in Europe and South Africa resulted in significantly better results. The truth however is that Irinotecan has not proven, as of this writing, that patients, even after 5-years, live a single day longer, and again the results only involve reduction of the tumor and statistical games.

In one study, which was published in July in the NEJM (New England Journal for Medicine) one can read that patients with colon cancer, who were given campto together with %-FU and leucovorin, died almost three times as frequently as patients who were given only 5-FU/leucovorin – and indeed the fatalities were due to the results of the therapy and not the cancer! In 2001, the NCI (National Cancer Institute/ USA) stopped two studies with campto.

An additional substance is tegafur, which is so to speak a "preliminary stage preparation" of 5-FU which only changes to 5-FU in the body. Here as well: Where are the studies that show significant advantages for longer life?

Xeloda and Orzel are also considered as "hopefuls". Orzel is a combination of Tegafur/Uracil (UFT). But the issues cited above apply here as well.

A peripheral comment. According to a study by the business consulting firm, Frost & Sullivan, the "market" for colon cancer in 2000 was estimated at 277.7 million USD, however it is projected to grow to 564.1 million USD by 2006. Whoever still believes that there are no financial conflicts of interest here must be from another planet.

And now folfox as well
I find that oxaliplatin, another very potent chemotherapy, is being used more and more frequently. Many doctors appear to be exited that oxaliplatin was able to show in a study (Journal of Clinical Oncology - 2000/Giacchetti) that 53% of all patients responded to this medication, while in the control group (5-FU and leukovorin) the number was only 16%. Also the time before the next tumor appeared was improved.

I am not surprised by these results from such a strong toxin. I can only hope however that your doctor will also tell you that the oxaliplatin patients in this study died EARLIER on average, than did those in the control group. In addition as the major Mosaik study (ASCO 2003, abstr. 1015) clearly proved, extreme side effects occurred like neutropenias, i.e. a lack of neutrophilic granulocytes, which can even prove fatal (41% instead of only 4.7%!!!).

Tragically this again demonstrates that tumor destruction and longer life do not follow a parallel curve. In the meantime the question comes up; "When did physicians and pharmaceutical companies jointly introduce the FLOICHMA protocol for colon cancer patients? (FLOICHMA = fluorouracil-leucovorin-oxaliplatin-irinotecan-cyclophosphamide-holoxan-methotrexate-anthra-cyline).

Irradiation

Irradiation actually take a subordinate role with colon cancer, as many conventional physicians no longer believe in its effectiveness for this type of cancer. Just how quickly one can be "deceived" is shown by the scandal in Hamburg, where more than 60 patients were "contaminated".

Often it is still being used for pain relief where the sense of this measure must be strongly questioned as it is precisely this measure which often leads to increased pain.

Another approach is preoperative radiation to afford better operating conditions by reducing the tumor. Here as well, meta studies (8507 patients, 22 randomized studies/Lancet 2001; 358:1291–304) have been able to show that a person will not live any longer through this treatment, neither will a person live any longer through pre-operative, or post-operative irradiation. However what is clearly shown in the studies is that the likelihood of dying of other illnesses is increased by 15%. This 15% represents a really significant number that every physician be aware of, before he advises his patients to undergo irradiation.

Additional therapies like hormones, antibodies, etc.w

Monoclonal antibodies
An immune preparation that is supposed to mark the cancer cells; e.g. the antibody 17 –1A. In a study with Dukes 3 patients under the direction of Professor Gert Riethmüller (Munich), 30% fewer metastases occurred in the post-observation period of 5 years (medication: panorex). A second, approved antibody is rituximab, which however was previously used for non-Hodgkin's lymphonomas and its effect is supposed to unfold through the binding to a protein called CD20-antigen. Since the middle of 2000 there have been warnings concerning the antibody Herceptin/trastuzumab, because 15 women died within 24 hours of the treatment. This example indicates that the use of antibodies has been prematurely approved, and that we are not even aware of the possible side effects when millions of people have been given antibodies.

Alcohol therapy
In this procedure 96% alcohol is injected directly into the tumor, and can thus contribute to the death of cancer cells. Although it sounds simple and logical, in reality it is very difficult to execute and is used only for a certain type of tumor.

Liver metastases
With colon cancer quite frequently additional tumors develop in the liver. Four therapies are listed below that could be used:
Chemotherapy-embolization
Here chemo medications are injected into the liver arteries and then the vessels which lead to the tumor are blocked in order to "dry out" the tumor. This therapy is also referred to as TACE=transaterial chemotherapy embolization.

Urea/creatine
See under therapies: Urea/creatine

LITT - laser induced thermal therapy or HITT
Here tumors in the liver are destroyed via laser or high-frequency waves. Usually this is only possible if the tumors are
less than 4 cm in size.

Frequency therapies
I have seen good results in treating liver disorders with frequency therapies like PapImi or the Aquatilis therapy.

Avastin/Bevacizumab
In July of 2003 the price of Genentech stock soared 36% in
one day due to the announcement of a new cancer medication
called Avastin. Avastatin is an antibiotic against the vessel
growth factor VEGF. Again the newspapers reported on the
great progress in the treatment of colon cancer – as usual!

However the fact is that Avastatin is nothing more than
another antiangiogenesis medication of which there are
already hundreds which have not exactly decreased the number of colon cancer fatalities. The sole (American) study has
previously only been able to show that patients have lived a
few weeks longer – in combination with chemotherapies. The
fact that the same medication previously failed the approval
process for breast cancer, and was already considered to be a
bankrupt medication, naturally was not communicated to
readers of most newspapers.

Corpus carcinoma

1. The allopathic definition:
Corpus carcinoma is also referred to as endometrial carcinoma, because it emanates from the mucous membrane of the uterus (endometrium).

2. How frequently does this type of cancer occur (incidence rate) in Germany (USA appr. x 3)?
Currently app. 11,000 women annually. Primarily older women after menopause are affected.

3. Subdivisions:
Corpus carcinomas are almost all adenocarcinomas (emanating from glandular tissue). The poorer the differentiation (see below) the greater the chance that squamous epithelial type parts will occur (adenosquamous tumors). Clear cell carcinoma also occur in very rare cases, primarily in very young women.

Stages:

IA: tumor limited to endometrium.

IB: invasion to less than one half of the myometrium.

IC: invasion to greater than one half of the myometrium.

IIA: endocervical glandular involvement only.

IIB: cervical stromal invasion.

IIIA: tumor invades serosa and/or adnexa and/or positive peritoneal cytology.

Stage IIIB: vaginal metastases.

Stage IIIC: metastases to pelvic and/or para-aortic lymph nodes.

IVA: tumor invasion of bladder and/or bowel mucosa.

Stage IVB: distant metastases, including intra-abdominal and/or inguinal lymph nodes

4. How is this type of cancer diagnosed by allopathic practitioners?
Unusual bleeding, abdominal pains, enlarged uterus, ultrasound, CT, magnetic resonance tomography, hysteroscopy (endoscopy of the uterus, curetting, i.e. tissue engineering).

What are the allopathic therapy concepts?

Surgery
See Uterine cancer and Cervical cancer

Chemotherapy
See Uterine cancer and Cervical cancer

Irradiation
See Uterine cancer and Cervical cancer

Additional therapies like hormones, antibodies, etc.
See Uterine cancer and Cervical cancer

Ependymoma

1. The allopathic definition:
Brain tumors that consist of the ventricle (brain chamber filled with cerebral spinal fluid) and the ependym which sheaths the central channel of the spinal marrow.

2. How frequently does this type of cancer occur (incidence rate) in Germany (USA appr. x 3)?
Incidence rate: 30-40 children per 100,000 under the age of 15. A total of 5% of all intracranial tumors are ependymomas. They comprise 9% of all gliomas. The ependymoma of the spinal marrow comprises 60% of all gliomas of the spinal marrow. Ependymomas of the cerebral hemisphere mainly occur in children and adolescents. Thereafter they mainly occur at age 35.

3. Subdivisions:
Statistically there are more benign tumors than there are malignant tumors. There are three groups of benign tumors: myxopapillary ependymomas (usually occurring in the backbone), papillary ependymomas (extremely rare, seated in the cerebellopontine area), and subependymomas (frequently found in the 4th ventricle, and that extend into a large area between the cerebellum and medulla). Anaplastic ependymoma is the malignant form of this tumor. Anaplastic means that more highly-differentiated cells (normal cells) transform into lesser differentiated cells (i.e. they become malignant).

Stages:
See WHO grading Astrocytoma. The ependymoma is usually

assigned to WHO stage 2. Anaplastic ependymomas however belong to level 3, and many are also assigned to level 4 (secondary glioblastoma), however with a better prognosis.

4. How is this type of cancer diagnosed by allopathic practitioners?
In addition to neurological examinations, imaging processes are used, primarily due to the many differential diagnoses: Electroencephalogram (EEG), evoked potentials (acoustically evoked potentials AEP, visually evoked potentials or VEP, sensory evoked potentials SEP), computertomogram (CT), blood tests (e.g. tumor markers), magnetic resonance tomography (MRT), angiography, positron emission tomography (PET), and naturally biopsies. Because ependymomas frequently block cerebral-spinal fluid discharge, there are specific symptoms of increased intercranial pressure.

Histologically the main criteria is the so-called pseudo-rosette around the blood vessels. The tumor cells are arranged with long fibrils around the vessels.

What are the allopathic therapy concepts?

Surgery
An operation is the first choice for treatment. In this process do not forget that the location of the tumor often only allows operations with an extremely high operation risk, and consequently any operation should be considered very carefully.

Allopathy usually assumes fundamentally that the tumor mass should be reduced, if at all possible from the operation/technical view. I fundamentally disagree with this argument, because my personal experiences with patients who have conquered their tumor without operation, offer compelling reasons to the contrary. In addition the high relapse rate after operations should not be forgotten.

Chemotherapy

Fundamentally we can say that all previous chemotherapy attempts have failed. There have been and there are trials with cisplatin, CCNU (lomustin), cyclophosphamide, carboplatin, methotrexate, vincristin and many more. - however the results have not been particularly promising and here the fundamental question can be posed as to whether chemotherapy is the right approach at all for ependymomas.

Unhappily this area is interesting to many oncologists and thus the chance that you or your child will get a chemotherapy, and one with the strongest toxins available in the field of oncology (cisplatin, cyclophosphamide and carboplatin), unfortunately are quite high. Be careful and do not allow yourself to be persuaded by human tests, which have not helped other people (to put it in charitable terms).

Because the prognosis for children with anaplastic ependymoma after operation and radiation is not very good, many oncologists recommend "a final therapy trial" with chemotherapy to the parents. I must clearly contradict this approach, as it is not a "final attempt", rather it is the last act of despair offered by an oncologist who has run out of Latin terminology. Here the statistics speak clearly and every thinking person must ask himself the question; "When will allopathic practitioners finally come to understand that chemotherapy is not the right approach for brain tumors.

Irradiation

Ependymomas are usually irradiated generously because there is fear of the so-called "drop metastases" (with the exception of children under 1 year of age). A usual structure is e.g.:

* Total cranium 30 Gy

* Total spinal cord 30 Gy

*   Boost: tumor region 20 Gy to 50 Gy

For more information about irradiation see Astrocytomas.

Additional therapies like hyperthermia, gene therapies, etc.

Please read the chapter on astrocytomas, since what is discussed there also applies to ependymomas.

Esophagus
(esophageal carcinoma)

1. The allopathic definition:
Tumor of the esophagus

2. How frequently does this type of cancer occur (incidence rate) in Germany (USA appr. x 3)?
Current incidence rate: for men 6 per 100,000, and for women 1-2 per 100,000 annually. Smoking, but also excessive alcohol, play a statistical role.

3. Subdivisions:
Usually (app. 90%) of esophageal carcinomas are squamous epithelial carcinomas. In rarer cases however they can also be adenocarcinomas (emanating from the glands), small cell carcinomas, adenoid cystic carcinomas, or mucoepidemoid carcinomas.

Stages:

TX: Primary tumor cannot be assessed

T0: No evidence of primary tumor

Tis: Carcinoma in situ

T1: Tumor invades lamina propria or submucosa

T2: Tumor invades muscularis propria

T3: Tumor invades adventitia

T4: Tumor invades adjacent structures

4. How is this type of cancer diagnosed by allopathic practitioners?

Swallowing disorders (dysphagia), pain, and weight loss are typical initial symptoms. In addition there are naturally many non-specific symptoms like: Pressure and the feeling of being full, nausea and vomiting, loss of appetite, eructation, bloody stool etc.

If the tumor in the stomach bleeds then this blood in the stool can be verified (e.g. fecal occult blood test). However a carcinoma can only be verified with certainty through a biopsy, or through microscopic examination. In addition endosonography, gastroscopy, x-ray examination with contrast agent, CT and explorative laparotomy play a role in better understanding the location of the tumor.

What are the allopathic therapy concepts?

Surgery

An operation represents the first option. The goal of surgical measures should be complete removal of the tumor in healthy tissue (R 0 resection). For T1 and T2 tumors the assumption is made that this goal can be achieved in most cases. Here a so-called transthorax oseophagectomy is performed, where in addition to the tumor, parts of the esophagus, lymph nodes, parts of the pleura and of the alimentary duct are also removed.

Many patients however have already been in T3 stage for a long time when they are diagnosed, and an operation for tumors of the upper esophagus is often no longer possible due to proximity to the trachea. In these cases many patients are then recommended to first have chemotherapy and/or irradiation, as they would for T4 tumors. This recommendation naturally has multiple disadvantages. First an operation after chemotherapy/irradiation is much more complicated than is an operation before chemotherapy/irradiation. Here you must be aware that according to official data (Siewert et.al.) every 20th patient will die within 30 days due to the effects of the operation. For patients with risk factors (heart, lung, or liver problems) this number is increased to every 6th to 14th patient.

In addition there is the issue as to how successful chemotherapy/radiation even is since tumors first become larger, and second they can show much more aggressive growth under such a therapy. Consequently the patient should consider this step very carefully. In addition there is the factor that biological therapies no longer "take" as well, or they cannot work at all, and thus the door to biological therapy is completely shut.

Also many patients do not know that there are several studies (Wang 1989, Schlag 1992, Girling 1992, Nygaard 1992, LePrise 1994, etc.) where it is clearly shown that particularly for T1 and T2 patients there is no survival advantage. For T3 patients there are studies (Stahl 1996, Walsh 1996) which show that patients who survived the operation, lived longer with a chemotherapy than those patients who were only operated on. However if the high operation risk is factored in then these data again look very negative.

For T3 tumors of the middle and lower esophagus usually an RO resection (complete removal of the tumor) is attempted. Patients should be aware that in many cases the larynx is removed, naturally with all the attendant negative consequences (speech).

Chemotherapy
Chemo preparations like 5-FU, mitomycin C, methotrexate, bleomycin, CCNU, etoposide, nindesin, and even cisplatin have been used, and are being used. Here at the outset the lowest common denominator is: There is absolutely no proof that you will live significantly longer through chemotherapy.

Any physician who maintains something different should submit his claims to you in writing. As of this printing there are no comparative studies. Many doctors say that there are good studies such as the RTOG study from America. But what is behind this study? In this case "only irradiation therapy" at 64 Gy was compared with a combination of irradiation at 50 Gy, plus chemotherapy with 4 cycles of cisplatin and 5-FU.

The result was that patients who were given the combination had fewer metastases and the tumors remained smaller. At first this sounds good. But in reality in this process the survival time was not extended, and the old trick of comparing two allopathic measures was used. If patients fewer metastases occurred in the group of the "only irradiation therapy", then the same allopathic practitioners would say that in the future patients should be irradiated with high quantities of radiation.

Irradiation

First even allopathic practitioners state that the present studies (RTOG, Okawa, Earlam, John etc.) speak against irradiation as the sole means of treatment, and secondly in my opinion patients are robbed of any chance of healing, indeed usually they are robbed of any chance of improvement through radiation as the sole means of treatment. For patients who can no longer be helped, the side effects are so enormous that they are not outweighed by the advantage of a possible chance of reducing the tumor. However what is most important for the patient, is that he will not live a day longer through irradiation of the esophagus according to present data.

Additional therapies like hormones, antibodies, etc.

Immune therapies with antibodies or cytokines do not play a role for esophageal cancer and although there have been and are frequent approaches, to this date not a single therapy has been developed.

Gall bladder cancer

1. The allopathic definition:
Gall bladder cancer is a malignant illness of the epithelial tissue of the gall bladder.

2. How frequently does this type of cancer occur (incidence rate) in Germany (USA appr. x 3)?
Current incidence rate: 5 per 100,000 people.

3. Subdivisions:
The tumors are differentiated according to their cell type, such as adenocarcinomas (glandular tissue), signet ring cells, sarcoma cells, etc.

Stages:

TX: Primary tumor cannot be assessed

T0: No evidence of primary tumor

Tis: Carcinoma in situ

T1: Tumor invades lamina propria or muscle layer

T1a: Tumor invades lamina propria

T1b: Tumor invades the muscle layer

T2: Tumor invades the perimuscular connective tissue; no extension beyond the serosa or into the liver

T3: Tumor perforates the serosa (visceral peritoneum) and/or directly invades the liver and/or one other adjacent organ or structure, such as the stomach, duodenum, colon, or pancreas, omentum or extrahepatic bile ducts

T4: Tumor invades main portal vein or hepatic artery or invades multiple extrahepatic organs or structures

4. How is this type of cancer diagnosed by allopathic practitioners?

Disorders of the upper stomach, jaundice, weight loss, nausea and vomiting, loss of appetite, ultrasound examinations, ERCP (endoscopic, retrograde-cholangiography). In this process a long mirror probe is introduced into the duodenum via the esophagus. From that point a contrast agent is sprayed into the bile duct/ gall bladder. The x-ray allows more precise evaluation of the bile ducts and the gall bladder.

Computertomography (CT), percutaneous transheptic cholangiography and drainage (PTCD) for unsuccessful ERC, gastroscopy with biopsy, sonography, tumor markers CA 72-4, Ca 19-9, CEA, possibly liver function test for jaundice.

Often patients will have a past history of gall stones. However to conclude from this fact (as stated in a lot of the literature) that gall stones are a preliminary phase of gall bladder cancer, or that they even trigger gall bladder cancer, I consider to be incorrect, in light of the fact that less than 2% of all patients with gall stones also develop a carcinoma.

What are the allopathic therapy concepts?

Surgery
Operation of the gall bladder is specified as the first and only indication for curative therapy and is even considered to be the sole standard therapy for carcinomas in situ (Tis), mucosa

carcinoma, and category T1b primary tumors (infiltration of the muscles).

For category T2 tumors usually the gall bladder bed is also removed with an approximately 3 cm wide seam, or anatomic liver resection (removal of segments IVb and V) with lymphadenectomy (removal of lymph nodes along the ligamentum hepatoduodenale. Often the passage between liver and gall bladder (ductus choledochus) is removed for a T3 tumor.

For larger operations it is possible that the duodenum and the spleen are also removed. However this means greater impact on the future quality of life and should be weighed very carefully. On the other hand, life without a gall bladder is quite possible without extensive changes.

Chemotherapy

Although there is not a single study that has been able to offer proof of life extension, chemotherapies are still being recommended for patients with gall bladder cancer. Thus for instance there are studies with oxaliplatin, 5-FU and leucovorin. Although we know today that the combination of 5-FU and leucovorin, in particular, can lead to premature death of the patient, the ethics commission repeatedly allows new human trials with these preparations. I have absolutely no understanding for this and can only warn against it.

Another approach is regional chemotherapy, which "naturally" offers itself in a closed system like the gall bladder. In this regard one must weigh the following points:

1. Usually gall bladder cancer is diagnosed in a stage in which the tumor is no longer limited to the bladder.

2. This theory assumes that tumor= cancer and that the tumor must be destroyed as quickly as possible.

In summary, one can say that up this point all chemotherapy approaches have failed and if this therapy is offered to you, then you must ask your doctor to please provide you with written documentation that demonstrates the contrary.

Irradiation
Collaboration with radiologists for gall bladder cancer is quite controversial, even among allopathic practitioners. In the literature or at conferences you can find almost any statement ranging from, "ineffective since the bladder is not sensitive to radiation", to, "one should always try to reduce the tumor mass with irradiation".

The fact is that radiation therapy is also recommended to patients time and again without any data that vouch for the effectiveness of this procedure. In summary, the same issues applies in this case that apply for chemotherapy. If this therapy is offered to you, then please demand that your physician provide you with written documentation, which demonstrates the contrary.

Additional therapies like hormones, antibodies, etc.w

Therapies like hormone blockades, interferons etc. are not prescribed for gall bladder cancer because the entire therapy basically concentrates on the operation. The great disadvantage, (or advantage depending on your point of view), is naturally the fact that gall bladder cancer occurs very rarely, and consequently it is not all that interesting for pharmaceutical companies to invest their money for studies in this field. Principally for this reason there are few studies, and those that do exist only involve chemotherapy combinations in comparison with other allopathic measures. Naturally these studies are not very interesting for patients, as they have been specified more by individual companies' marketing concepts, or to get research money "in circulation".

Glioblastoma

1. The allopathic definition:
Brain tumor of blastomatosic, mesenchymal, and glial portions. Usually occurs in the hemispherical medullary layer.

2. How frequently does this type of cancer occur (incidence rate) in Germany (USA appr. x 3)?
In Germany 8-10 people out of 100,000 get glioblastoma annually. Primarily these are children under 10 years of age, and adults between 60-75.

3. Subdivisions:
Glioblastomas look different in different stages and consequently are not always easy to diagnose. Line-shaped necrosis (dead cells) for example are an indicator that a glioblastoma is involved.

Stages:
See WHO grading Astrocytoma.

4. How is this type of cancer diagnosed by allopathic practitioners?
In addition to the neurological examinations, primarily due to the many differential diagnoses, imaging processes are used for the most part: Electroencephalogram (EEG), evoked potentials (acoustically evoked potentials AEP, visually evoked potentials or VEP, sensory evoked potentials SEP), computertomogram (CT), blood tests (e.g. tumor markers), magnetic resonance tomography (MRT), angiography, positron emission tomography (PET), and naturally biopsies.

What are the allopathic therapy concepts?

Surgery

According to allopathic literature operation is the only causal therapy. Concurrently however all the literature describes that glioblastomas return 100% after an operation. Often operations are not even possible because the tumor is too large, or the oncologists believe that an operation would no longer be effective, if for example the tumor has broken into the basal ganglia.

Allopathy usually assumes that the tumor mass should be reduced, if at all possible from the operation/technical view. I cannot agree with this argument, especially when I consider the previous recurrence rates of 100% In addition my personal experiences with patients who have conquered their tumor without operation, also speak against this form of argument.

There is something else that is very unsettling. If you speak with an allopathic practitioner about glioblastoma, then he will not hold out much hope for you. In my opinion this is not because glioblastomas are much more aggressive than are other tumors, but rather because the allopathic approach, which views tumor destruction as the sole chance of healing tumors in the brain, is destined to fail. Until there is a shift in thinking, glioblastomas will never be treated successfully allopathically.

Chemotherapy

Usually chemotherapy is only offered to young patients whose health is generally good. Usually the following chemo protocols are used: VM-26, ACNU, BCNU and a combination of procarbazine, CCNU and vincristin (PCV). High-dose therapies with MTX (methotrexate) are also possible. As of this printing there is not a single clear proof for a significant advantage relative to survival time.

Instead of finally accepting that chemotherapies for glioblastomas are the wrong approach, "experts" have gone over to generously exploiting this experimental field. How far this can go is indicated by the MTX high-dose study in which people are persuaded to undergo such a therapy with the argument that there is no therapy for glioblastoma. If you ever speak with such a doctor, then make sure you ask him whether he just means that there is no allopathic therapy, or whether he means that there are none whatsoever. It is not just Dr. Burzynksi in Texas who has demonstrated time and again that there are some very effective therapies.

Irradiation
Treatment with ionizing radiation plays a much more significant role than does chemotherapy. Today electron accelerating devices (teletherapy) are used almost exclusively. In the meantime cyclical accelerators (betratron) have been displaced by linear accelerators.

The fundamental distinction is between total brain irradiation and irradiation of the tumor only. You must realize that with total brain irradiation these rays primarily destroy cells that are well-supplied with oxygen (healthy cells). However as we know (see Cancer theories) this is not the case for cancer cells and consequently the side effects (like increased edema formation) are never foreseeable. Interestingly enough accelerated tumor growth is one of these side effects. I emphasize this point because physicians often do not tell their patients this, unfortunately.

In the meantime there are a wide variety of irradiation techniques like stereotactic irradiation, "internal" irradiation with radionuclides like radium 226, iridium 192, Cesium 137, cobalt 60, gold 198 or iodine 125. Catheters are operatively implanted in the tumor via bore holes in the skull (overloading process) and for seed implantation radionuclides (seeds) are "worked into" the tumor tissue as small pellets or rods.

There are studies where patients in the irradiation research arm have lived longer; usually this is also communicated to every patient. In addition to the previously-mentioned arguments, however the fact that these patients lived a maximum of a few weeks longer and that they incur the risk that their tumor grows, speaks against the use of radiation therapy as the sole treatment. Moreover there is still the issue of whether it is possible at all to be healed after irradiation.

Additional therapies like hormones, antibodies, etc.
See under astrocytoma.

Kidney cell carcinoma

1. The allopathic definition:
Malignant tumor of the epithelial cells of the kidney parenchym.

2. How frequently does this type of cancer occur (incidence rate) in Germany (USA appr. x 3)?
Current incidence rate: 6.7 per 100,000.

3. Subdivisions:
Usually kidney tumors are differentiated according to cell type (basophilic, eosinophilic, spindle cell, clear, chromophobic, etc.), histologic structure (acinar, compact, papillary, cystic etc) and malignancy grade (how malignant = G1, G2, and G3).

Stages:

In stage I, the tumor is 7 centimeters or smaller and is found only in the kidney.

In stage II, the tumor is larger than 7 centimeters and is found only in the kidney.

In stage III, cancer is found: in the kidney and in 1 nearby lymph node; or in an adrenal gland or in the layer of fatty tissue around the kidney, and may be found in 1 nearby lymph node; or in the main blood vessels of the kidney and may be found in 1 nearby lymph node.

In stage IV, cancer has spread: beyond the layer of fatty tissue around the kidney and may be found in 1 nearby lymph node; or to 2 or more nearby lymph nodes; or to other organs, such as the bowel, pancreas, or lungs, and may be found in nearby lymph nodes

4. How is this type of cancer diagnosed by allopathic practitioners?
Pain, blood in urine, palpable tumor, anemia, fever, liver disorders. Ultrasound, CT, pielography, x-ray, angiography, MRT (magnetic resonance tomography) , PET (positron emission tomography).

What are the allopathic therapy concepts?

Surgery
Operation is always the first choice for nerve cell carcinomas. In this regard there is a distinction between organ-saving operations and total operations. If no metastases is present, then all surgeons usually suggest a radical operation. Naturally this is based on the approach: "Let's cut out the tumor and that will do." This is very dangerous and usually results in relapses automatically. Please don't fall for this error.

Interestingly enough there are studies in which survival times for patients who had metastases with the first diagnosis and who had an operated, were no different than they were for those patients who did not have an operation (e.g. Patel and Lavengood 78). Different studies also showed that the number of metastases had no influence on survival time (Brandscheid 92). These studies again demonstrate that the tumor mass, or removal of the tumor is not nearly as important as it is consistently made out to be.

Chemotherapy
First: There is no chemotherapy that can extend life in the case

262

of kidney cell carcinoma. There have been, and there are attempts with vinblastin, lonidamine, high-dose with tamoxifen or with carmustine und lomustin, but they were always just attempts, which never could prove that patients lived a single day longer because of these therapies. Consequently I do not understand why patients are still being offered chemotherapies.

Irradiation
Although to this date there are no hard facts confirming that irradiation contributes to people living significantly longer, this therapy is still offered frequently. And it is offered even though kidney cell carcinomas generally are viewed as "not sensitive" to radiation. This may be true. However, what is not true is that the kidney is not susceptible to radiation in general – on the contrary.

Palliative irradiation
Neither do I agree with palliative irradiation therapy, since if one assumes that the patient will die soon anyway, why should that patient be subjected to all the suffering associated with radiation therapy.

Often improved quality of life through irradiation is discussed, e.g. for bone metastases. Here you must be aware that where pain is concerned, allopathic practitioners often are only familiar with pain medication in the form of pills and irradiation. Both therapies naturally offer significant disadvantages for a patient in his last days and in this case non-conventional pain therapies (for instance coffee enemas and low-dose analgesics or lactic acid) should really be considered, or those involved should at least talk to an allopathic practitioner who can prescribe more than medication for pain.

Additional therapies like hormones, antibodies, etc.

Hormonal therapies

Because higher estrogen receptors were measured in the normal kidney tissue for a small percentage of people with kidney cancer, the thought was to use estrogen blockers such as tamoxifen for therapy. Other than the pharmaceutical companies, to this date these therapies have not been a benefit to anyone.

Cytokine

Messengers like interferon or interleukin appear to play an important role with kidney cancer and thus there are several approaches involving both substances. In studies there were higher remissions than there were in the comparison groups without cytokines. Unfortunately there are still too few "hard facts" that would allow us to say today whether interferon alpha or interleukin-2 , could help, or whether a different cytokine could help, nor is there any indication of which quantities might prove helpful. More extensive studies are necessary in this regard. And do not forget that cytokines induce severe side effects, such as heart disorders, for many patients.

A different approach, which has been pursued in Italy for many years by Dr. Pizza, is the use of cytokines in extremely low doses. In this process cytokines are injected directly into the lymphatic system (see Transfer factors).

Chemoembolization for liver metastases

Here chemo medications are injected into the liver arteries and then the vessels which lead to the tumor are shut off in order to "dry out" the tumor. This therapy is also referred to as TACE=transarterial chemotherapy embolization.

Urine/creatine therapy for liver metastases
See under Therapies: Urine/creatine

LITT - laser induced thermal therapy or HITT
Here tumors in the liver are destroyed via laser or high-frequency waves. Usually this is only possible if the tumors are less than 4 cm in size.

Frequency therapies
I have seen good results in treating liver disorders with frequency therapies like PapImi or the Aquatilis therapy. Both therapies are described in detail in this book.

Laryngeal carcinoma
(Cancer of the larynx)

1. The allopathic definition:
The laryngeal carcinoma represents malignant epithelial growth of cells that emanate from the larynx.

2. How frequently does this type of cancer occur (incidence rate) in Germany (USA appr. x 3)?
Pharyngeal and laryngeal cancer: app. 7,200 men and 2,500 women annually. Men over 60 are most frequently affected.

3. Subdivisions:
Depending on the locatoin of the carcinoma: Supraglottis, subglottis or glottis.

Depending on the type of cancer: in up to 95% of cases squamous epithelial tumors are involved. Small cell tumors, adenocarcinomas, or carcinosarcomas are quite rare.

Depending on the type of cellular differentiation: (i.e. similarity to healthy cells): G1 (highly differentiated), G2 (medium differentiation), G3 (poorly differentiated).

Supraglottis
T1: Tumor limited to one subsite* of supraglottis with normal vocal cord mobility

T2: Tumor invades mucosa of more than one adjacent subsite* of supraglottis or glottis or region outside the supraglottis (e.g., mucosa of base of tongue, vallecula, medial wall of pyriform sinus) without fixation of the larynx

T3: Tumor limited to larynx with vocal cord fixation and/or invades any of the following: postcricoid area, pre-epiglottic tissues, paraglottic space, and/or minor thyroid cartilage erosion (e.g., inner cortex)

T4a: Tumor invades through the thyroid cartilage, and/or invades tissues beyond the larynx (e.g., trachea, soft tissues of the neck including deep extrinsic muscle of the tongue, strap muscles, thyroid, or esophagus)

T4b: Tumor invades prevertebral space, encases carotid artery, or invades mediastinal structures

Glottis
T1: Tumor limited to the vocal cord(s) (may involve anterior or posterior commissure) with normal mobility

T1a: Tumor limited to one vocal cord

T1b: Tumor involves both vocal cords

T2: Tumor extends to supraglottis and/or subglottis, and/or with impaired vocal cord mobility

T3: Tumor limited to the larynx with vocal cord fixation and/or invades paraglottic space, and/or minor thyroid cartilage erosion (e.g., inner cortex)

T4a: Tumor invades through the thyroid cartilage and/or invades tissues beyond the larynx (e.g., trachea, soft tissues of neck, including deep extrinsic muscle of the tongue, strap muscles, thyroid, or esophagus)

T4b: Tumor invades prevertebral space, encases carotid artery, or invades mediastinal structures

Subglottis
T1: Tumor limited to the subglottis

T2: Tumor extends to vocal cord(s) with normal or impaired mobility

T3: Tumor limited to larynx with vocal cord fixation

T4a: Tumor invades cricoid or thyroid cartilage and/or invades tissues beyond the larynx (e.g., trachea, soft tissues of neck, including deep extrinsic muscles of the tongue, strap muscles, thyroid, or esophagus)

T4b: Tumor invades prevertebral space, encases carotid artery, or invades mediastinal structures

4. How is this type of cancer diagnosed by allopathic practitioners?

Groups at risk are smokers, and particularly people who smoke, and who drink excessive amounts of alcohol. Difficulty swallowing, hoarseness, nodes, and pain. Laryngeal inspection, laryngoscopy, fiberendoscopy, CT or magnetic resonance tomography, stroboscopy (to evaluate vocal cord vibration), sonography, x-ray, ultrasound, bone scintigraphy.

What are the allopathic therapy concepts?

Surgery

Operation is the absolute first choice. In this process first the attempt is made to save the larynx. Here stripping of one or both vocal cords (decortitation) can be used, or the vocal chords can be removed completely (cordectomy). In addition only parts of the larynx, or the entire larynx can be removed (laryngectomy). For this major intervention the end of the trachea is sowed into the skin of the neck and the pharynx is closed.

More and more physicians are starting to operate from the inside, primarily for smaller tumors, in order to spare the patient as much damage as possible. Here the chance speech restoration remains intact, and the patient does not have to suffer an artificial breathing opening (tracheotomy), which has a major effect on the quality of life. Basically any operation involves a great risk of later and greater readjustments relative to speech and breathing. Just breathing through the artificial breathing opening, represents a great challenge for many patients. Since there is no data that radical operations produce a significant improvement of survival time, the consequences should be weighed very carefully prior to such intervention.

Chemotherapy
Although to this date there is not a single study that can demonstrate a significant extension of life through a chemotherapy (combination), this therapy is still being offered to patients. Often it is offered with palliative (alleviating) afterthoughts. In these cases every physician and every patient should ask themselves whether chemotherapy really is the right way for a person to spend the last days of his life. I cannot agree with this opinion.

Usually patients are offered a sole chemotherapy with cisplatin, carboplatin, (both have the most serious side effects), 5-FU, or mitomycin, or they are also offered a combination of the previously-cited preparations. Every doctor who recommends chemotherapy to his patients, should either justify in writing, that the chemotherapy he uses has demonstrated successes relative to extension of life (not reduction of the tumor!) or he should make it clear to his patients that the measure is being employed for palliative purposes. This is the only way to give the patient a chance to protect himself

269

against such a therapy. Otherwise the psychological pressure placed on the patient would be much too high, and this is neither in the interest of the physician nor the patient. If your physician should have a different opinion here, then request a detailed discussion in this regard and ask him what his motivations are.

Supraglottis carcinomas have a particularly extensive lymphatic network, and for this reason lymph node metastases are very frequent here, often even on both sides. In this case patients are also recommended to undergo a neck dissection (cleaning out the neck with removal of the lymph nodes).

Irradiation
In my experience irradiation is recommended for almost all patients in later stages. However if a person sifts the medical literature, there are few hard facts which can prove that irradiation contributes to significant extension of life for people with laryngeal carcinomas. Usually in these cases this means that through irradiation (with 60-70 Gy) better voice quality can be achieved; that it would be advantageous to irradiate the lymph drainage areas and naturally that this can prevent metastasis. But where are the proofs for these theories? Which studies show that irradiation really offers major advantages relative to survival time in comparison with "operation only treatment"?

Additional therapies like hormones, antibodies, etc.

Hormonal therapies, but also other therapies like cytokine therapies (Interleukin, Interferon ... or monoclonal antibodies) either do not play a role, or to this date have not supplied proof of being an effective alternative. If one of these therapies is offered to you, then be aware that you are being offered a chance to participate in a study.

(Primary) Liver tumor

1. The allopathic definition:
Epithelial tumors like the hepatocellular carcinoma, the chloangiocarcinoma or a mixed type of both carcinomas. In addition: mesenchymal tumors like the angiosarcomas or early tumors like the hepatoblastoma.

2. How frequently does this type of cancer occur (incidence rate) in Germany (USA appr. x 3)?
Maximum of 3% of all carcinomas occurring in Germany.

3. Subdivisions:
The hepatocellular carcinoma is the most frequent carcinoma.

Stages:

TX: Primary tumor cannot be assessed

T0: No evidence of primary tumor

T1: Solitary tumor without vascular invasion

T2: Solitary tumor with vascular invasion or multiple tumors none more than 5 cm

T3: Multiple tumors more than 5 cm or tumor involving a major branch of the portal or hepatic vein(s)

T4: Tumor(s) with direct invasion of adjacent organs other than the gallbladder or with perforation of the visceral peritoneum

4. How is this type of cancer diagnosed by allopathic practitioners?

Initially stomach pains on the upper right side of the stomach (epigastrium). In rarer cases also with fever. The alpha-feto-protein is usually sharply increased (500-700 ug/ml). Imaging processes like CT, MRT, sonography, scintigraphy, coeliaco-mesentericography, portography, and biopsies.

What are the allopathic therapy concepts?

Surgery

Is employed in all stages and is certainly the first option. Here the following operations are employed:

A: Partial resection for tumor mass reduction, which can be quite effective, or removal of the tumor.

B: Liver transplant. This can quickly contribute to healing, however it is very expensive, and it is not possible for every patient, due to a lack of donors. Please be aware that in this case naturally only the tumor, and not the base illness of cancer, are treated. This is very important because our experience shows that if patients rely only on the transplant, the tumors come back quite frequently and quite quickly.

Chemotherapy

1. Systemic chemotherapy with Adriamycin or Doxorubicin have failed up to this point. Even if this therapy did result in a reduction of the tumor, survival time was not significant influenced positively through this measure. Since both of these chemotherapies have the most serious side effects, use of this therapy should be carefully considered.

2. Also regional chemotherapies, e.g. via the arteria hepatica, offer no proof to this day that patients live significantly longer due to the therapy.

In general it can be said that chemotherapies severely stress the liver which is already damaged, and that this approach, understandably cannot function.

Radiation

In my opinion, using irradiation for liver tumors is even more difficult to understand than is the chemotherapy approach. In my opinion, the use of radioactive marked microspheres as so-called "internal radiation therapy" is also predestined to fail, as they increase liver toxification.

Additional therapies like alcohol, LITT, etc.

Alcohol therapy

In this procedure 96% alcohol is injected directly into the tumor, and can thus contribute to the death of cancer cells. Although it sounds simple and logical in reality it is very hard to execute, and to this day it has not been crowned with particular success.

Chemo-embolization

Here chemo medications are injected into the liver arteries and then the vessels which lead to the tumor are shut off in order to "dry out" the tumor. This therapy is also referred to as TACE=transarterial chemotherapy embolization.

Gene therapy/structure proteins

For example attempts with apoptin, so-called structure proteins, to this date have not been able to demonstrate any advantages for humans.

Urea/creatine
See under therapies: Urea/creatine

LITT - laser induced thermal therapy or HITT
Here tumors in the liver are destroyed via laser or high-frequency waves. Usually this is only possible if the tumors are less than 4 cm in size.

Frequency therapies
I have seen good results in disorders of the liver/bile ducts using frequency therapies like PapImi, or the Aquatilis therapy. Both therapies are described in detail in this book.

General information about liver cancer
The liver is the number one detoxification organ and it plays an extremely significant role. This is not just due to its detoxification functions, but is also due to its influence on all metabolic processes, like fat metabolism or the metabolic restructuring of sugar. This is why all types of detoxification measures play a more important role relative to liver illnesses than they do for all other types of cancer. Consequently do everything necessary to exclude or avoid toxins.

Allopathic practitioners still wonder why all therapies for liver cancer fail. But they do not ask whether the highly toxic therapies (anesthetics during the operation, chemotherapy, and irradiation), contribute to deterioration. Particularly for liver cancer, the focus should not be placed on destruction of the tumor, but rather 100% on detoxification.

Malignant melanomas

1. The allopathic definition:
For malignant melanomas the discussion involves malignant new cell formation of pigment forming skin cells.

2. How frequently does this type of cancer occur (incidence rate) in Germany (USA appr. x 3)?
Currently app. 100,000 illnesses annually.

3. Subdivisions:

The following groups are primarily differentiated:

SSM   Superficial spreading melanoma

NM   Nodular melanoma

LMM   Lentigo-maligna melanoma

ALM   Acrolentiginous melanoma

Stages:

IA: The tumor is not more than 1 millimeter thick, with no ulceration. The tumor is in the epidermis and upper layer of the dermis.

IB: The tumor is either: not more than 1 millimeter thick, with ulceration, and may have spread into the dermis or the tissues below the skin; or 1 to 2 millimeters thick, with no ulceration.

IIA: Tthe tumor is either: 1 to 2 millimeters thick, with ulceration; or 2 to 4 millimeters thick, with no ulceration.

IIB: The tumor is either: 2 to 4 millimeters thick, with ulceration; or more than 4 millimeters thick, with no ulceration.

IIC: The tumor is more than 4 millimeters thick, with ulceration.

In stage III, the tumor may be any thickness, with or without ulceration, and: has spread to 1 or more lymph nodes; or has spread into the nearby lymph system but not into nearby lymph nodes; or has spread to lymph nodes that are matted (not moveable); or satellite tumors (additional tumor growths within 2 centimeters of the original tumor) are present and nearby lymph nodes are involved.

In stage IV, the tumor may be any thickness, with or without ulceration, may have spread to 1 or more nearby lymph nodes, and has spread to other places in the body

4. How is this type of cancer diagnosed by allopathic practitioners?
The diagnosis can only be ensured through a biopsy (cell removal). Otherwise the doctors follow the ABCD rule:

A: Asymmetry

B: Border irregular

C: Colorit (color) varying within the lesion.

D: Diameter greater than 5 mm

What are the allopathic therapy concepts?

Surgery

Operation is the therapy for melanoma. In this process the attempt is always made to cut into healthy tissue, and basically to cut "generously" in the process. Likewise affected lymph nodes are also removed.

Because particularly in the initial stages of the melanoma, surgical measures are the easiest for the patient/ doctor, and the statistics look good, the assumption is always made that an operation, possibly with an additional interferon therapy would be sufficient. However the good statistics look as good as they do because melanomas are usually detected in an early stage. Non-conventional therapies also have very good statistics for this reason. Thus the Chipsa Clinic in Mexico published a study in which (mainly through the Gerson therapy) 100% of all patients with a T1 melanoma survived 5 years. To the best of my knowledge this is by far the most successful study that has ever been published about melanoma patients.

However this study also shows that melanomas detected early on do not grow nearly as fast as they are reported to grow in most of the literature. This is also confirmed by the cases I have documented of patients with melanomas who did not undergo any kind of therapy and whose tumors only became larger after many years. As patient do not be deceived into thinking that with removal of the tumor, the cancerous event has been operated out.

Chemotherapy

Usually dacarbazin (DTIC), but also BCNU, vincristin, vindesine, fotemustine, bleomycin and even cisplatin are used. In a test with DTIC there were indeed remissions, however there were also fatalities through acute liver toxification (Ceci, G. Cancer 61, 1988-1991). * To this day there are no meaningful studies that demonstrate that you will live significantly longer through any combination, or single treatment, of chemotherapeutic medications. (Multiple studies showed no positive effect – F. J. Lejeune, S+S 1986 – 549-559.)

Because it is so important: To this day there is not a single study that can prove that patients with melanoma live longer, when they undergo chemotherapy. The doctor who suggests chemotherapy for you also knows this, and you can be sure 99% of the time that you will be taking part in some kind of study in this case.

Unfortunately there are doctors who even suggest high-dose chemotherapy for their patients. In this regard you should know that even the NCI (National Cancer Institute, USA) which normally recommends chemotherapies, has distanced itself from high-dose chemotherapy with autological bone marrow transplants, because patients do not live longer through this therapy. If your doctor should recommend this therapy to you, then please ask him why he is doing so.

Irradiation
Irradiation is mainly recommended for patients, for whom operations (e.g. near the eyes) are very difficult, or for large surface melanomas on the face. In addition, the assumption is frequently made that bone marrow metastases or patients with a lot of pain should be irradiated. However the fact is, that to this day there is no study that has been able to show that patients with melanomas live a single day longer through irradiation.

Additional therapies like hormones, antibodies, etc.

Cytokine therapies
In recent years cytokine therapies with interleukin and interferon have established themselves, however to this day there has been no breakthrough success, although this is frequently

stated in the media and in medical journals. What was still viewed as cancer therapy in the 80s, today is viewed more rationally by more and more oncologists because to this day there are no studies to prove that patients live significantly longer due to this therapy. While there are indeed studies showing high "response rates" (reduction of the tumor and longer periods that are recurrence-free), where are the studies that prove that patients also live longer due to these therapies?

Even the argument that cytokines improve the response rate of chemotherapies (e.g. Tilgen 1995) must be considered as third rank, as in this case as well, there are no studies as of this writing that can prove that patients live significantly longer. In this regard the side effects of the cytokine therapy should not be forgotten nor should the associated high costs, which are usually paid by the health insurance companies. Consequently the value, particularly of interferon therapies, is being more frequently questioned, even among allopathic practitioners.

Fever therapy
The use of fever therapies (endogens through bacteria) has been proven positive in my opinion for all malignant melanomas, and should be taken into consideration for all cases.

Hormonal therapies
There are studies, for instance with tamoxifen, but to this date they have only helped stockholders, they have not helped patients.

Dendrite cells
Currently there are studies underway at many universities involving dendrite cells, the results however can only be evaluated in several years

Mesothelioma

1. The allopathic definition:
A malignant tumor emanating from the mesothelial cells of the pleura.

2. How frequently does this type of cancer occur (incidence rate) in Germany (USA appr. x 3)?
Current incidence rate: 1.2 per 100,000.

3. Subdivisions:
In general there is a distinction between diffuse pleural mesothelioma, diffuse malignant pleuramesothelioma, and malignant mesothelioma. Here the mesothelial cells of the pleura or of the peritoneum can be affected.

Stages:

I: Disease confined within the capsule of the parietal pleura (i.e., ipsilateral pleura, lung, pericardium, and diaphragm).

II: All of stage I with positive intrathoracic (N1 or N2) lymph nodes.

III: Local extension of disease into the following areas, e.g., chest wall or mediastinum, heart or through the diaphragm or peritoneum, with or without extrathoracic or contralateral (N3) lymph node involvement.

IV: Distant metastatic disease.

4. How is this type of cancer diagnosed by allopathic practitioners?
Pains in the chest area, coughs, biopsies (careful – this naturally involves a significant risk of spreading), x-ray, spirometry – lung function diagnostics.

What are the allopathic therapy concepts?

General
Many allopathic practitioners see the diagnosis of pleuramesothelioma as fundamentally incurable. Even if they do not say it, this is still what the patient "feels". Free yourself from this self-fulfilling prophecy. If you do not believe that you will return to health then who else will? If your physician holds out no hope for you, then look for this hope in yourself first, and then in other people around you. Learn to understand that you do not have to die of this illness – regardless of what your doctor tells you!.

Naturally I am familiar with the official statistics. In contrast to most allopathic practitioners, however I am acquainted with people who have been living with this diagnosis for many years, and they have been living very well. Basically I agree with allopathic opinion that here there is no allopathic therapy and that every patient must immediately ask himself the following question after the diagnosis: "Why do I need a physician who clearly tells me that he knows of no therapy for my illness.

Surgery
The extent to which an operation can help is a very controversial issue, even among allopathic practitioners. Some authors say that pleural mesotheliomas are basically inoperable, and others write that it is strictly necessary to operate, since most patients die because of their primary tumor and not because of the metastases.

Likewise my personal opinion is split. On one hand I have often observe that a patient can gain time through reduction of the tumor mass, on the other hand the immune system is weakened for months through such a massive intervention, and self-healing forces are withdrawn. Consequently I believe that the decision for an operation can be only be made on a case by case basis.

Chemotherapy

First: There is no chemotherapy that can extend life in the case of a pleuramesothelioma. There have been and there are attempts with adriablastin, cisplatin, carboplatin, cyclophosphamide, doxorubicin, 5-FU, methotrexate and even gemcitabin, but they were always just attempts, attempts which never could prove that patients lived a single day longer because of these therapies. For this reason I do not understand why patients are still being offered chemotherapies.

Radiation

That which has been said about chemotherapy also holds true for irradiation In 1992 when more than 100 patients were treated, no survival advantage could be determined (Mattson et al., 1992). Often palliative irradiation is discussed. I cannot agree here, as the side effects of such irradiation are significant.

Additional therapies like hormones, antibodies, etc.

Other allopathic therapies like monoclonal antibodies or hormonal therapies are not used in for pleuramesotheliomas. The entire therapy revolves around destruction of the tumor, but this undertaking is naturally destined to fail with such an aggressive tumor. A legitimate question is; "Why aren't there any new approaches up to this point". There are many reasons for this, most likely the main reasons are that there are simply too few cases, and that pharmaceutical companies simply do not have a compelling motivation to do something in this direction.

How ignorant this is today is evidenced with the example of the IAT therapy (see IAT). When Dr. Burton first reported on the successful treatment of 11 patients with mesotheliomas he was immediately dismissed as a quack. Even in 1999, when a team appointed by the American government these cases jointly with our organization and confirmed them, nothing was done.

The only physician in Germany who used IAT many years ago had his practice closed by the authorities after the fact was made known. Although he fought hard for this treatment and applied for all approvals, he was never successful in obtaining them. Given the fact that allopathy does not have a single therapy for this disease, and that Dr. Burton demonstrably had many patients who survived for many years, thanks to his therapy, (some of them for more than 20 years), then it is not hard to see the efforts that are undertaken to prevent non-conventional therapies from being introduced on the market – particularly those therapies with few side effects.

Morbus Hodgkin's
Lymphogranulomatosis

1. The allopathic definition:
Malignant system disease characterized by the presence of single nucleus and multinucleated Hodgkin cells and Reed-Sternberg giant cells.

2. How frequently does this type of cancer occur (incidence rate) in Germany (USA appr. x 3)?
Current incidence rate: 2-3 per 100,000 people

3. Subdivisions:
There are 4 different histological groups:

* LP (Lymphocyte Predominance, app. 3%)
* NS (Nodular Sclerosis, app. 80%)
* MC (Mixed Cellularity, app. 15 %)
* LD (Lymphocyte Depletion app. 2%)

Stages:

WHO/REAL classification

Classical Hodgkin's lymphoma.

Nodular sclerosis Hodgkin's lymphoma.

Mixed cellularity Hodgkin's lymphoma.

Lymphocyte depletion Hodgkin's lymphoma.

Lymphocyte-rich classical Hodgkin's lymphoma.

Nodular lymphocyte-predominant Hodgkin's lymphoma.

4. How is this type of cancer diagnosed by allopathic practitioners?

First, through the presence of Hodgkin and Reed Sternberg cells through removal of a lymph node (biopsy). X-ray of the chest area, ultrasound and CT, bone centigram, bone marrow biopsy, often the spleen is removed (however this is also controversial among allopathic practitioners due to the hazard of bacterial complication).

What are the allopathic therapy concepts?

Surgery

Operations do not play a major role with Morbus Hodgkin, but rather are only used when lymph nodes cause major physical problems like congestion, or for obtaining tissue samples.

Allogenic bone marrow transplant / stem cell transplant:

In this therapy, bone marrow / stem cells are removed from the patient and, after administering a high-dose chemotherapy (usually with cyclophosphamide, melphalan, BCNU, Ara-C, methotrexate und etoposide) the bone marrow / stem cells is/are returned to the patient. Usually this therapy is only offered to young patients, because in the first place it is extremely expensive, second, for older people there is too great a risk of fatality through the therapy, and third the successes are quite modest, as only app. 50% of the survivors of this procedure reach a standstill, and this success remains stable for only 30-50% of this group over a period of years.

With the allogenic bone marrow / stem cell transplant, the patient gets stem cells from a donor, and with the peripheral blood stem cell transplant the blood of the patient is channeled through a machine, which removes the stem cells from the blood and then returns the blood into circulation (also referred to as leukopheresis). The stem cells thus acquired are armed with cancer-killing medications and re-infused into the patient.

Chemotherapy and radiation

For Morbus Hodgkin there are studies showing that the combination of irradiation and chemotherapy produces major successes. For this reason holistic-oriented physicians hardly trust themselves to treat patients with this diagnosis. There are no comparative studies with non-conventional therapies, and the question as to whether patients have become healthy because of a therapy, or in spite of a therapy, remains unanswered. Here as well I would like to avoid any misunderstanding: I do not want to speak in negative terms about the successes of allopathy, rather my interest is to critically examine why people become healthy.

Usually patients are irradiated according to the EF (Extended Field) or the IF (Involved field) scheme with 30-40 Gy. There are breaks in the process so that the bone marrow can better recover.

In addition there are chemotherapies in accordance with the COPP scheme (COPP-ABVD and COPP-ABV-IMEP). COPP stands for cyclophosphamide, vincristin, procarbazine und prednison, and ABVD consists of the following toxins: adriamycin, bleomycin, vinblastin and dacarbazine. The MOPP (M=mechlorethamine) scheme, which was used previously is not used very much today.

Additional therapies like hormones, antibodies, etc.

An antibody, which has been used for Morbus Hodgkin, was for instance MAb BerH2. In Germany the Cologne University Clinic has used this antibody, however without significant advantages relative to survival.

Another antibody is the immune toxin or Ki-4.dgA. This is an antibody that is aligned against the CD25 antigen on the Hodgkin /Reed Sternberg cells. The cell toxin, which is coupled on the Ki-4 antibody is called Ricin-A. Looking beyond the immense side effects, there is no study that has even come close to showing that patients with Morbus Hodgkin have lived even a single day longer through the use of this medication.

Other therapies are not used for Morbus Hodgkin. From my personal experience I would like to say that I have only met a few patients with this clinical picture, since the therapy rests completely in the hands of conventional medicine, and here there are also massive legal conflicts. But when it comes to recurrences allopathy unfortunately has little to offer, and only at this point do patients ask whether there are other therapies. Unfortunately by this time these patients have reached such a labile condition both physically and mentally that it is difficult for any therapist to have a positive effect.

I do not say that it is impossible because I know a person quite well who returned to health in this stage using non-conventional therapies, and who today even leads a cancer organization. What I really want to communicate is that even with Morbus Hodgkin, each patient must precisely consider the extent to which he will allow his body to be destroyed. Naturally I don't have a standard solution for this problem either. But I say it because I have often experienced that, even for recurrences, only those therapies that have failed in the past are used again, and at this point I think a paradigm shift would be beneficial.

Multiple myeloma
(Plasmacytoma)

1. The allopathic definition:
Multiple myeloma (MM) involves malignant, monoclonal plasma cells (plasma cells mature from white blood corpuscles that are called lymphocytes) and consequently they are assigned to the low-malignancy non-Hodgkin's lymphomas.

Often MM is also referred to as plasmacytoma or Morbus Kahler. Strictly speaking this is incorrect because plasmacytoma actually designates an illness without bone marrow infiltration, which is not the case with MM.

2. How frequently does this type of cancer occur (incidence rate) in Germany (USA appr. x 3)?
Current incidence: 4.5 per 100,000. What is evident in this regard is that the incidence among blacks is twice the incidence among the white population.

Studies of risk factors are cited in many text books:

* Chronic antigen stimulation of the immune system (e.g. through IL-6 induction as stimulator of B-cell differentiation)

* Viral or bacterial diseases, immunizations (BCG, diphtheria, scarlet fever, whooping cough), allergies or auto-immune disorders.

* Radiation exposures (interesting here is that on one hand the prevailing opinion is that low-dose radiation exposure poses no disadvantages, and on the other hand it is precisely this low radiation exposure, e.g. in the case of radiologists or

employees of nuclear companies, which is made out to be (co-) responsible for MM, as studies demonstrate).

* Herbicides and insecticides

* Metals (lead, arsenic, cadmium, copper dust, nickel, etc.)

* Hair dying agents

* Genetic factors or chromosomal anomalies like 14q+

* Oncogenes like c-myc mRNA or bcl-1- und bcl-2 ...

3. Subdivisions:
Morphological classification according to cell type:

* Marschalko

* Small cell

* Cleaved

* Polymorphous

* Asynchronous

* Blastic

In addition these categories are often grouped in prognostic degrees:

1. Low-grade malignancy

2. Intermediate grade malignancy

3. High grade malignancy

4. How is this type of cancer diagnosed by allopathic practitioners?
The diagnosis of multiple myeloma is considered to be assured if two of the following "Ossermann criteria" are satisfied:

A: Verification of more than 10% partially atypical plasma cells

B: Verification of an M-protein in the serum and/or urine

C: Verification of at least one osteolysis
(Decomposition of bone tissue)

Protein chemistry
Immunoglobulins in the serum and urine, beta-2 microglobulins, albumin, C-reactive protein, various cytokines.

Labeling index
This index indicates the percentage of myeloma cells with an H-thymidin scan.

Additional examinations
X-ray (for evaluating the bones), magnetic resonance tomography, bone density measurement, bone marrow biopsy.
A differential diagnosis must always exclude monoclonal gammopathy of uncertain significance (MGUS).

Stages:
Stage I multiple myeloma means all of the following:

Hemoglobin >10 g/dL.
Normal serum calcium.

Normal bone structure.
Low M-protein production as shown by:
IgG <5.0 g/dL.
IgA <3.0 g/dL.

Stage II multiple myeloma means multiple myeloma that fits in neither stage I nor stage III.

Stage III multiple myeloma means 1 or more of the following:

Hemoglobin <8.5 g/dL.
Serum calcium >12.0 mg/dL.
More than 3 lytic bone lesions.
High M-protein production as shown by:
IgG >7.0 g/dL.
IgA >5.0 g/dL.

In addition the stages in A (normal kidney function) and B (limited kidney function) are subdivided.

Additional differentiations:

Isolated plasmacytoma of the bone
Only a single-cell plasma tumor is found in the bones.

Plasmacytomas outside of the bone marrow (extra-medullar Plasmacytoma)
Here plasma cell tumors are only found outside of bones and bone marrow in the soft parts, usually in the tonsils, or the tissues around the nose.

Macroglobulin anemia
Plasma cells that produce a certain type of M proteins and often result in swollen lymph nodes or spleen and liver enlargement.

Monoclonal gammopathy of unknown origin.
M-proteins are found in the blood, but the patient does not have symptoms.

Treatment-resistant plasmacellular neoplasia
In spite of allopathic therapies the plasmas cells do not decrease.

What are the allopathic therapy concepts?

Chemotherapy
Multiple myelomas represent a chemotherapy stronghold. Here however there is something to be aware of.

1. MM cannot be healed through conventional chemotherapy. All attempts in recent years (mainly with melphalan/prednison = MP) have failed. Also the use of cyclophosphamide in the usual doses has not resulted in the successes that were expected.

2. Today's gold standard was arrived at based on studies by Jagannath, Barlogie, Vesole, Attal, and others, and it is: High-dose chemotherapy with autologic blood stem cell transplant.
    Within this protocol however there are still differing views relative doses, combinations (with total body irradiation, with cyclophosphamide, Busulfan and Idarubicin or Anthracyclines) and frequency. This therapy is basically suggested for patients who are younger than 60.

3. What patients must know is that in most studies (again) the discussion primarily involves "high response rates", "remission rates", and "recurrence-free intervals". If the data relative to quality of life and extension of life are considered then the numbers are significantly more sobering. Thus number of patients, which cannot be underestimated (up to 17%)

die due to the therapy (blood poisoning, general immune weakness etc.) and in many studies the survival time was only a few weeks/months. This is significant because this therapy decreases the quality of life for months and one should never forget that the therapy can kill you. However there are also studies which demonstrate that patients who received high-dose chemotherapies have lived longer compared to those patients who received normal dose chemotherapies. Unfortunately to this day there is not a single study that compares chemotherapies with therapies that do not include chemotherapies.

4. There are also high-dose therapies involving melphalan without stem cell transplant, however in these studies too many people died due to the excessive suppression of the bone marrow. For this reason the tendency today toward therapies with autologic or allogenic bone marrow/blood stem cells.

5. One alternative to autologic bone marrow transplant (BMT) is donation of bone marrow from an HLA (Human Leucocytes Antigen) identical donor. However the fatality rate within three years is over 40% with this therapy.

In summary one can say that for patients under 60 years of age the high-dose combination with stem cells or the dual high-dose therapy at 6-month intervals has established itself. Usually physicians in Germany follow the Munich-Bolzano high-dose protocol (VAD = vincristin, adriamycin und dexamethasone or IEV = ifosfamide, epirubicin und etoposide).

For patients over 60 years of age, the Alexanian protocol is always used (i.e. melphalan and prednisone) although the results here are anything but convincing.

ATTENTION
Patients in stage 1 are usually not given a therapy, as studies (Durie/Salmon) have shown that patients derive no advantage

from a therapy. But I consider it to be a major error to believe that one should do nothing, or to wait until everything gets worse! Do not make this mistake, start today with the 3E program.

Irradiation

Allopathic practitioners also view irradiation therapies for MM differently. On one hand, studies such as the one by Björkstrand (1996) show that patients really only experience disadvantages from total body irradiation, on the other hand, irradiation has almost established itself as the gold standard. Many doctors are also starting to use irradiation only in cases of osteolysis or bone pain. In this case the usual response is high-doses (8-10 Gy).

Since there are few hard facts to demonstrate that irradiation can contribute a longer life for patients with MM, it is certainly "remarkable" that this therapy has been established as standard in so many clinics.

Additional therapies like hormones, antibodies, etc.

Interferon

Similar to the situation with irradiation therapy I also find it "remarkable" that a therapy that involves interferon has established itself in so many hospitals, although in this case as well there are no hard facts confirming that patients live significantly longer due to these therapies. Considering the side effects of this therapy and how expensive it is, this is astounding (maybe not so astounding when the financial aspect is considered).

There are indeed studies that attempt to show survival advantages for patients, who after a high-dose therapy, had a complete remission (Powels 1995), but here as well one must be very careful, as this data could also be evaluated differently.

Bisphosphonates
Bisphosphonates are similar to pyrophosphoric acid and they can contribute to bones being resistant to decomposition. Known medications are bondronate or aredia. Usually the patient gets an infusion in three-week intervals.

When giving bisphosphonates for treatment of bone metastasis I notice again and again that many doctors do not distinguish between decomposition processes (lysistic) and constructive processes (neoplastic). Here any shadow shown by an imaging process is designated as bone metastases regardless of whether this "metastases" is now eating a hole into the bone, whether it has settled on the bone. For this reason many physicians prescribe bisphosphonates, even for neoplastic processes. I cannot agree with this opinion and consequently recommend that you ask your physician to explain precisely what type of bone metastases you have.

Thalidomide/revimide/CC5013
Today many people still remember thalidomide due to the Contergan scandal. For MM there are studies in which thalidomide given together with chemotherapy was able to achieve extended life times. However more recent studies show that the side effects are more serious than was originally assumed. These side effects include thrombosis, heart and skin disorders, and significant nerve damage.

Bortezomib / Velcade
In May 2003 in America (and 2004 in Germany) the chemotherapy medication bortezomib (a proteasome inhibitor) was approved for treatment of MM. This was done prematurely, as the medication was not approved because MM patients have been lived significantly longer, rather it was approved due to an American law which regulates the sale of "medications that promise success". In one study, 188 patients were injected with bortezomib, and 52 patients experienced an

improvement, which on average was maintained for only 12 months. The remaining 136 patients experienced only disadvantages. By the way, the medication was approved precisely due to this study, and for your information it costs 20,000 Euro just for the first four months.

Myelodysplastic syndrome

1. The allopathic definition:

This is a overarching term for various bone marrow diseases that primarily occur in patients in the second part of life. Basically this involves symptoms that do not fit into other cancer types like leukemias, and thus they are included under this term.

Moreover the myelodysplastic syndrome is a "side effect" of multiple medications such as cytostatic agents.

2. How frequently does this type of cancer occur (incidence rate) in Germany (USA appr. x 3)?

Incidence rate: 3.5-12 per 100,000 annually.

3. Subdivisions:

Usually doctors use the FAB (French-American-British) division which distinguishes 5 different morphological subgroups.

Morphological subtype	Blast percentage in the blood	Blast percentage in the bone marrow	additional changes
Refractory Anemia (RA)	≤ 1 %	< 5 %	
RA with ringsideroblasts (RARS)	≤ 1 %	< 5 %	>15% Ring-sideroblasts in BM
RA with an abundance of blasts (RAEB)	< 5 %	5–20 %	
Chronic myelomono cytic leukemia	< 5 %	5–20 %	peripheral Monocytosis (Multiplication of the monocytes)
RAEB in transformation (RAEB/T)	≥ 5 %	21–30 %	Facultative Auer rods

4. How is this type of cancer diagnosed by allopathic practitioners?

Final diagnosis can only occur through the microscope. Bone marrow smears or core needle biopsies are required for this. Although often pancytopenia (reduction of the blood cells) is found in the blood, many patients do not have any symptoms. Others in turn have an increased susceptance to infection, bleeding, or they have symptoms of anemia. With chronic myelomonocytic leukemia (CMML) frequently a splenomegalia (enlarged spleen) is also found.

Differential diagnostically MDS must be distinguished from reactive-conditioned changes in the hemograms and bone marrow. First, lack of folic acid or vitamin B12, or infectious processes, must be excluded. Increased blast counts in the bone marrow indicate a starting, acute leukemia. The probability that MDE will develop into acute leukemia is 30 – 60% for patients with RAEB or RAEB-T (leukemic MDS).

What are the allopathic therapy concepts?

Here we must say that there is no basic therapy system. This means naturally that myelodysplastic syndrome is actually not an illness, but rather a collection of various symptoms, which are manifest differently in every patient. This is why treatment of the symptoms is also the priority. In addition, the advanced age of many patients is another consideration.

Initial measures often include blood transfusions and avoidance of medications that can disturb the bone marrow. Steroids also are still being used. Concerning blood transfusion, it must be stated here that there are many unknown risks and known risks that can disturb the immune system. In addition this causes an overload of iron, so that binding the iron through so-called iron chelation may be necessary.

Bone marrow transplant
Depending on the source of the transplanted bone marrow (or of the stem cells) there are two types:

1. Allogenic bone marrow transplant / stem cell transplant: Here the patient receives stem cells from a donor.

2. Autologic bone marrow transplant / stem cell transplant: with this therapy bone marrow/stem cells are removed from the patient and after administering a high-dose chemotherapy it/they are readministered.

For myelodysplastic syndrome, allogenic bone marrow/stem cell transplant is used for younger patents (those under 50 years of age). Many doctors consider this to be the only curative therapy.

Chemotherapy
For many years the chemotherapy was a low-dose treatment with cytosin-arabinosid (low-dose Ara-C). I still do not understand this mistake, even if there are many explanations put forth for it, because it is precisely this therapy that suppresses the hemogram. It is easy to understand why this therapy is really not used so often today (usually only for leukemic MDS (RAEB, RAEB-T). Thus be careful if this therapy is offered to you.

While chemotherapies can indeed achieve short-term remissions, relapse is pre-programmed and the poor results clearly speak for themselves. Unfortunately there is a tendency to use aggressive therapies, particularly for RAEB, RAEB/T und AML-MDS. In most case the protocols are derived from the usual standard protocols for acute myeloic leukemias. This fact indicates that there is no allopathic concept for myelodysplastic syndrome and the despairing attempt is made to use whatever comes closest. But the actual problem is that research efforts to determine the cause of this illness have failed, and consequently people are "doctoring around with the bone marrow symptom" as best they can. Please do not misunderstand. There are no statistics that prove you will live significantly longer if you undergo chemotherapy.

Irradiation
Irradiation really should not play any role for MDS. Nevertheless I am aware of individual cases where this therapy instrument has been integrated in a treatment protocol.

Additional therapies like hormones, antibodies, etc.

Growth factors
So called haemopoetic (blood-forming) growth factors play a major role in treating MDS. Here the approach is: Let's treat the symptom (too little blood) and the patient will get better. Naturally this approach is doomed to fail over the long term, however it is used because it brings short-term symptom improvements.

Currently in use are primarily DGM-CSF, G-CSF, erythropoietin and interleukin 3. GM-CSF and G-CSF, which result in an increase of neutrophilic granulocytes, these however quickly decline when the medication is no longer taken. At the same time however there is danger of an increased tendency to bleeding, since thrombocyte production can decline when using this medication. In one study involving 102 patients, no advantage could be determined relative to extension of life, or to be more precise, patients even died sooner with this treatment. This makes me even more concerned that this therapy is still being used frequently.

The results with Interleukin and Erythropoietin are even worse. If these therapies are offered to you as standard therapies for MDS, then please request that your doctor give you a written list of those studies that prove you will live significantly longer through this treatment – I could not find these studies.

Vitamins, interferons and others
There are studies in progress ,and there have been studies with derivatives of vitamin A and Vitamin D3, as well as with interferons alpha and interferon gamma. But none of these studies have resulted to this point in any advantages for MDS patients, they have however proven beneficial for stockholders.

Caution
Because allopathy does not have a therapy concept, the chance that you will be asked to participate in a study is naturally quite high.

Non-Hodgkin's lymphoma

1. The allopathic definition:
Non-Hodgkin's lymphomas (NHL) are malignant cells of the lymph system, the B-cells and the T-cells.

2. How frequently does this type of cancer occur (incidence rate) in Germany (USA appr. x 3)?
Current incidence rate: 15 per 100,000.

3. Subdivisions:

REAL/WHO Classification

B-cell neoplasms:
* Precursor B-cell neoplasm: precursor B-acute lymphoblastic leukemia/lymphoblastic lymphoma (B-ALL, LBL).
* Peripheral B-cell neoplasms.
* B-cell chronic lymphocytic leukemia/small lymphocytic lymphoma.
* B-cell prolymphocytic leukemia.
* Lymphoplasmacytic lymphoma/immunocytoma.
* Mantle cell lymphoma.
* Follicular lymphoma.
* Extranodal marginal zone B-cell lymphoma of MALT type.
* Nodal marginal zone B-cell lymphoma (± monocytoid B-cells).
* Splenic marginal zone lymphoma (± villous lymphocytes).
* Hairy cell leukemia.

* Plasmacytoma/plasma cell myeloma.
* Diffuse large B-cell lymphoma.
* Burkitt's lymphoma.

T-cell and putative NK-cell neoplasms:
* Precursor T-cell neoplasm: precursor T-acute lymphoblastic leukemia/lymphoblastic lymphoma (T-ALL, LBL).
* Peripheral T-cell and NK-cell neoplasms.
* T-cell chronic lymphocytic leukemia/prolymphocytic leukemia.
* T-cell granular lymphocytic leukemia.
* Mycosis fungoides/Sézary syndrome.
* Peripheral T-cell lymphoma, not otherwise characterized.
* Hepatosplenic gamma/delta T-cell lymphoma.
* Subcutaneous panniculitis-like T-cell lymphoma.
* Angioimmunoblastic T-cell lymphoma.
* Extranodal T-/NK-cell lymphoma, nasal type.
* Enteropathy-type intestinal T-cell lymphoma.
* Adult T-cell lymphoma/leukemia (HTLV 1+).
* Anaplastic large cell lymphoma, primary systemic type.
* Anaplastic large cell lymphoma, primary cutaneous type.
* Aggressive NK-cell leukemia.

What are the allopathic therapy concepts?

General
NHL is a stronghold of allopathic therapies like chemotherapy and irradiation. There are also statistics in this regard which show that a high percentage rate (fluctuating between 20% to over 60%) have survived the five-year barrier with these therapies. Naturally what many patients do not know is that there are only few patients who have not been treated allopathically with this therapy, and naturally the question again arises, do patients survive because of or in spite of the

therapy? Another point is also "forgotten" with regards to allopathic therapy recommendations. After a therapy involving chemotherapy and irradiation, which as we know, is carcinogenic itself, there is no return to holistic therapy, because the damage caused by this therapy combination cannot be restored by any holistic therapy. In practical terms this means that the patient must decide for one direction or the other. The option of, "let's test this first, and if it fails then we will pursue a different path", is not possible in 99.9 % of the cases.

Operation
Operations do not play a major role with NHL, rather they are only used when lymph nodes cause major physical problems like congestions.

Bone marrow transplant
Depending on the source of the transplanted bone marrow (or of the stem cells) there are two types:

1. Allogenic bone marrow transplant / stem cell transplant: Here the patient receives stem cells from a donor.

2. Allogenic bone marrow transplant / stem cell transplant: with this therapy bone marrow/stem cells are removed from the patient and after administering a high-dose chemotherapy are readministered.

Even among allopathic practitioners there is no clear decision for allogenic or autologic therapy forms. Naturally one must say that both therapies are based on the theory that the "degenerated" cells must be killed, and as we know today this is only a symptomatic approach.

Chemotherapy and radiation
For NHL therapies one must first change the paradigm,

because many physicians tell their patients that the more aggressive the illness the better it can be treated. This means that highly-malignant lymphomas respond the best to therapies. Naturally this perspective is only valid because there are only two possible therapies. Chemotherapy and irradiation. Naturally both therapies are best at killing rapidly growing cells, and consequently this approach applies today.

The CHOP system has established itself as standard therapy for highly malignant lymphomas. CHOP is short for cyclophosphamide, doxorubicin, prednison and vincristin. Usually after 3-5 chemotherapies, irradiation is prescribed as an additional measure. The standard in this regard is 20-30 irradiations at 2 Gy each.

Irradiation is at the top of the list for intermediate and low-malignancy lymphomas. In this process the primary tumor regions and neighboring lymph nodes are irradiated. More extensive areas are also irradiated if there is an affection of multiple lymph nodes. However these therapies fail in advanced stages (3 and 4) and the procedure then is just a palliative (alleviating) approach. I disagree totally with this and consequently recommend that patients in this stage carefully consider which path they want to pursue.

In addition patients are unfortunately still being offered the "wait and see therapy". Distance yourself as quickly as possible from a physician who only suggests this therapy to you. If you have NHL, then you cannot simply wait – even if I believe that this therapy is still better than a palliative prescribed chemotherapy with subsequent irradiation. Ask your doctor what you are supposed to be waiting for. Does he want you to wait for a miracle or to wait until you get worse?

Please excuse these hard words, but I consider it absolutely irresponsible to tell a cancer patient to continue on as he has done in the past. This is precisely the path which allowed the NHL to occur. Do not make this mistake and stick with the 3E program.

In general one can say that there are hard facts which show that patients particularly with highly-malignant NHL survive 5-years with allopathic therapies. However I cannot agree with the opinion that this is due primarily to irradiation. We should not forget that MDS (myelodysplastic syndrome) occurs in increased incidence, for irradiated NHL patients, but not only for these. MDS, which can be considered a type of preliminary stage leukemia, which can develop into acute myeloic leukemia. These statistics alone are sufficient to demonstrate the carcinogenic effect of irradiation.

You see, all these main effects of irradiation are "trivial-ized" and as patient you must understand that the chance is high, that you will exchange one illness for another within a few years. I cannot let the argument: "At least I would still have some good years that I would not have had without the chemotherapy", go without comment because you cannot know what would happen to you if would undergo a holistic therapy. This will only be possible when at last studies are available involving non-epithelial types of cancer where holistic therapies are compared with allopathic therapies. Unfortunately we are still decades away from such studies.

Additional therapies like hormones, antibodies, etc.

Monoclonal antibodies
For several years now there have been approaches with so-called monoclonal antibodies, e.g. with anti-CD 20. Unfortunately these therapies have not delivered what the pharmaceutical companies have been promising, and conse-quently these therapies must be also be grouped under the study category.

Furthermore, in June 2000, one manufacturer of mono-clonal antibodies , (Genentech), was compelled to send a warning letter to all physicians in the USA, warning of serious side effects, because 15 women died (within 24 hours of infusion) through therapies with monoclonal antibodies.

Interferon
The use of interferons is still controversial, because here there are no meaningful studies and many people consider this area to be nothing more than a way to make money.

Non-small cell
bronchial carcinoma

1. The allopathic definition:
Bronchial carcinomas involve an epithelial tumor, emanating from the alveoli, bronchia, or the trachea.

2. How frequently does this type of cancer occur (incidence rate) in Germany (USA appr. x 3)?
For men bronchial carcinoma is the most frequently occurring tumor, and the incidence rate for men is 75 per 100,000, and for women it is 35 per 100,000. This means app. 45,000 new illnesses in 2001.

3. Subdivisions:
Histologically three types are distinguished:

* Squamous epithelial carcinoma

* Large cell and small cell carcinoma

* Adenocarcinoma

Stages:
See Small cell bronchial carcinoma

4. How is this type of cancer diagnosed by allopathic practitioners?
Coughing or coughing up blood. Pain in the chest area. Often metastases are also found before the primary tumor is detected. X-ray, CT, lung function diagnostics, like spirometer,

blood gas analysis, or perfusion scintigraphy. Moreover often mediastinoscopy (inspecting the superior mediastinum) and punction are performed.

What are the allopathic therapy concepts?

Surgery
See the division listed under small cell bronchial carcinoma.

Chemotherapy
* Usually cisplatin, cyclophosphamide, mytocin and methotrexate are used.

* To this day there are no substantiated studies that you will live significantly longer through any combination or single treatment of chemotherapeutic medications. All previous studies, even in the most positive case, show only a slight improvement in survival time, which must be paid for with major side effects, particularly for chemotherapies that include cisplatin.

* For almost 20 years the chemotherapy treatment for lung cancer has been described as significantly important for the survival time of patients. It is also true that there are studies in which patients, lived longer in comparison with patients who received no treatment at all. But what does "lived longer" mean? In most studies the extension was between 1.1 month and a maximum of 34.9 weeks. 34.9 weeks was clearly the best study to date (Fuks, J. Z. JCO 1983). For all others it was usually a few days or a few weeks. Here you must know that this extension was only achieved with significant damages, because cisplatin, (one of the chemotherapy medications with the most serious side effects) was used in this case.

Iressa
Even the manufacturer, Astra Zeneca, writes (2005) on their
Internet site (www.iressa-us.com) that lung cancer patients get
no clinical advantage with this approved medication. Why is
it even on the market?

Radiation
The information cited for chemotherapy also applies for irradiation. In this case patients are constantly being told how
much their chances of survival would be increased through
irradiation. But let's take a closer look at the numbers.

* A study published in 1998 (Port Meta study) involving 2128
patients with non-small cell bronchial carcinoma proved that
after two years 7% fewer patients were alive than were alive
in the comparison group. This needs serious consideration. It
is not just the fact that patients were irradiated, with all the
side effects, not just the fact that these patients were given
such a treatment in their last months of life, but in addition on
average they even died earlier. If you are advised to undergo
radiation therapy then make sure to ask your oncologist
whether he is aware of any better data.

* In ten studies single chemotherapies were compared with
chemotherapies combined with irradiation. None of these
studies showed the combination offered a survival advantage
for patients with non-small cell lung tumors.

Additional therapies like hormones, antibodies, etc.

* See under small cell bronchial carcinoma.

* The inhibiting of signal transduction through protein C
alpha inhibitors is supposed to help in combination with

chemotherapies. Protein kinases play a role in abnormal cell growth in tumors and are formed in increased quantity with some tumors, as they are with bronchial carcinomas.

Through the use of so-called antisence substances like LY900003 (Affinitac) formation of pathogenic proteins is supposed to be suppressed. In June 2003 during the ASCO meetings in America a study was presented involving 616 patients. This study showed that there were neither advantages in survival time, nor in the response rates of chemotherapies.

Oropharynx carcinoma

1. The allopathic definition:
Tumors of the oral part of the pharynx.

2. How frequently does this type of cancer occur (incidence rate) in Germany (USA appr. x 3)?
Incidence rate: 2-5 per 100,000 for men, and 0.5-1 per 100,000 for women. Alcohol and smoking are listed as causes in many books, however there are no proofs of this.

3. Subdivisions:

Histologically there are the following distinctions:
* Epithelial tumors (the majority of tumors)

* Lymphoepithelial tumors

* Salivary gland carcinomas

Depending on the location three tumors are usually differentiated:

* Palatal tonsils

* Root of the tongue

* Soft palate

Stages:

TX: Primary tumor cannot be assessed

T0: No evidence of primary tumor

Tis: Carcinoma in situ

T1: Tumor =2 cm in greatest dimension

T2: Tumor >2 cm but =4 cm in greatest dimension

T3: Tumor >4 cm in greatest dimension

T4a: Tumor invades the larynx, deep/extrinsic muscle of tongue, medial pterygoid, hard palate, or mandible

T4b: Tumor invades lateral pterygoid muscle, pterygoid plates, lateral nasopharynx, or skull base or encases carotid artery

Since almost all tumors are detected relatively late, in most cases metastases are already present, usually in the lymph nodes. Afterwards metastases are found, particularly in the lungs.

4. How is this type of cancer diagnosed by allopathic practitioners?
Difficulty swallowing, and sore throat with emanations in the ear, bad breath (foeter ex ore), lockjaw, blood in the saliva, voice has a nasal sound (rhinolalia), swelling of the neck lymph nodes. Reflection, biopsy as main criteria, CT, MRT, sonography, x-ray.

What are the allopathic therapy concepts?

Surgery
Operation is the absolute first measure. Usually it is combined with irradiation, or irradiation and chemotherapy, because in most cases it is not possible to remove the tumor completely.

Basically you must know that here patients often are offered an operation that will affect the quality of their life. These recommendations are based on the principle that a tumor must be completely removed, otherwise healing cannot occur. Most surgeons view tumor mass reduction on its own as "not enough".

I have no doubt that a complete removal of the tumor is advantageous. However the decision to cut away half of the face with subsequent attempt at plastic surgery reconstruction is serious, and in my opinion a partial resection of the tumor can also improve the immune system. However if the immune system is damaged after the operation with irradiation and chemotherapy, then even a partial resection cannot help – here I agree with the allopathic practitioners.

In addition to the usual tumor removals, removal of the tonsils, and the root of the tongue usually the so-called neck dissection (removal of the lymph nodes of the lateral neck area) is also prescribed.

Chemotherapy
5-FU (Fluorouracil), Cisplatin, Mitomycin C and Carboplatin are preferred. Particularly in the case of epithelial tumors this approach is destined to fail, and it has not been proven to help patients live longer in comparison to non-conventional therapies. All the studies that have been published (again) only compare conventional therapies with other conventional therapies (Byfield, Kish Marcial). Logically one of the combinations (cisplatin, 5-FU and leucovorin with irradiation) did better than irradiation only (Wendt 1998).

The "study possibilities" here even go so far as to compare whether an irradiation therapy prior to, during, or after the chemotherapy comes out better. (Adelstein 1990). Interestingly enough the results of this study are often indicated in two-year, or three-year survival rates, and not in 5-year survival rates which are the norm. I leave evaluation of this circumstance up to you.

Irradiation
Because often complete operations are not possible, and allopathic practitioners view destruction of the tumor as the highest priority of cancer therapy, irradiation therapies represent a stronghold for oropharynx carcinomas. Irradiation is almost always recommended, even as early as T2. But here you must be aware that oropharynx carcinomas are rarely detected in the T1 stage.

For many years patients have been treated with the "usual" irradiation system (30-35 x 1.8-2 Gy). When patients died in spite of this, or because of this, (Marks 1978, Meoz-Mendez 1978, Mendenhall 1987), it was not the radiation therapy that was called into questioned, but rather it was the administration. Then "experts" came up with the idea that the cells, which do not die immediately can recover between irradiation treatments, and consequently a patient should be irradiated more than once a day.

For this reason in recent years the "hyperfractionation" or "acceleration" of radiation therapy has become established. For the patient this means that he will be irradiated at least twice a day, however with at a lesser dose.

Assuming that this theory is correct, then all radiologists who only irradiate their cancer patients once a day, would be considered as absolute neophytes. Pursuing this logic, why irradiate only two times a day, the dose could be reduced even more and the patient could be irradiated 5 times a day, for example. And if this theory were correct then why don't the patients live any longer (Nguyen 1988, Horiot 1992) – and why do they have significantly more serious side effects?

To what extent irradiation, which allopathy considers to be carcinogenic, reduces the chance of healing, and promotes the progress of the disease is a question that apparently nobody is pursuing. Given the one-sided view that cancer equals tumor, and that tumor must be destroyed under any circumstances, all other precautionary measures are swept under the rug.

Particularly in the case of tumors of the root of the tongue, allopathic practitioners should take a better look at the statistics and consider whether more therapy is really needed here.

Additional therapies like hormones, antibodies, etc.

Treatment of oropharynx carcinomas rests completely in the hands of surgeons and radiologists. In addition since the number of cases is not particularly high, greater investments do not make economic sense for pharmaceutical companies. Cytokines (interferon, Interleukin) or hormone therapies do not play a role here.

Ovarian carcinoma
(fallopian tube cancer)

1. The allopathic definition:
A malignant disease of one of the fallopian tubes, or both fallopian tubes.

2. How frequently does this type of cancer occur (incidence rate) in Germany (USA appr. x 3)?
Currently app. 8,000 women annually.

3. Subdivisions:
The principle distinction is between epithelial tumors, the so-called carcinomas, the sex cord stromal tumors, like thecacell or granulosa tumors, and the lipoid cell or germ cell tumors like the teratomas, chorion carcinomas, or dysgerminomas.

Epithelial tumors account for more than 90%. Here as well there are subdivisions like endometriode, serous, mucosa etc. which are a lot less important for the therapy than they are for the pathologists.

Stages:
IA: Tumor limited to 1 ovary; capsule intact, no tumor on ovarian surface. No malignant cells in ascites or peritoneal washings.*

IB: Tumor limited to both ovaries; capsules intact, no tumor on ovarian surface. No malignant cells in ascites or peritoneal washings.*
IC: Tumor limited to 1 or both ovaries with any of the following: capsule ruptured, tumor on ovarian surface, malignant cells in ascites or peritoneal washings. [8]

317

IIA: Extension and/or implants on the uterus and/or fallopian tubes. No malignant cells in ascites or peritoneal washings.

IIB: Extension to and/or implants on other pelvic tissues. No malignant cells in ascites or peritoneal washings.

IIC: Pelvic extension and/or implants (stage IIA or stage IIB) with malignant cells in ascites or peritoneal washings.

IIIA: Microscopic peritoneal metastasis beyond pelvis (no macroscopic tumor).

IIIB: Macroscopic peritoneal metastasis beyond pelvis =2 cm in greatest dimension.

IIIC: Peritoneal metastasis beyond pelvis >2 cm in greatest dimension and/or regional lymph node metastasis.

Stage IV ovarian cancer is tumor involving 1 or both ovaries with distant metastasis. If pleural effusion is present, positive cytologic test results must exist to designate a case to stage IV. Parenchymal liver metastasis equals stage IV.

4. How is this type of cancer diagnosed by allopathic practitioners?
Stomach pains, bloating, unusual bleeding, severe weight loss with concurrent enlargement of the stomach circumference.

Transvaginal (through the vagina) sonography, tumor markers CA 12-5, CSS and CEA, x-ray with contrast agent enema, CT. Since ovarian carcinomas also occur more often as second tumors of other primary tumors such as breast or stomach tumors, naturally examinations are prescribed which are based on these tumors.

Surgery

Is employed in all stages and is certainly the first option. Usually a so-called "total operation" is undertaken, in which the uterus, the fallopian tubes and parts of the abdominal viscera (tissue covering within the stomach area) are removed. Usually lymph nodes are also removed. Fertility-saving operations are actually only performed for rare germ cell tumors such as the granulosa cell tumor, as these tumors also have a high, 10-year survival rate, even for "moderate" operations (between 70-90%).

Clearing out the lymph nodes is also a controversial procedure even among allopathic practitioners, as there is no data that can show that patients live significantly longer through this procedure.

For patients in stage 1a who want to have children an ovary-saving operation can also be considered, since the radical operation offers no advantage relative to illness-free survival (Colombo et al.; 1994).

Often surgeons deem it necessary to also remove the intestinal and bladder parts. Since this has major effects on the quality of life, or represents a greater operation risk, this step should naturally be considered carefully.

In stage 4 all allopathic measures apply as only palliative measures (alleviating) and consequently an operation is not performed. From the perspective that a reduction in tumor mass offloads the immune system, naturally this measure is quite doubtful.

Frequently doctors also prescribe a "second look operation". The objective of this operation is to determine whether the tumor has come back (which in turn usually means more chemotherapy).

Chemotherapy

Ovarian carcinomas are considered to be sensitive to chemotherapy, and consequently chemotherapy is offered to all patients, except those in stages 1a and 1b. Studies have also clearly demonstrated that tumors get smaller when treated with preparations that contain cisplatin, or in combination with taxol. Since publication of the GOG 111 study of the Gynecologic Oncology Group (GOG), there has been promotion for a combination of platinum-containing chemo preparations and Taxol. Usually carboplatin is preferred over the preparation cisplatin, but not because it is more effective, but rather because fewer side effects were demonstrated in one study.

Amidst all the allopathic enthusiasm there are several points that you as patient should not forget. First, this combination was better in comparison to cisplatin with cyclophosphamide (again only chemotherapies were tested), second, it primarily showed better response rates i.e. only slightly better survival times, and third, many physicians do not know that the studies naturally look so good because all the patients who broke-off the therapy due to intolerable side effects were not included in the study. Patients must be aware that this combination can only be administered with the most serious side effects, like kidney and nerve damage, hearing loss, and much more.

Basically it can be said that there have been studies in which patients with carboplatin/taxol have lived longer in comparison to the previously-used chemotherapy combinations with cyclophosphamide, chlorambucil and doxorubicin. The additional days (not years!) however have been purchased at a very high price, significant reduction in quality of life, and the risk of dying directly or indirectly because of the therapy.

The ICON study published in 2002 however demolished the therapy suggestions which had been highly praised for years. In this study 2074 women were observed over a five-year period in four countries. This is the most extensive study on ovarian cancer. The study demonstrated that patients who were given taxol did not live a single day longer, but they did have to deal with more side effects. There is still discussion as to how the studies which previously were so positive came about (take a guess!). If your doctor suggests taxol, then tell him a little about the ICON study.

High-dose therapies

High-dose therapies show (naturally) high response rates, however this area is still clearly considered to be experimental, and I can only warn against these human experiments today.

Irradiation

Although today there are no hard facts confirming that irradiation contributes to women living significantly longer, this therapy is still considered part of the standard program. Particularly from the perspective of its "palliative character". Since blood-forming bone marrow is in the target area of the irradiation, frequently there are serious complications or side effects.

Consequently I cannot agree with the opinion of palliative irradiation, and when the side effects are considered, then each patient and each doctor must very carefully consider whether a patient should be irradiated in the last days of life.

Additional therapies like hormones, antibodies, etc.

Since in recent years operation and chemotherapy have been established as the standard therapy, other therapies like hormonal therapies or cytokine therapies do not play a role. This is difficult to understand considering that the success rate of conventional therapy for advanced ovarian cancer (usually ovarian cancer is detected in an advanced stage) is under 13%, according to official statistics.

Pancreas carcinoma
(pancreatic cancer)

1. The allopathic definition:
Pancreatic cancer is a malignant disease of the epithelial tissue of the pancreas.

2. How frequently does this type of cancer occur (incidence rate) in Germany (USA appr. x 3)?
Current incidence rate: 9-10 per 100,000. Smoking appears to have a negative effect, as the incidence of this disease is three times higher among smokers.

3. Subdivisions:
The main distinctions are based on the location of the tumor. Approximately 70% of all tumors are in the head, 20% in the middle, and 10% in the tail of the pancreas.

Almost all tumors emanate from exocrinal (outward secretion) epithelial tissue, and in app. 80% of the cases ductal adenocarcinoma is involved (ductal= within a duct and adeno = gland). In rare cases other epithelial tumors such as squamous carcinoma, the mucinous carcinoma, or the cystadenocarcinoma are involved. Tumors such as sarcomas or lymphomas rarely occur.

Stages:

TX: Primary tumor cannot be assessed

T0:   No evidence of primary tumor

Tis: Carcinoma in situ

T1:   Tumor limited to the pancreas, =2 cm in greatest dimension

322

T2:   Tumor limited to the pancreas, >2 cm in greatest dimension

T3:   Tumor extends beyond the pancreas but without involvement of the celiac axis or the superior mesenteric artery

T4:   Tumor involves the celiac axis or the superior mesenteric artery (unresectable primary tumor)

4. How is this type of cancer diagnosed by allopathic practitioners?
Upper stomach pains, slow weight loss, diarrhea, occurrence of diabetes mellitus, enzyme tests like amylase, GOT, GPT, LDH, tumor markers like: CEA, CA 19-9, CA 494, SPAN-1 and DUPAN-2, ultrasound, EUS (endoscopic ultrasound), CT (computer tomography), ERCP (endoscopic retrograde cholangiopancreatiography), restriction enzyme mismatch PCR (for ras-oncogenic. These are certain oncogenic – tumor-generating – which can be found in app. 60% of all pancreatic carcinomas).

What are the allopathic therapy concepts?

Surgery
Is particularly employed in stage 3, and it is certainly the first option. Unfortunately most pancreatic carcinomas are inoperable, because they are detected at such a late stage. In the so-called Whipple operation, the pancreas head, a part of the small intestine, parts of the stomach, the gall bladder, and additional adjacent tissue is removed. This is supposed to ensure that insulin and digestive enzymes can continue to be formed. In the operation, the intestinal loop is sewed onto the rest of the stomach or pancreatic duct.

    If the tumor is located in the tail of the pancreas then only the tail and the spleen are removed. Usually an operation is recommended if this is possible. In any event you should discuss tumor mass reduction with the surgeon, i.e. if a classic operation is not possible, as partial removal of the tumor could offload the immune system.

Chemotherapy
Primarily a treatment with 5-FU (fluorouracil) in combination with other chemo preparations is prescribed. In addition there are studies with mitomycin C, ifosfamide and cisplatin. Since the mid 90s gemcitabine (Gemzar) has been used with increasing frequency.

However the fact remains that as of this writing, there are no sure tests to indicate that you will live longer through any combination or chemotherapies, or through any single chemotherapy. There are even studies (such as Frey with 152 patients) in which the patients who were given a chemotherapy combination (5-FU + CCNU) died earlier.

Also the use of gemcitabine is not convincing today, although my research has shown that this medication has established itself as a standard in Germany. The present data are only involve comparison with 5-FU, and these data (MSB. 1996; 18 (12):1) also show life extension of only 6 weeks, in the best case, in comparison to 5-FU. In other words this study says that patients who took Gemzar instead of 5-FU, in this study, lived 6 weeks longer. Unfortunately there is no study with information relative to whether patients who were not given any chemotherapy would have lived longer than those who took either 5-FU or Gemzar.

Here again we can see how powerless allopathy is when it comes to dealing with certain types of cancer. Although according to official statistics 99% of all patients who were given this therapy die within 5-years (most of these die within one year), nevertheless it is mainly this therapy that is recommended to patients. The discussion usually involves palliative (alleviating) therapy approaches. But why should a therapy with such serious side effects be used, when even in the best case they will only live a few days longer, and much of that time will be wasted in the hospital?

What has to happen in order for other therapy approaches to be recognized for this type of cancer. This question should be posed to your doctor as well as to your health insurance company, which is prepared to pay for chemotherapies, but which rejects demonstrably more successful therapies like Gerson, Budwig, or Gonzales.

Irradiation
Basically irradiation does not play a role for pancreatic carcinomas. Nevertheless we experience again and again that it is offered to patients as "trial therapy". What is being "tested" here is always explained with reference to palliative symptom control or combined radio-chemotherapy. I am absolutely opposed to this and every doctor should ask himself whether he really should be suggesting such therapies to his patients.

General
In most cases pancreatic cancer is diagnosed in a very late stage of the disease and unfortunately it has a poor prognosis. The patient's collaboration is encouraged, particularly for this illness. Our research and our experience show that healings are only possible for this type of cancer with very intensive change in life. Primarily the use of a chemotherapy should only occur when the objectives are clearly defined, since today we must assume that, first the patient will not live significantly longer through the use of chemotherapy, and secondly the quality of life will clearly decline in the process. In addition in my opinion through chemotherapy any chance of a cure (not extension of life!) is definitively destroyed.

With this diagnosis you will not be able to avoid confronting your future intensively and having to make decisions for a specific direction of therapy. Due to the low life expectancy, in this case you cannot "try this first and if it does not help then try …". Right from the start you should decide on a direction of therapy.

There is another consideration in this regard. Many allopathic practitioners view the diagnosis of pancreatic cancer as fundamentally incurable. Even if they do not say it, this is still what the patient "feels". Free yourself from this self-fulfilling prophecy. If you do not believe that you will return to health then who else will? If your physician holds out no hope for you, then look for this hope in yourself first, and then look for it in those around you. Learn to understand that you do not have to die of this illness – regardless of what your doctor tells you!.

Who survives?
An intensive detoxification therapy in combination with high-dosed enzyme/vitamins (see Nutrition therapy, or also Dr. Nicholas Gonzales), together with a change in diet (Dr. Budwig / Dr. Gerson / Dr. Salzborn…) in addition to Professor Hackethal, were the only documented cases of healings or long-term survivals that I could find for pancreatic carcinomas.

Since the pancreas plays a major role in digestion, nutritional therapy is very important. We know that experts always say that there are no cancer diets, nevertheless we cannot get around the fact that the data I have gathered clearly confirms the contrary.

Because it is so important: In my opinion allopathic therapies do not result in healing for pancreatic carcinomas. The only people who have a chance of being healed are those who are prepared to consistently pursue a 100% holistic concept.

Ukrain
See under Ukrain.

Penis carcinoma

1. The allopathic definition:
A malignant disease of the penis

2. How frequently does this type of cancer occur (incidence rate) in Germany (USA appr. x 3)?
Currently app. 1% of all malignant diseases (0.4 to 1 per 100,000 annually).

3. Subdivisions:
The penis carcinoma is histologically (biopsy) a cornificated, usually well-differentiated squamous epithelial carcinoma. In principle there are only high differentiation and low diffrention carcinomas. Only 10% are non-differentiated carcinomas.

A special form is the so-called "spindle cell carcinoma", which can easily be mistaken for a sarcoma through light and optics. If in doubt its squamous epithelial origin can be verified using immune immunohistochemy (keratin antibodies).

Histological classification:

1. Epithelial:
1. Benign
*   Condyloma accuminatum
*   Intermediate (pre-cancerous)
*   Interepithelial neoplasia (erythroplasia/Morbus Bowen) Grade I to III
*   Morbus Paget

2. Malignant
*   Squamous epithelial carcinoma

a) Verrucous carcinoma
b) Spindle cell carcinoma
* Basalioma
* Melanocytic tumors
* Mesenchymal tumors
* Tumors of the lymphatic tissue

Information: Melanomas can be immunohistochemically (specific antibodies) excluded or confirmed.

Stages:

Stage I penis cancer is cancer limited to the glans and the fore-skin, not involving the shaft of the penis or corpora cavernosa.

Stage II penis cancer has invaded the corpora cavernosa of the penis but has not spread to lymph nodes on clinical exam.

Stage III penis cancer has clinical spread to the regional lymph nodes in the groin. Cure is related to the number and extent of nodes involved.

Stage IV penis cancer is invasive cancer that has caused extensive and inoperable involvement of lymph nodes in the groin and/or distant metastases

4. How is this type of cancer diagnosed by allopathic practitioners?
Reddening, itching, nodes on the glans or on the transition to the penis shaft. Here there must always be a differential diag-nostic explanation against different various changes like Morbus Bowen, erythroplasia Queyrat etc.. Palpable large lymph nodes, hardening, and edema of the entire penis, disor-ders when urinating. Certain determination however can only be made through a biopsy.

What are the allopathic therapy concepts?

Surgery
Basically where allopathy is concerned, tumor = cancer, and when the tumor is removed then the cancer is gone as well. Unfortunately this one-sided view of cancer has resulted in the situation that attempts will be made destroy the tumor through invasive therapies (OP, chemotherapy, and irradiation). Consequently for penis carcinomas many men are counseled to undergo a partial or total penis amputation. Although this intervention has a significant impact on the later situation in life, as of this printing there are no studies that demonstrate whether there is an alternative therapy in this case.

I only mention that every man should make this decision very carefully because I know that many physicians only spend a few minutes discussing this very important subject with their patients.

For carcinoma in situ (TIS), erythroplasia Queyat and Morbus Bowen an organ-saving operation with 5 mm safety clearance in healthy tissue is usually undertaken. Alternatively operations are performed with lasers, however medical specialists are confronted here with problems involving a lack of histological reconditioning possibilities of the tissue. If the carcinoma has infiltrated then either a partial or total penectomy will be recommended depending on the stage.

Chemotherapy
The following cytostatic agents are used for penis carcinoma: bleomycin, methotrexate, cisplatin, 5-FU(fluorouracil) and vincristin. The general context is that chemotherapy should only be used if metastases are present, and in the case of relapses. However here you should know that there are absolutely no proofs that you will live significantly longer through chemotherapy. If your physician should maintain something else then please have him show you this in writing.

Irradiation
Since surgical intervention involves excessive stress for many patients, many oncologists are starting to use irradiation instead. Do not forget here that behind the approach there is the concept: Tumor gone = cancer gone.

From a technical point of view interstitial implantation (T1 to T3 tumors), usually with iridium, and percutaneous radiation therapy are primarily used. Here a high dose of radiation up to 40 Gy is employed.

Likewise irradiation is recommended for affection of regional lymph nodes. In the literature however one can read that this is even disputed among allopathic practitioners, as there are no studies that demonstrate that this therapy has a significant advantage relative to survival time, and moreover this therapy has many side effects. The same applies for irradiation after a penectomy.

Additional therapies like hormones, antibodies, etc.

Hormonal therapies and cytokine therapies with Interferon or Interleukin do not play a significant role for penis carcinoma. Hormonal therapies are also useless.

HPV (human papilloma viruses)
There are studies which establish a connection primarily between HPV type 16 and penis carcinomas. The causal relationship however is still seriously questioned.

Prostate carcinoma

1. The allopathic definition:
Prostate cancer is a disease of the prostate gland.

2. How frequently does this type of cancer occur (incidence rate) in Germany (USA appr. x 3)?
Current incidence rate: 47 per 100,000.

3. Subdivisions:
The primary distinction is between carcinomas that do not cause complaints, carcinomas which are detected asymptomatically, e.g. due to metastases, and classic carcinomas, which are detected due to tumor marker increase or complaints.

Stages:

TX: Primary tumor cannot be assessed

T0: No evidence of primary tumor

T1: Clinically inapparent tumor not palpable nor visible by imaging

T1a: Tumor incidental histologic finding in =5% of tissue resected
T1b: Tumor incidental histologic finding in >5% of tissue resected

T1c: Tumor identified by needle biopsy (e.g., because of elevated PSA)

T2:   Tumor confined within prostate

T2a: Tumor involves 50% of =1 lobe or less

T2b: Tumor involves >50% of 1 lobe but not both lobes

T2c: Tumor involves both lobes

T3:   Tumor extends through the prostate capsule

T3a: Extracapsular extension (unilateral or bilateral)

T3b: Tumor invades seminal vesicle(s)

T4:   Tumor is fixed or invades adjacent structures other
       than seminal vesicles: bladder neck, external
       sphincter, rectum, levator muscles, and/or pelvic wall

**4. How is this type of cancer diagnosed by allopathic prac-
titioners?**
Complaints when urinating, increased tumor marker (PSA) –
see chapter: Diagnosis. Often a benign enlargement of the
prostate occurs beforehand, lower stomach pains, rectal examination with the finger, transrectal ultrasound examination
(TRS), biopsy.

What are the allopathic therapy concepts?

Surgery
The so-called radical operation is a frequent operation and is
usually recommended if no metastases or lymph nodes are in
evidence. In this procedure the entire prostate with seminal
vesicles and spermatic ducts is removed, as are the nearby

lymph nodes and part of the bladder neck. Your physician will list possible incontinence (incapability of holding urine) and impotence as "side effects". These side effects however can affect the rest of your life and they should be weighed very carefully. My experience has shown me that almost all men become impotent after an operation, because of operation-caused injuries of the sphincter muscle, which in turn bring problems of impotency along with them. What does not sound all that bad, in truth has serious consequences.

Physicians frequently throw out percentages. Only "?? %" of those who are operated on are incontinent after the operation. Only "??%" remain impotent etc. Excuse me Mr. Doctor. Where do these numbers come from? I read the same books, I go to the same conferences, and I speak with all the patients years after the operation. I cannot confirm these numbers and you should be very careful when considering which intervention to perform. In this regard please read the German books by Professor Julius Hackethal (for example Operation – ja oder nein (Operation – Yes or No?), or Der Meineid des Hippokrates (The False Oath of Hippocrates). I cannot evaluate whether an operation is necessary for you at this point or not. In any event haste is not recommended (counted in weeks) and you should take your time and do the research. Be aware of the risk the operation involves, and the possible significant effect on your life.

Read the books written by Professor Hackethal carefully and ensure that you include other therapies in your considerations. Do not forget that a high percentage of men over 70 with a prostate carcinoma die and it is not because of a carcinoma. The lifetime risk of a 52 year old man developing a prostate carcinoma is currently app. 42% as calculated by Dr. W.F. Whitmore. The risk of dying from it however is only 3%. There is probably no other type of cancer that is even close to being as non-aggressive as prostate cancer. According to an estimate calculated in 2003 by Dr. R.M. Hoffman this means that approximately 44% of all patients in whom prostate cancer was detected were "over diagnosed", i.e. they would never have died of this disease if it had simply not been detected. Professor Hackethal for this reason always spoke about a harmless house cancer, and he was right, as the numbers confirm.

Often removal of the testes (orchiectomy) is also recommended to patients. This is done because app. 90% of the testosterone (male hormone) is formed in the testes and this hormone can have negative influences on the cell growth of carcinoma cells. Testosterone can be found in highly-increased concentration in the inner gland of the prostate. In this regard you must know however that through this intervention your voice pitch can change, which often can also represent a major change in your life.

Chemotherapy
Actually chemotherapy plays an absolute subordinate role, as the OP and hormonal therapies are always in the forefront. There were approaches with xenobiotic suramin, however these were quickly abandoned. If your doctor recommends a new chemotherapy then make sure that you request a list of documented successes in writing and read them yourself! Often a palliative (alleviating) chemotherapy is mentioned when other therapies fail. I do not agree with this approach and I cannot understand doctors who inflict this on their patients in such a situation.

In October 2004 Professor Dieter Hölzel from the Großhadern Clinic in Munich published the data on prostate cancer, which he had collected since 1987. What is frightening is that the survival time for men with metastasized prostate cancer was 19 months in the period from 1987 – 1993, and in the period from 1994 – 2002 it was only 18 months. We hear so many positive things about the progress of oncology. In 17 years of research and utilization of the most modern chemotherapies the final result is that thanks to these new therapies which have been marketed so successfully for years, on the average men die 1 month sooner than they did in 1987. When I consider what I have had to listen to because I have warned mainly older men about chemotherapy for prostate cancer, then I can only say that I do not know whether to laugh or cry when I read this study.

Irradiation
Although to this date there are no hard facts that irradiation contributes to men living significantly longer, this therapy is still considered part of the standard program. It is usually recommended that up to 70 Gy be administered in rotation technique or multi-field technique, usually over a 6-8 week period. Doctors forget frequently in this case that due to the breadth and duration of the irradiation almost total irradiation of the hemogram occurs, since the rays penetrate the body, as is known. Even healthy people would have an increased risk of getting cancer many times over after such torture.

Additional therapies like hormones, antibodies, etc.

Hormonal therapies play a major role in prostate cancer. Here so-called Lh-Rh analogues are used. Although this might sound complicated, in reality this just means that these medications in the hypophysis inhibit certain hormones (gonadotropins) which have a strong influence on the gonads.

Another method is direct blockade of steroid receptors through Flutamide for instance, and consequent blockade of the androgen receptors of the prostate and the hypophysis. Both therapies are often combined and thus a total blockade is attempted.

Without doubt the hormone blockade plays an important role. Here however we should not forget that most patients die in spite of this therapy – which again demonstrates the relative importance of the therapy. There is another factor that plays an important role in prostate cancer. Many patients who do (did) absolutely nothing live for a very long time with this type of cancer. This is why one should take a good look at many statistics, as nobody knows how important the therapy was.

Naturally all good numbers are ascribed to the therapies, but let's be honest: How do the doctors actually know this? How can we explain the fact that so many older men have prostate cancer without complaints? Why are so many alternative therapies so successful for prostate cancer etc. In this case you really should review the article: The because-of /in-spite of theory, as there is no area where it applies so well as it does for prostate cancer.

Leibowitz triple blockade
Dr. Robert Leibowitz is a physician in California who has achieved a certain renown, even among conventional oncologists, with his so-called triple blockade. His treatment protocol includes a therapy with enantone/trenantone or zoladex, 150 mg casodex and proscar (finasteride) as maintenance therapy over 13 months. He recommends 750 mg flutamide as an alternative to casodex (if too expensive).

Dr. Leibowitz published several studies (www.prostate-web.com/publications.html) in which he compares the triple blockade with the usual hormone blockades. If these studies are correct then his protocol does much better than the usual hormone blockades. Unfortunately his results have not been independently evaluated and an objective assessment consequently is difficult. In my view he mixes his therapy with different chemotherapies noticeably often, which makes the evaluation even more difficult. Also questions need to be asked concerning Proscar as maintenance therapy, because it has been shown in studies that prostate cancer becomes noticeably more aggressive through Proscar if it is taken for a long time, as demonstrated in a 2003 study published in the

New England Journal of Medicine (10.1056/ NEJMoa030660). In the study 37% of all patients who took Proscar over 7 years had a Gleason value over 7. In the placebo group however the number was only 22.2% after 7 years.

Professor Julius Hackethal

Prof. Dr. Julius Hackethal has been pursuing an independent way of hormone blockade since 1985, by daily injecting Buserelin (profact) a so-called hormone blocker (GnRh), in high doses (20-40x higher than recommended). Usually Buserelin was given for 6-24 weeks and thereafter for 3-6 months with pauses. I was the first person who investigated more than 30 cases and documented 13 cases before the clinic had to close its doors.

Because Professor Hackethal had a holistic approach it is hard for me to evaluate whether his successes should be ascribed to his type of hormonal blockade or whether they are due to all of the other therapies (detoxification, nutrition, BCG, light, psychological care, etc.). The fact that he was able to demonstrate successes, however cannot be disputed.

Saliva gland cancer

1. The allopathic definition:
Malignant disease of a salivary gland.

2. How frequently does this type of cancer occur (incidence rate) in Germany (USA appr. x 3)?
Current incidence rate: 1 per 100,000.

3. Subdivisions:
1. Depending on the structure of saliva glands in acinus cells, ductal cells, and myoepithelial cells.

2. According to the WHO division there are 18 different saliva gland carcinomas. The most frequently occurring are:

* Adenocarcinoma (emanating from glandular tissue)
  This subgroup is rare (4%) and is usually located in the Glandula Parotis.

* Squamous epithelial carcinoma
  Rare tumor (2%) which primarily affects older men.

* Adenoid cystic carcinoma
  Likewise a rare tumor, which usually occurs in the gum area and affects the glandula submandibularis. A more slowly growing tumor.

* Acinus cell carcinoma
  Slow-growing tumor which occurs more frequently in women and usually affects the parotid gland.

* Non-differentiated carcinoma
Fast-growing tumor, with which distant metastases frequently occur.

* Mucoepidermoid carcinoma
Up to 70% of these tumors develop in small glands of the gum and also occur in young patients.

* Carcinoma in the pleomorphic adenoma
Usually a tumor of the parotid glands. Occurs primarily in patients over 70 years of age.

Stages:

TX: Primary tumor cannot be assessed

T0: No evidence of primary tumor

T1: Tumor 2 cm or less in greatest dimension without extraparenchymal extension

T2: Tumor more than 2 cm but not more than 4 cm in greatest dimension without extraparenchymal extension

T3: Tumor more than 4 cm and/or tumor having extra parenchymal extension

T4a: Tumor invades skin, mandible, ear canal, and/or facial nerve

T4b: Tumor invades skull base and/or pterygoid plates and/or encases carotid artery

4. How is this type of cancer diagnosed by allopathic practitioners?

Palpation, function test of the facial nerve, biopsy – which however does not always permit a precise evaluation. Benign tumors, non-epithelial malignomas and metastases of other primary tumors must be explained differential diagnostically.

What are the allopathic therapy concepts?

Surgery

From the allopathic perspective the operation is the first and the most important therapy. For all operations the major issue is whether it is possible to save nerves such as the facial nerve. In many cases unfortunately this is not possible and leads to greater impact on the quality of life. Frequently the lymph nodes are also removed (e.g. neck dissection).

Statistically viewed operation is by far the most important therapy, as irradiation and chemotherapy do not hold particular promise of success. Nevertheless, the scope of intervention must be considered very carefully as a life without facial nerves represents a significant handicap.

Chemotherapy

Chemotherapies actually do not play a role in the treatment of saliva gland cancer. There have been, and there are still repeated approaches, primarily for recurring tumors, to control these tumors, but as patient you must know that this is nothing more an than act of despair on the part of the oncologist. There is absolutely no evidence that patients will live a single day longer through the use of chemotherapy.

If your doctor maintains the contrary then please have him confirm this in writing.

Irradiation

Irradiation is part of the prevailing therapy although here as well there are no studies that can confirm a significant extension of life. In the studies there are (again) only "tumor control rates" (Borthne 1986), "improvement of recurrence rates" etc., however there is no information about living longer, and there is no information about comparisons with biological therapies. The low value of irradiation therapy is also demonstrated by a study (Buchholz 1992) which shows that there is not even a control rate of 26% for irradiation as sole therapy.

Additional therapies like hormones, antibodies, etc.

Gene therapies
In the media there are always reports about successful gene therapies for cancer. For example: *Researchers at the Vienna University of Veterinary Medicine, and from the University of Rostock have achieved major successes for inoperable saliva gland cancer. They were able to stop tumor growth for 20 weeks and even achieve a significant reduction of tumors, without special side effects. As only approximately 15% of the patients with saliva gland cancer respond to conventional therapies, this could open an application area for gene therapy.*

Reports like this one really must be read between the lines because sentences that sound good like "stop tumor growth for 20 weeks", or "significant reduction of the tumor" say absolutely nothing about the quality of the therapy, and absolutely nothing relative to whether the patients live a single day longer because of the therapy.

However what is interesting in this report is the sentence: "Since only approximately 15 percent of patients with salvia gland cancer respond to conventional therapies". When the objective is to have your own therapies appear in a better light, then you mention that conventional therapies are not nearly as successful as they are always made out to be.

Small cell bronchial carcinoma

1. The allopathic definition:
Bronchial carcinomas involve an epithelial tumor, emanating from the alveoli, bronchia, or the trachea.

2. How frequently does this type of cancer occur (incidence rate) in Germany (USA appr. x 3)?
For men bronchial carcinoma is the most frequently occurring tumor and the incidence rate for men is 75 per 100,000, and for women it is 35 per 100,000. This means app. 45,000 new illnesses every year.

3. Subdivisions:
Histologically three types are distinguished:

* Squamous epithelial carcinoma

* Large cell and small cell carcinoma

* Adenocarcinoma

For small cell bronchial carcinoma, 3 additional groups are differentiated:

* Oat cell (similar to lymphocyte, also called oat cell carcinoma)

* Intermediate cell type

* Combined type with large cell parts or adeno or squamous epithelial parts

Stages:

TX: Primary tumor cannot be assessed, or tumor is proven by the presence of malignant cells in sputum or bronchial washings but is not visualized by imaging or bronchoscopy

T0: No evidence of primary tumor
Tis: Carcinoma in situ

T1: A tumor that is =3 cm in greatest dimension, is surrounded by lung or visceral pleura, and is without bronchoscopic evidence of invasion more proximal than the lobar bronchus (i.e., not in the main bronchus). The uncommon superficial tumor of any size with its invasive component limited to the bronchial wall, which may extend proximal to the main bronchus, is also classified as T1.

T2: A tumor with any of the following features of size or extent: >3 cm in greatest dimension. Involves the main bronchus and is =2 cm distal to the carina. Invades the visceral pleura. Associated with atelectasis or obstructive pneumonitis that extends to the hilar region but does not involve the entire lung

T3: A tumor of any size that directly invades any of the following: chest wall (including superior sulcus tumors), diaphragm, mediastinal pleura, parietal pericardium; or, tumor in the main bronchus <2 cm distal to the carina but without involvement of the carina; or, associated atelectasis or obstructive pneumonitis of the entire lung

T4: A tumor of any size that invades any of the following: mediastinum, heart, great vessels, trachea, esophagus, vertebral body, carina; or, separate tumor nodules in the same lobe; or, tumor with a malignant pleural effusion.

4. How is this type of cancer diagnosed by allopathic practitioners?

Coughing or coughing up blood. Pain in the chest area. Often metastases are also found before the primary tumor is detected. X-ray, CT, lung function diagnostics, like spirometer, blood gas analysis or perfusion scintigraphy. Moreover mediastinoscopies (inspecting the superior mediastinum) and punction are often performed.

What are the allopathic therapy concepts?

Surgery

Is employed in all stages and is often the first option. Here the distinction is made between wedge resection (removal of a small portion of the lung), lobectomy, (removal of a lobe), and pneumectomy (removal of a lung). However lasers, cryosurgery, photodynamic therapy (light in combination with cytostatic agents, are frequently employed.

Here there must be fundamental understanding that removal of a lung lobe is a major intervention, and it is also a dangerous intervention, which at least one in 20 patients, and at most one in 10 patients, do not survive (Goldstraw 1994). Removal of a complete lung is even more dangerous and is even more invasive relative to quality of life. Operations play a major role in lung cancer treatment, because often serious breathing disorders can occur. Also lasers are being used more and more frequently for partial destruction of the tumor and for improved breathing.

Chemotherapy

* Usually epi-adriamycin, vincristin, cisplatin, etoposide and cyclophosphamide are used. Also topotecan and gemcitabine are being used more frequently.

* Small cell bronchial carcinomas are considered to be sensitive to chemotherapy and thus chemotherapy is offered to almost all patients. It is possible that your doctor will say that you will live three times longer with chemotherapy, than you would without chemotherapy, and that he will refer to several studies. He is right, it is correct that in two studies patients lived three times as long as patients in the compare group, who received no treatment (Green 1969 / Wittes 1991 / Malik 1986).

But let's take a closer look at the numbers. In the study published in 1969 by Green the survival time was 16 weeks instead of 6 weeks. Doctors then say that with cyclophosphamide (name of the chemotherapy) one can live almost three times as long. The truth however is that in the best case you will live 10 weeks longer, and you will live with the most serious side effects of chemotherapy like nausea, bleeding bladder inflammations and much more.

Also other studies have only been able to prove that patients have lived a maximum of several weeks longer, at the cost of enormous effects on their quality of life. What is not said is that there are also studies (Brower 1983) in which patients have not lived longer.

* Moreover you must know that many studies look good only because those patients who had to stop the therapy due to "intolerable side effects" are not included in the study.

* High-dose therapies show high response rates (naturally), however this area is still clearly experimental, and I can only warn against these human experiments today.

* For almost 20 years treatment of small cell lung cancer with chemotherapy has been described as significantly important for the survival time of patients. But as of this writing there is no study that compares chemotherapies for lung cancer with

biological therapies. Why oncologists tell their patients over and over again about the great successes of chemotherapy for small cell lung cancer, remains (conditionally) a puzzle for me as there are no studies that justify such a procedure.

What can be explained is really just the sentence: "For small cell bronchial carcinomas we have many more chances than we do for non-small cell bronchial carcinomas." This is due to the fact that there no successful studies at all for non small cell bronchial carcinomas.

Irradiation

The information cited for chemotherapy also applies for irradiation. In this case patients are constantly being told how much their chances of survival would be increased through irradiation.

* A study published in 1998 (Port Meta study) with 2128 patients with non-small cell bronchial carcinoma proved that after two years 7% fewer patients were alive than were alive in the comparison group.

* The present data for small cell bronchial carcinoma exclusively compare irradiation with various chemotherapies, or with combinations. In one study published in 1975, patients with irradiation as sole treatment survived 218 days as compared to 87 days for patients who had chemotherapy as the sole treatment (Laing 1975). Now do not make the mistake of believing that undergoing chemotherapy and irradiation is required in order to achieve longer survival times. Unfortunately this is not possible as multiple studies have shown.

Additional therapies like gene therapy, transfer factors, etc.

Gene therapies
Gene therapies, or cytokine therapies just with Interleukin-2, have not been able to bring forth any proofs that would be worthy of mention, although this is always represented differently in the media.

Transfer factors
See under transfer factors Dr. Pizza/Bologna

General information about lung cancer
Next to our liver, our lungs play the most important role in detoxification. On one hand the lungs are exposed to major "hazards" like nicotine, air pollution, etc., and on the other hand they must exhale waste substances (carbon dioxide) generated by the energy production processes. Considered from a holistic perspective, this is why detoxification measures play a primary role.

Conventional medicine's focus on destruction of the tumor should not obstruct your holistic perspective of the problem. Naturally the unpleasant symptoms of lung cancer require acute medical care and here medicine has also made great progress. Unfortunately all too often I experience, particularly with lung cancer, that everything only revolves around these symptoms and that many patients and physicians forget the importance of detoxification, or of a fundamental holistic approach to treatment.

Soft tissue sarcoma

1. The allopathic definition:
Tumors of the connecting tissue and the musculature.

2. How frequently does this type of cancer occur (incidence rate) in Germany (USA appr. x 3)?
Current incidence rate: 2 per 100,000.

3. Subdivisions:
Sarcomas are first categorized according to the tissue from which they emanate, thus: Fatty tissue, vessels, muscles, or nerve sheaths. The following categories are differentiated:

1. Fibrosarcoma
Connective tissue, which however is only rarely diagnosed. The prognosis for grade 1 is very good because in this stage the tumor does not tend to metastasize. Grade 3 is considered to be a very aggressive tumor.

2. MFH (malignant fibrous histiocytoma)
Is viewed as a primitive mesenchymal and partially fibroblastic (connective tissue cells) tumor. Usually a combination of spindle cells and multinucleated cells. Graduation from 1-3.

3. Aggressive fibromatosis/desmoid (benign connective tissue tumor)
Although this tumor is considered to be benign, it can cause problems after the operation due to its rapid return. Histologically it is differentiated from a fibrosarcoma by uniform maturation with collagen formation and lack of a "mitotic activity" which means that it does not divide so aggressively.

4. Liposarcoma

Tumor from the fatty tissue. Here four groups are differentiated:

4a   Highly differentiated lipoma-like liposarcoma G1

4b   Myxoides (myxo = mucous) liposarcoma G2–G3

4c   Round-cell liposarcoma

4d   Pleomorphic liposarcoma

5. Leiomyosarcoma

There are cutaneous leiomyosarcomas that emanate in erector pili musculature, and deep leiomyosarcomas that emanate from vascular musculature; in part including the vessel walls.

6. Rhabdomyosarcoma

High grade malignant tumor which primarily occurs in childhood years.

7. Vascular tumors

There are three groups in this category:

7a   Malignant haemangiopericytoma
Growth of the perivascular cells, however not the endothelial cells.

7b   Kaposi's sarcoma
Idiopathic haemorrhagic sarcoma = vessel tumor.
Often occurs in conjunction with HIV.

7c   Malignant haemangioendothelioma
Well-differentiated tumor cells.

8. **MPNST**
Malignant peripheral nerve sheath tumors
Previously was also called fibrosarcoma. The cells
are variously differentiated and extend from
fibroblasts to Schwann cells.

9. **Extra skeletal chondrosarcoma**
(chondro = cartilage)
There are two types:

9a   Extra-skeletal myxoid chondrosarcoma

9b   Mesenchymal chondrosarcoma

10. **Malignant tumors without clear differentiation**
The following tumors are assigned to this subgroup:
Alveolar Soft-tissue sarcoma, epitheloid sarcoma,
clear cell sarcoma, extra-skeletal Ewing's sarcoma,
malignant extra-renal rhabdoid tumors or the synovial
sarcoma.

4. How is this type of cancer diagnosed by allopathic practitioners?
Tumor formation, pain, x-ray, CT, MRT etc. For differential
diagnosis however a biopsy is always required.

What are the allopathic therapy concepts?

Surgery
Many surgeons say when operating on a sarcoma, the surgeon
should never see the tumor. In other words this means the
operation should extend quite far into healthy tissue, since
sarcomas cannot be precisely delimited from healthy tissue.

I do not confirm to this opinion, because it is based on the approach: "Let's cut out the tumor and that will do." We can see where this approach has brought modern oncology, by observing how "generously" (5 cm in healthy tissue) operations are performed for sarcomas, and particularly with young people. Here legs or arms are amputated, and eyes are removed – always with the hope that this will stop the growth. But how many sarcomas do not return after such operations? My experience does not show that radical operations are any more promising of success than are normal tumor removals. If your surgeon should have a different opinion then please ask him in detail which studies he is basing his statements on, and ask him to show you these studies in writing (see also chapter: When do I have cancer, according to the Foundation for Bone Tumor - Reference Center).

Chemotherapy

As of this printing there is not a single clear proof for a significant advantage relative to survival time. Nevertheless chemotherapies are still considered to be the primary allopathic concept for sarcomas. Usually doxorubicin, cyclophosphamide, methotrexate, ifosfamide, but also vincristin, etoposide or ifosfamide are used.

Because chemotherapies for sarcomas do not supply appropriate response rates (or only supply them in high doses), this is a fertile area for studies not only in Germany. Thus the chance that that you will be requested/asked/forced to participate in such a study is relatively high. If your doctor tells you however that there are no other therapies, then make sure you ask him whether he means that there are no other allopathic therapies, or whether he does not know of any others.

Due to this failure of all chemotherapy combinations, universities also more and more involved in studies of chemotherapies in combination with hypothermia.

Irradiation

Although even with this form of therapy, no hard facts exist at this time that irradiation can contribute to people living significantly longer, this therapy still is part of the standard program for many oncologists. This is even more amazing because there are many studies, which show that there is absolutely no advantage that can be expected from additional irradiation (e.g. Suit et. al. 1985).

Since usually a large volume capture of the tumor area is attempted for sarcomas, many patients also get a very high quantity of radiation. Isn't it precisely this quantity of radiation that permits a new tumor to occur?

Additional therapies like hormones, antibodies, etc.

In the initial stages of the therapy, sarcomas are strictly in the provenance of the surgeon. Although this perspective does not work, as is demonstrated simply by the high relapse quotas, there is still no rethinking of sarcoma treatment, and other approaches like monoclonal antibodies or cytokine therapies play virtually no role in allopathic treatment of sarcomas.

Fever therapies

My previous researches show that fever therapies (see also Coley's toxin) bring good results with sarcomas, and it is imperative that they be included in the therapy consideration. To my knowledge, the use of fever-generated bacteria and/or hyperthermia (exogen-generated fever) in particular is a successful alternative.

Stomach cancer

1. The allopathic definition:
Epithelial tumors of the stomach mucous membrane.

2. How frequently does this type of cancer occur (incidence rate) in Germany (USA appr. x 3)?
Currently app. 19,000 new illnesses per year.

3. Subdivisions:
Primarily the distinction is made between early carcinoma, which only affects the mucous membrane, and advanced carcinoma, which also infiltrates the muscle layers.

In addition the so-called Laurén classification is used, which has special significance for the dimensions of an operation. The Laurén classification differentiates:

Interstinal type
The cancer grows like a mushroom (polyp) into the stomach lumen is well-delimited.

Diffuse type
The cancer grows in the stomach wall and is poorly delimited.

Mixed type
The cancer grows both in the direction of the stomach lumen, as well as sideways into the stomach wall.

Histologically there is the following division according to the international WHO scheme.

* Papillary adenocarcinoma

* Tubular adenocarcinoma
* Mucinous adenocarcinoma

* Signet ring cell carcinoma

* Adeno-squamous carcinoma

* Small cell carcinoma

* Non-differentiated carcinoma

Stages:

TX: Primary tumor cannot be assessed

T0: No evidence of primary tumor

Tis: Carcinoma in situ: intraepithelial tumor without invasion of the lamina propria

T1: Tumor invades lamina propria or submucosa

T2: Tumor invades the muscularis propria or the subserosa

T2a: Tumor invades muscularis propria

T2b: Tumor invades subserosa

T3: Tumor penetrates the serosa (visceral peritoneum) without invading adjacent structures

T4: Tumor invades adjacent structures

4. How is this type of cancer diagnosed by allopathic practitioners?
A bacteria, the helicobacter pylori, that nests in the mucous membrane of the stomach, and causes inflammation of the stomach lining (gastritis), is considered to be responsible for

more than 90% of early stomach carcinomas in Germany. The risk of getting a stomach lymphoma is increased with a helicobacter pylori infection by a factor of 6. In my opinion here the cause and effect are reversed. Most of the people in whom Helicobacter pylori can be demonstrated, namely do not develop a carcinoma.

Naturally, in addition there are many non-specific symptoms like: Pressure and the feeling of being full, nausea and vomiting, loss of appetite, weight loss, and eructation, swallowing disorders, bloody stool, etc.

If the tumor in the stomach is bleeding, then this blood in the stool can be verified with a test (e.g. haemoccult test), anemia, tumor markers CA 72-4 and possibly CA 19-9 and CEA.

However a carcinoma can only be verified with certainty through a biopsy, or through microscopic examination. In addition endosonography, gastroscopy, x-ray examination with contrast agent, CT and explorative laparotomy play a role in better understanding the location of the tumor.

What are the allopathic therapy concepts?

Surgery
An operation is the first option. A subtotal gastrectomy means that, tumor, neighboring tissue, and nearby lymph nodes, are removed. However for the most part the stomach remains intact.

With total gastrectomy the stomach, parts of the esophagus, the small intestine, and the adjacent tissue/lymph nodes are removed. Possibly the spleen is also removed.
Fundamentally a total gastrectomy has a major impact on quality of life and must be well considered. Even if new operation techniques, such as creating a new stomach using the small intestine, or by interponation of a piece of the intestine, do represent improvements over the existing condition, nei-

ther of these measures are a real replacement. Particularly reflux of food into the esophagus is a major complication and should be prevented through these measures.

Surgical measures should have complete removal of the tumor in healthy tissue (R 0 resection) as their goal. Sufficient safety clearance in this case depends on the type of growth and is 5 cm for intestinal type 5, and 8 cm for diffuse type 8.

Photodynamic therapy
With photodynamic therapy a dye is administered to the patient, which reaches the tumor cells in the stomach via the blood. The particularity of this dye is its reaction to light at certain wavelengths, which transforms it into a cell killing substance. If a surface stomach cancer is exposed to laser light at the required wave length several days after administering the dye, then a substance is formed from the dye, which kills the tumor cells at the illuminated tumor region. The light at a certain wavelength, which is required for this chemical reaction is conducted to the right location by an endoscope.

Chemotherapy
Chemo preparations like 5-FU, doxorubicin, 4-epidoxoru-bicin, etoposide, mitomycin, irinotecan, taxotere and even cis-platin are used for stomach carcinomas. Here, even at the outset, the lowest common denominator is: There is absolutely no proof that you will live significantly longer through a chemotherapy.

Thus Dr. Dent compared patients who received therapy with 5-FU and irradiation, with groups that received a therapy with thiotepa, and with a placebo comparison group. There were no differences in survival time. Dr. Kingston published a much more extensive study one year later. In the Kingston study the first group received 5-FU plus MeCCNU and the second group was given a placebo. Interestingly enough the results in this case were almost the same. The placebo group even did a little better, i.e. those in the control group lived longer! If your doctor suggests a chemotherapy for you, then speak with him in detail and make sure that you ask him to confirm his statements in writing.

Even the results of the highly praised studies involving FAMTX, FAM, ELF and ECF must be considered very critically. In these studies (again) various chemotherapy combinations were compared, and then the combination with which the patients survived the longest was highly praised, in this case FAMTX. However particularly with FAMTX (5-FU, adriamycin, methotrexate) there are very significant side effects. In addition there is no proof that the patients really live longer. Moreover the use of preoperative chemotherapies, usually with cisplatin, have not been able to show, to this day, that patients live significantly longer because of these therapies.

Irradiation
Irradiation is often recommended to patients in the case of inoperable tumors and after operations in which the tumor could not be completely removed. The main arguments against irradiation however are that patients are robbed of any chance of healing, indeed in most cases they are robbed of even a chance at improvement, and for patients who cannot be helped the side effects are so significant that they are not offset by the advantage of a possible chance for a reduction of the tumor. However what is most important for the patient is the fact that he will not live a single day longer through irradiation of the stomach.

Additional therapies like hormones, antibodies, etc.
Immune therapies with antibodies or cytokines are not used for stomach cancer.

Testicular cancer

1. The allopathic definition:
Germ cell tumors of the testes.

2. How frequently does this type of cancer occur (incidence rate) in Germany (USA appr. x 3)?
Current incidence rate: 4-8 per 100,000 men, usually between 20-40 years of age.

3. Subdivisions:
Histologically there are four different types of testicular cancer:

* Malignant germ cell tumors

* Stromal tumors (e.g. Sertoli or Leydig cell tumors)

* Tumors of the epidydimus, the seminferous tubuals of the testes (rete testis), spermatic duct (ductus deferens) of the testicular capsules and the blister-shaped adnexa

* malignant lymphomas and metastases

In addition there is a division in:

* Seminomas (tumors emanating from the germinal tissue)

* Non-seminoma

* Teratoma (mixed tumor of the three germ layers)

Stages:

pTX: Primary tumor cannot be assessed

pT0: No evidence of primary tumor (e.g., histologic scar in testis)

pTis: Intratubular germ cell neoplasia (carcinoma in situ)

pT1: Tumor limited to the testis and epididymis without lymphatic/vascular invasion; tumor may invade into the tunica albuginea but not the tunica vaginalis

pT2: Tumor limited to the testis and epididymis with vascular/lymphatic invasion, or tumor extending through the tunica albuginea with involvement of the tunica vaginalis

pT3: Tumor invades the spermatic cord with or without vascular/lymphatic invasion

pT4: Tumor invades the scrotum with or without vascular/lymphatic invasion

4. How is this type of cancer diagnosed by allopathic practitioners?
Palpation, impotency problems, swelling of the testes, enlargement of the breast (gynaecomastia), blood tests like AFP, HCG, LDH, H-PLAP, etc., ultrasound, chest x-ray, CT, urography, lymphography.

What are the allopathic therapy concepts?

Surgery

The removal of the affected testes is the absolute first therapy, and is undertaken from the curative perspective (healing is the aim).

Chemotherapy and radiation

Seminomas:

Carboplatin is preferred as monotherapy for seminomas in stage 1. But the studies (Dieckmann 1993, Oliver 1990) are no better than those studies with irradiation as sole treatment, so that usually irradiation of the lymph nodes (BWK 11 to LWK 4) is with app. 26 Gy is preferred. What is interesting in this regard is the fact that the survival rate with a "wait and see strategy" (i.e. no therapy at all) is just as high as it is with radiation therapy (Ramakrishan 1992, Thomas and Williams 1992). And in this case the probability of relapse is app 20%.

I will say this again because it is so important: Whether you undergo radiation therapy, or do not undergo radiation therapy, has no influence on survival time. The question could be asked, "But then why are patients even offered irradiation?" This question cannot be answered with reference to testicular cancer, rather here you must consider the total issue confronting oncology, if you want to make some headway with this issue.

In stage 2a and 2b lymph nodes are usually irradiated with app. 35 Gy, and from stage 2c primary chemotherapy is the first choice. Here the PEB plan (Platinum-Etoposide-Bleomycin) or alternatively PEI (I=ifosfamide) are most frequently used. Here it is interesting to note that mono chemotherapies, e.g. with carboplatin, were able to achieve similar results (Horwich), and here as well the question arises; why do patients have to suffer the much greater side effects, and why do all of us have to bear the much greater costs?"

Non-seminoma, teratoma, and Leydig cell tumors
In these cases as well the use of irradiation in stage 1 can be questioned, as survival times are not improved by this therapy (for example Roth 1987). Starting in stage 2a, operating on the lymph nodes plus chemotherapy is considered to be the standard. Studies made by the Testicular Cancer Interstudy Group however have shown that if the chemotherapy was not administered, 51% had no relapse within 5 years. In other words, more than half the patients get chemotherapy for no absolutely no reason whatsoever. Chemotherapy is the absolute standard from stage 2c, and for teratomas.

Leydig cell tumors and also Sertoli cell tumors do not respond as well to chemotherapies. Here an operation and the removal of lymph nodes is prescribed. Irradiation plays almost no role at all here.

Additional therapies like hormones, antibodies, etc.

Antibody therapies or hormonal therapies are not used for testicular cancer. There is something more that must be noted here. The best statistics in all chemotherapy studies are those for testicular cancer. What I have noticed however is that the studies again only compare the more recent chemotherapy protocols with those of 30-40 years ago, and again we do not know whether additional, less-toxic, therapies are available. There is no doubt that this data sounds good initially, but it should not be forgotten great healings have been shown for testicular cancer, primarily in the initial stages with "just an operation". Naturally questions about the danger of this type of cancer come up immediately. Please do not misunderstand. I do not want to trivialize testicular cancer in any way. But basically, if we can believe the statistics, then there is no other type of cancer which can be handled as well in the operating room.

Moreover due to the legal aspects, there is no holistic physician who would trust himself to treat testicular cancer. This is why there are no comparative data, which could provide me with any more elucidation about the real success of chemotherapy. In the meantime I know several people who have healed testicular cancer without chemotherapy. This reinforces my belief that testicular cancer can be treated alternatively, even if current data speak quite positively for chemotherapy.

Thyroid gland carcinoma

1. The allopathic definition:
Thyroid gland carcinoma is a disease of thyroid gland epithelial tissue.

2. How frequently does this type of cancer occur (incidence rate) in Germany (USA appr. x 3)?
Currently app. 2,400 new illnesses per year.

3. Subdivisions:
Here tumors are differentiated which emanate from the follicular cells (anaplastic, papillary, and follicular) and from the parafollicular (para=adjacent) cells (medullar) (follicles are small blisters/vesicles, that are clad with epithelial tissue). Thyroid gland hormones are formed in these follicles. Between the follicles there are C-ells, which form the hormone, calcitonin.

App. 65% of all tumors are papillary tumors. For patients under 40 this number increase to app. 90%. Follicular carcinomas usually occur in people who are over 50.

Details about the individual types

Anaplastic tumors
These tumors are considered to be very aggressive from the allopathic perspective, as they often grow over different organs. Under the microscope they appear as large spindle-shaped cells. In addition, there are many dead cells and there is rapid cell division.

Here the patient must free himself from the self-fulfilling prophecies of many physicians. Naturally it is true that this type of thyroid cancer grows very quickly. However I consider it to be a catastrophic error for the patient to prematurely speak of short life times (see the chapter on care). The poor prognosis results namely (also) from the fact that allopathic practitioners unfortunately still apply chemotherapies and irradiation exclusively for fast growing epithelial tumors. Today this form of therapy has not been proven to be successful, nevertheless it is suggested as the only therapy in most cases. For this reason I view psychological care or intensive mental therapy as absolutely necessary for anaplastic carcinomas.

Please take this point very seriously. If you believe the words and the official statistics then you will suppress your immune system in ways that are perhaps decisive for therapy.

Medullar (C-cell) carcinoma
These tumors spread out in a nest shape and store amyloid (protein sugar complex). They are supposed to be strewn over the lymph system and usually a clear enlargement of the C-cells can be demonstrated.

Follicular carcinoma:
These tumors tend to encapsulate themselves. They are also supposed to spread themselves over the lymphatic system and in the blood as well.

Papillary carcinomas
These carcinomas can grow encapsulated, invasive, or non-encapsulated. Under the microscope there are large nuclei in the cell. They as supposed to spread over the lymph system, however distant metastases are rarer.

Stages:

TX: Primary tumor cannot be assessed

T0: No evidence of primary tumor

T1: Tumor =2 cm in greatest dimension, limited to the thyroid

T2: Tumor >2 cm but =4 cm in greatest dimension, limited to the thyroid

T3: Tumor >4 cm in greatest dimension limited to the thyroid or any tumor with minimal extrathyroid extension (e.g., extension to sternothyroid muscle or perithyroid soft tissues)

T4a: Tumor of any size extending beyond the thyroid capsule to invade subcutaneous soft tissues, larynx, trachea, esophagus, or recurrent laryngeal nerve

T4b: Tumor invades prevertebral fascia or encases carotid artery or mediastinal vessels

4. How is this type of cancer diagnosed by allopathic practitioners?
Enlargement of the thyroid gland (over-excitability and under-excitability, pressure feeling, pain, cold thyroid nodules, ultrasound, biopsy (sometimes very difficult), calcitonin determination, scintigraphy, x-ray.

What are the allopathic therapy concepts?

Surgery
With the exception of anaplastic or non-differentiated carcinoma, operation is clearly the first priority and represents a

curative therapy. In this process the thyroid as well lymph nodes are removed (thyroidectomy). This intervention also applies for anaplastic carcinomas that are limited to the thyroid gland. From the allopathic perspective naturally a subsequent radioiodine therapy can only be considered promising if the thyroid is completely removed.

Small papillary carcinomas (<1 cm) represent an exception. In these cases a portion of the thyroid gland is usually removed, since with these tumors there is no radio iodine therapy after the operation.

Since thyroid gland hormones (T3= L-triiodo-thyronin and T4+ L-thyroxin) can no longer be formed after an operation, these must be substituted daily. Also iodine plays a major role here as iodine is a major component of T3 and T4.

Chemotherapy
Basically there is no data for all thyroid gland carcinomas that prove extension of life. Even allopathic practitioners exclude chemotherapies for all differentiated carcinomas. Doxorubicin is used solely for anaplastic carcinomas. The data however are also negative in this case and most physicians understand the use of chemotherapies to be only palliative (alleviating).

I cannot agree with this procedure, since the use of doxorubicin robs the patient of the chance of holistic therapy, and thus the next steps are prescribed. Nor do I accept the argument of "strengthening the sensitivity of the irradiation", since the success of irradiation does not depend on administration of additional toxins, as many studies prove.

Because the current approach of combined chemotherapy and irradiation therapy results in an extremely low survival rate, naturally the question arises as to why doctors are still suggesting this approach. To say nothing about the quality of life for the person who pursues this therapy.

Another point is also "forgotten" with this allopathic therapy recommendation. After therapy with chemotherapy and irradiation, which as we know fails in almost 100% of the cases, there is no longer a possibility of returning to a holistic therapy, because the damages caused by this therapy combination cannot be restored by any holistic therapy. In practical terms this means that the patient must decide for one direction or the other. The option of "let's test this first, and if it fails then we will pursue a different path", is not possible for anaplastic carcinomas.

Irradiation
For thyroid gland cancer there are two types of irradiation:

1. The radio iodine therapy, in which iodine is radioactively enriched.

2. External irradiation.

Radio iodine therapy
With the exception of C-cell carcinoma and the anaplastic carcinoma, carcinoma tissue of the thyroid gland stores iodine. If one now enriches iodine with radioactive material, then this material supposed to destroy the remaining cancer cells. Naturally this theory presupposes that the metastases theory is correct, otherwise there is no way to explain this therapy. Usually it is recommended 4-6 weeks after the operation. Often annual repetitions are also recommended.

Patients are told again and again that there is no damage to other cells, since the iodine is absorbed only by the metastases. But what happens if these are not even present? Why are there so many cases involving the most serious bone marrow damage? Why do so many patients die if the theory cited above is correct? Doubtless it is possible to more precisely destroy cancer cells through the storage of iodine in thyroid gland cells, in this case than is the case in other organs. Nevertheless one must reexamine radio iodine therapy, which is considered as the highest standard, particularly when no metastases can be verified, because such a therapy represents a major stress for our organism – and this stress occurs at a time when we really need all of our immune capability. Also you should not forget that for this therapy means that you must be in a sealed room which you cannot leave for app. 2 weeks. All of your feces must be considered as radioactive waste and no one may be near you. Do you also find it paradoxical that on one hand we can read that this therapy is not hazardous for other organs in the body, and on the other hand, such extensive precautionary measures are required?

External irradiation:
External irradiation plays more of a subordinate role, as usually the radio iodine therapy is used. However for carcinomas where this is not possible, external irradiation is often used, in order to at least reduce the tumors in theory. I say in theory, because it is also possible that tumors can grow very rapidly under the irradiation, or shortly thereafter. Although hard facts are missing to confirm that external irradiation can contribute to longer life, particularly for medullar carcinomas, it is still being recommended for this type of tumor.

Additional therapies like hormones, antibodies, etc.

Hormonal therapies
Usually L-thyroxin is substituted for the rest of the patient's life, in order to block TSH (thyroidea stimulating hormone), which is considered to be a growth factor for thyroid gland cells. Otherwise to this date there are no successful therapies like antibodies etc.

Urinary bladder carcinomas

1. The allopathic definition:
Malignant tumors of the urogenital system.

2. How frequently does this type of cancer occur (incidence rate) in Germany (USA appr. x 3)?
Current incidence rate: 20 per 100,000. Here age plays a significant role, as the incidence rate for people under 20 years of age is only 0.2 per 100,000, and for people over 80 years of age, the incidence rate is 200 per100,000. Also the influence of aniline dyes is described over and over again. But chemotherapies like cyclophosphamide are also mentioned as the cause of bladder cancer.

3. Subdivisions:
The primary distinction here is between epithelial tumors and non-epithelial tumors:

Epithelial tumors:

Benign:
Transitional cell papilloma (special form diffuse papillomatosis), inverted transitional cell-papilloma, squamous epithelial papilloma.

Malignant:
Urothelial carcinoma (localized with squamous epithelial and/or glandular metaplasia) squamous epithelial carcinoma, adenocarcinoma, undifferentiated carcinoma.

Non-epithelial tumors:

Benign:
Leiomyoma, neurofibroma, haemangioma, granular cell tumor.

Malignant:
Rhabdomyosarkoma, leiomyosarcoma, fibrosarcoma, osteosarcoma.

Other tumors:
Phaechromocytoma, lymphoma, carcinosarcoma, malignant melanoma

4. How is this type of cancer diagnosed by allopathic practitioners?

Palpation of the renal bed and the lower stomach, urine analysis and urine culture: Primarily blood in the urine, serum creatinine, ultrasound, urethrocytoscopy, biopsy, usually a transurethral electro-resection (TUR) is performed for the parts removed from the tumor base and from the tumor edges. The resection of the tumor base should also include the bladder musculature.

Staging: MRT (magnetic resonance tomography), CT, X-ray overview of the thorax, clarification of liver metastases with ultrasound, liver values like alkaline phosphatasis, LDH etc., bone scan scintigraphy.

What are the allopathic therapy concepts?

Surgery

TUR
Since frequently urinary bladder carcinomas are still locally limited when detected, they can frequently be completely removed by a relatively simple intervention, the transurethral

electro-resection (TUR). This measure alone results in a good 5-year survival period for non-invasive tumors. However this statistic also shows how non-aggressive urinary bladder carcinomas are, and how slowly they grow.

Radical cystectomy
For men, intervention includes removal of the urinary bladder, prostate, and seminal vesicles. In this process the erectile capability is sought to be maintained, however this does "not always occur". It is possible that lymph nodes in the pelvic area (pelvine lymphadenectomy) are also removed.

For women, the intervention includes removal of the urinary bladder, uterus, and two thirds of the urethra with adjacent section of the front vaginal wall.

Since patients with T4 tumors only have a 5-year survival rate of 0-6% after radical cystectomy, this operation can only be viewed as palliative (alleviating).

Attention: After a radical cystectomy, usually out-of-action large or small intestine segments are used in conjunction with "collection systems" outside of the body for urine discharge. Naturally this has a significant effect quality of life and should be considered most carefully.

Chemotherapy
Because the bladder is a hollow organ, the possibility exists for local and systemic applications of cell toxins. Primarily doxorubicin, mitomycin C, adriamycin, 5-FU, methotrexate, vinblastin, carboplatin and cisplatin are used. There are multiple studies, which have attempted to determine whether using one, or multiple chemotherapies concurrently, would result in better success. In general it can be said that there are indeed results, which demonstrate that longer remission rates are achieved through a combination of dichloromethotrexate with cisplatin for example, but the consequent influence on sur-

vival time is insignificant. Moreover the additional days (not years!) were purchased with extensively greater side effects.

In an Australian study, cisplatin was compared to cisplatin with methotrexate, in this case there were not even any advantages relative to survival time. Also a study in which cisplatin was compared with CISCA chemotherapy, resulted in no significant differences in remission rates, remission interval, or survival time. I found more than 150 studies with chemotherapies for bladder cancer just on the Internet alone. However it is forgotten that in this case as well there are only studies which compare one toxin with one, or with several other toxins. Logically one toxin will always come out looking better than another. What is apparent here however is that not a single active agent really contributed to people living any longer.

Any doctor who maintains that patients with urinary bladder carcinoma live significantly longer through chemotherapy should prove this to his patients in writing.

Irradiation

1. Prior to an operation:
Even among allopathic practitioners preoperative irradiation, particularly prior to cystectomy is quite controversial, because studies clearly confirm that nobody lives any longer due to this therapy. The only verifiable advantage would be if the tumor became smaller through irradiation, thus enabling performance of an organ-saving operation.

After an operation:
Here the primary factor is whether the lymph nodes are also affected or not. Accordingly, either "just" the bladder, or the entire pelvis is irradiated. Particularly with the latter technique, naturally almost all of your blood is also irradiated. It is interesting to note that according to the statistics success depends more on the operation, than it does on the irradiation, because the successes of irradiation can be measured by the

success of the operation. This means the more radical the operation, the better the survival chances.

Instead of an operation:
Based on the statistics that indicate primarily that those patients who had radical operations live longer, patients are only irradiated instead of undergoing an operation, if the operation is too dangerous (due to age, general condition, etc.).

Additional therapies like hormones, antibodies, etc.
Hormonal therapies and cytokine therapies with Interferon or Interleukin do not play a significant role for urinary bladder cancer. However the following therapies are used:

Laser therapy of the surface urinary bladder carcinoma
This therapy destroys the surface tumor or slightly infiltrating tumors with an Nd-YAG laser.

Photodynamic therapy of the surface urinary bladder carcinoma
In this process photosensitizer (e.g. photofrin) is injected intravenously. The main side-effect however is often a contracted bladder. Consequently many physicians have gone over to the active agent 5-aminolevulinc acid. Irradiation is usually administered 4-6 hours after the injection. A dye laser, which is positioned centrally in the bladder, is often used as the light source.

Ukrain
See under Ukrain.

Uterine cancer
(uterine carcinoma)

1. The allopathic definition:
A group of tumors whose mesenchymal tissue is malignant, either exclusively or in combination with epithelial cells of the uterus.

2. How frequently does this type of cancer occur (incidence rate) in Germany (USA appr. x 3)?
Currently app. 11,000 women annually.

3. Subdivisions:
Here the main distinction is based on the tissue types, thus carcinosarcomas, leiomyosarcomas, endometrial stromal sarcomas (sarcoma = tumor emanating from mesenchymal tissue.

Stages:

Stage I
Cancer is found only in the main part of the uterus (it is not found in the cervix).

Stage II
Cancer cells have spread to the cervix.

Stage III
Cancer cells have spread outside the uterus but have not spread outside the pelvis.

Stage IV
Cancer cells have spread beyond the pelvis, to other body parts, or into the lining of the bladder (the sac that holds urine) or rectum.

4. How is this type of cancer diagnosed by allopathic practitioners?

Unusual bleeding, abdominal pains, enlarged uterus, ultrasound, CT, magnetic resonance tomography, hysteroscopy (endoscopy of the uterus, curetting, (tissue engineering).

What are the allopathic therapy concepts?

Surgery

Is employed in all stages and is certainly the first option. Usually a total operation is performed. In this process the uterus, as well as the lymph nodes in the pelvis, are removed. Usually the entire cervix, both fallopian tubes, both ovaries, the pelvic lymph nodes and parts of the abdominal viscera (tissue covering within the stomach area) are removed (Wertheim-Meigs-operation). Cleaning out the lymph nodes is even disputed among allopathic practitioners, as there are no studies proving that patients live any longer through this measure (Hannigan et. al.; 1992, as well as Leibsohn). Considering that the side effects however are clearly greater, this option should be discussed with the surgeon in any event.

For patients in stage 1 who desire children, a uterus-saving operation can be considered, since the radical operation offers no advantage relative to illness-free survival, as Connors and Norris showed in their 1990 study. For endometrial stromal sarcoma the opinion is clearly that a total operation will be performed, because these tumors show a great estrogen receptor expression and Berchuk published in a 1990 study, that patients without removal of the fallopian tubes had a 100% relapse (with removal the number was only 43%).

Chemotherapy

All chemotherapy approaches for uterine cancer have failed in the past and must be ranked as experiments on humans. In spite of this I hear again and again that patients are being treated with cyclophosphamide, vincristin, ifosfamide, etoposide, mitoxantrone, piperazinedion, doxorubicin and dacarbazin. For carcinosarcomas many physicians even suggest chemotherapies with cisplatin, in spite of the enormous side effects.

Every patient and every physician should ask themselves the following question: "Would no chemotherapy at all be better than another attempt with one of those preparations, which as of this writing, only brought suffering and pain to patients? Instead of accepting the fact that chemotherapies are the wrong approach for uterine cancer, experts generously exploit this experimental field. There is really no other way to explain why so many women get so many useless chemotherapies. In any other field people would ask: "Why should I undergo a therapy, which in the first place cannot extend my life, and in the second place is so painful?" However where chemotherapies are involved, apparently we must just realize that it is totally proper to act without thinking.

Another point is that with cisplatin, you are possibly taking a chance with healing, as you damage your bone marrow so strongly, that you do not recover from the damage, or you die because of the therapy. This point is happily forgotten although countless people die through chemotherapy each year.

Irradiation

Everything that I have written about chemotherapies also applies for irradiation of uterine cancer. Particularly, irradiation is still considered to be the therapy for inoperable uterine cancer. However today no one has succeeded in proving that this therapy contributes to a significantly longer life for patients. The outdated concept is still assumed, that people live longer if tumors are smaller, e.g. through irradiation, although we have known for a long time that this is not the case.

Although there are no hard facts to this day to confirm that irradiation contributes to women living significantly longer, nevertheless it is again and again suggested to women, even from the perspective of its "palliative (alleviating) character". I cannot agree with the opinion of palliative irradiation, and considering the side effects, every patient and every doctor must precisely consider whether a patient should be irradiated in their final days of life.

For more about irradiation see Cervical cancer.

Additional therapies like hormones, antibodies, etc.

Since in recent years operation has established itself as the standard therapy, other therapies like hormonal therapies or cytokine therapies do not play a role. See Cervical cancer for more information relative to hormonal therapies.

Cancer treatments for children

I have two children, and with the exception of my wife, there is nobody in the world who I come even close to loving as much as I love my children. This is why I can at least imagine what it means when children are sick or close to death. Unfortunately for children who are ill with cancer there are several factors that come together at the same time, which make treatment more difficult. I would like to briefly discuss these factors before sharing my opinions on the specific types of cancer.

1. First, the courts. When children are involved, the German judicial system is not the only judicial system that is very strict in the interest of children. But who actually determines what is in the interest of a child? In the case of sick children these are medical associations, and government agencies who are responsible for children's welfare, and behind these organizations there are pharmaceutical companies that tell us parents what is good for our children. Usually we do not want to accept the fact that it is very important for these companies to satisfy their shareholders, because what which cannot be true, should not be true.

If this means that children will be taken away from their parents, then that is what will happen, even if we all know that it is certainly not in the interest of a child. But such a procedure is not the only "false interest" that can occur when your child is sick.

2. When the lives of children are at stake, all the energies in our brain are suddenly on the right creative side, and only a small amount of energy remains in our rational, left brain hemisphere. This is "normal" considering our great love for children. But is it also necessary? My experience here clearly says no. When our child is sick, we should keep a cool, clear head so that we can make vital decisions. Unfortunately this is easier said than done when children are sick, and so we (parents) make too many decisions based on emotions.

3. I have been privileged to experience the positive, even life-saving influence, that parents can have on their children, on many occasions. Unfortunately most people today do not understand anything about the positive energy that they can transmit, and believe that if they love their child adequately, this should suffice. Here however my experience speaks a different language. Even if you understand what I am saying, I still request that if you would like to help your child with your energy, then ensure that you create the mental program described in this book for your child and for yourself, or follow the 3E program in general. I know that you do not have cancer, I know that your child does. Please trust me and help your child by ensuring that your further development as well is healthy.

What have you got to lose? The worst that can happen is that you will eat healthier, and thus begin each day to visualize that your child is healthy again. You do not know me, and I understand that it would be hard to trust my statement that such a procedure can help your child. I understand this challenge, however I would like to repeat: What have you got to lose, other than time?

4. We are happy to believe the words of doctors and studies when they are "good". This is certainly the case for illnesses like leukemia, as here there are studies showing that children have lived long either because of, or in spite of, allopathic measures. However this does not mean that you can rely on these studies. In medicine there is hardly a field that is more "unscientific" than oncology, as you will understand after reading this book.

5. From a holistic perspective cancer for children is an acute to chronic toxification or stress situation of a still-young body. Should you now believe that it is just not possible for such young people, then unfortunately I must disappoint you. There are children who enter this world in a toxic condition through their mother's toxins, and consequently detoxification measures and nutrition therapies play a major role. And something else: I am 100% certain that a seriously ill child cannot permit himself to eat the poor food offered in a hospital on a daily basis.

6. Many parents do not want to understand or they cannot understand that the food served in a hospital could have anything to do with the illness of their child. I can readily understand this attitude. But will it help your child?

Please do not misunderstand me. Guilt or innocence is not the issue here, the issue is how you can help your child. I would like to cite an example. A seven-year old child had leukemia and the parents took their child to a holistic physician in Holland because they were afraid of losing their child through chemotherapy. The therapist spoke "only" with the parents and he found out that the father of the child was a pilot and that the mother was an on-call stewardess. This meant that the mother would be called-in to work 1-3 times a week on short notice and the son would be hurried over to the grandmother who lived nearby. As "first therapy measure" the therapist asked the mother to immediately stop this "frequent leaving of her son" and to tell him this on the same day. Within a week the leucocytes declined by approximately 50%, and within 3 weeks they were almost within normal range. Thereafter the son suffered no relapse and remained healthy.

From an allopathic perspective such cases are viewed as spontaneous remissions, but only because allopathy does not grasp (for a wide variety of reasons), that we not only have a body, but we also have a psyche. I share this story with you for one reason only: It is bad enough for doctors to make this mistake – in the interest of your child YOU should not make this mistake!

On the following pages I describe a few of the important types of cancer for children. I do not deal with this subject in extensive detail in this book. This is not due to lack of interest, on the contrary I am extremely interested in this field, but I know that in this area the pharmaceutical lobby is so powerful that you can really get your fingers burned, without bringing about any changes.

I can only recommend that parents form their own view of the (apparent) progress made in the field of children's oncology, and in the process that they remain critical relative to all statements whether alternative or allopathic. Make sure that you have the courage to ask critical questions, and to insist on answers, in your child's interest.

If I may give you a tip along the way, it is this: children have incredible powers of visualization. Harness these powers and use what you learn in this book with your children.

Info: The word tumor is used frequently in this book. Naturally a tumor is something different than a leukemia. However from a holistic perspective it represents every bit as much of an energy disorder. Consequently I have not written tumor/malignant cells each time like with leukemia or lymph cancer, but rather I have just used the word tumor.

Acute lymphatic leukemia (ALL)
For children

The allopathic definition:
Malignant degeneration and dysmaturity of white blood cells.
Here the body produces immature white blood corpuscles
(lymphocytes), the so-called blasts.

**2. How frequently does this type of cancer occur (incidence
rate) in Germany (USA appr. x 3)?**
Currently app. 600 illnesses annually.

3. Subdivisions:
L-1, l-2, and l-3 blasts are differentiated morphologically. L-1
blasts are small and have a homogenous nucleus.
Approximately 20% of all blasts have a large nucleus with
indentations, and in general they are heterogeneous (different
types). L-3 blasts are all large and homogenous (same type).

Stages:
As opposed to solid tumors, there is no stage division for
acute lymphatic leukemia. The type of treatment depends on
the age of the patient, the patient's hemogram, and whether
the patient is undergoing the first, second, or third therapy.
The following groups are differentiated:

Untreated children
Untreated acute lymphatic leukemia (ALL) means that to this
point no treatment, other than treatment of accompanying
symptoms has been offered. There are too many white blood
cells in the blood and in the bone marrow. Moreover other
signs and symptoms of a leukemia can be present.

Remission
Remission means that a treatment has taken place and that the number of white blood cells and the other blood cells in the blood and in the bone marrow is normal. The patient has no symptoms.

Relapse/recurrence/treatment-resistant
Relapse/recurrent means that the leukemia has reoccurred after a remission. Treatment-resistant means that the leukemia has not gone into remission after a treatment.

4. How is this type of cancer diagnosed by allopathic practitioners?
Fatigue, fever, subcutaneous bleeding (ecchymosis), paleness, bone pain, general neurological symptoms, joint pain. Bone marrow punction, (blast count higher than 25%), blood tests (leucocytes, Hb, thrombocytes, measuring the size of the liver and spleen, testicular examination, ultrasound, CT. Basically every physician should undertake a precise differential diagnosis of rheumatic disease or of osteomyelitis (bone marrow infection). In detail such a diagnosis should also be made for neuroblastomas, rhabdomysarcomas, and naturally lymphomas. Cytogenetic changes of individual chromosomes are evident in approximately 50% of the patients. The translocation of the cABL protooncogene (paternal chromosome 9q34) designated as "Philadelphia chromosome" and the BCR (breakdown cluster region/maternal chromosome 22q11) is present in 4% of incidences of childhood ALL, and 20% of incidences of adult ALL.

What are the allopathic therapy concepts?
In most therapeutic centers there are 4 steps for an ALL treatment. These are:

1. In the remission-generating initial therapy a lot of chemotherapy is used in order to kill as many leukemia cells as possible and to bring the cancer disease into remission. While earlier only cortisone and vincristin was used, today only mega-doses of a wide variety of chemotherapies are given in combination with cortisone and irradiation. Today primarily the following medications/chemotherapies are used: methotrexate, cyclophosphamide (mustard gas), vincristin, cortisone, daunorubicin, asparaginase, thioguanin, 6-mercaptopurin, cytosin-arabinosid, teniposide (VM 26). Today this treatment protocol has established itself as a gold standard.

2. In the second phase, termed the central nervous system (CNS) prophylaxis, the assumption is that that cancer cells must be prevented from settling in the brain or in the spinal chord marrow, even if no cancer has been found there yet. The whole procedure is offered as prevention and includes high-dosed chemotherapies with methotrexate, plus very strong irradiation of the (healthy) brain. The amount of radiation can be more than 10 times that which is given to adults to destroy other types of cancer tumors. This shows in the most brutal manner that allopathy is solely concerned with treatment of the symptoms.

3. In the third treatment phase, the so-called consolidation and intensification phase the attempt is made to kill leukemia cells which may possibly still remain, using more chemotherapies.

4. The fourth phase, the maintenance phase consists of giving children chemotherapies over years to avoid recurrence, (here the question arises, particularly after the experience with AIDS, whether it is precisely this therapy itself is suitable to generate cancer.

Bone marrow therapies (BMT)

A. Allogenic bone marrow transplant / stem cell transplant:
Here the patient receives stem cells from a donor. First high doses of chemotherapy are administered with or without supplemental irradiation, to destroy all the bone marrow in the body. Then healthy bone marrow is taken from a different donor. The healthy bone marrow of the donor is then injected into the patient, and this is then supposed to replace the destroyed bone marrow of the patient.

A. Autologic bone marrow transplant / stem cell transplant:
In this therapy, bone marrow / stem cells are removed from the patient, then the bone marrow is treated with medication to kill all cancer cells, and after high-dose chemotherapy it is returned to the patient. The bone marrow is frozen for storage. The patient then receives a high-dose chemotherapy with or without supplemental radiation therapy to destroy all the remaining bone marrow. The stored, frozen bone marrow is thawed and then injected back into the patient. Naturally one should not forget that bone marrow transplant involves a high risk of the patient dying due to the therapy. Neither of these therapies is without controversy, even among allopathic practitioners. For this reason think twice before deciding whether or not you would like to subject your child to this.

Irradiation:
The use of irradiation plays a major role in the CNS phase. Here the belief is that possibly present cancer cells will be killed off through strong irradiation. For better understanding: No doctor knows whether this is true or not. This is pure theory and due to this theory children are exposed to cancer-generating irradiation.

Additional therapies like hormones, antibodies, etc.

Although there are approaches with Interferon, other therapies like cytokine therapies or monoclonal antibodies, are not used for ALL, because in addition to testicular cancer and AML, ALL is *the* stronghold of chemotherapies.

General

If you have read the lines above about the treatment of ALL, and if you realize that there are many children who get this therapy when they are two to four years old, then sooner or later you might ask yourself the following question: Assuming that over a two year period a healthy child regularly gets 6-10 different chemotherapies, as well as high-dosed irradiation of the still-growing brain, and that the child must stay in a hospital with all the bacteria, viruses and the poor food, and then in addition must survive a bone marrow transplant = how many healthy children would die of this therapy?

Certainly a few, would most likely be your response. For this reason I permit myself to point out again and again, that we do not know whether children die because of these therapies, or in spite of these therapies. I am very much aware, that this question must be shocking for some parents and particularly for many oncologists.

On the other hand, it does not help, if we act as if we knew the answer to this question – nobody can answer this question and whoever claims he can is lying. Physicians often say that if ALL was not treated with chemotherapies then the children would have to die. However I would like to contradict this statement for several reasons:

1. In old medical text books you can read that in the past ALL was not always viewed as the fatal illness. Now, were all of these doctors quacks or lay people? The main argument was always that "blood-forming disorder" regulates itself. Do you really think that physicians would have written that if all their patients had died of ALL.

2. I have personally documented cases in which children with ALL did not die, either because they did not get chemotherapy, or although they did not get chemotherapy.

3. Not to undergo chemotherapy is not the same thing as doing nothing and waiting. Also children in particular should go through a detoxification regime e.g. maintain the oil protein diet and particularly they should participate in mental "happiness training".

4. Almost all children in Germany with ALL get chemotherapy. How do all the doctors know that children will die without chemotherapy?, as it is known that there are no comparative studies and there never were any comparative studies.

5. How many children do the doctors in Germany know, who have survived ALL without chemotherapy? None, one or two? Probably none, because the child would be immediately taken from its parents if the parents would not allow their child to undergo mandatory chemotherapies.

The legal point unfortunately is a very serious one. As parents we must know that authorization to bring up a child can be withdrawn, or is almost always withdrawn if the parent desires that the child be treated holistically. This is the fundamental reason why there is hardly a physician in Germany who would dare treat children without chemotherapy. The last doctor who dared to do this was Dr. Hamer and for this (and other reasons) he went to prison. The following German book is recommended if you want to read more about ALL and Dr. Hamer: Vermächtnis einer Neuen Medizin (Legacy of a New Medicine) / pages 482–484. Allopathic practitioners consider Hamer's statements to be the pure nonsense of a crackpot and they will tell you in detail why every point cannot be true. Why should they react any differently. I am the last person who does not understand this. Nevertheless we cannot get around the fact that we can only dismiss Hamer's words when the opposite of what he maintains has been proven.

Until then I permit myself, just as Dr. Hamer does, to question again and again, whether a therapy that can kill healthy children is really the right therapy for our sick children.

CAUTION: Here as well I would like to avoid any misunderstanding: For purely legal reasons I do NOT recommend that you not have your child treated (i.e. simply wait), regardless of whether the treatment is according to Dr. Hamer or whether it is allopathic. Dr. Hamer's therapy does not just consist of waiting, rather he explains to his patients or the parents in detail what they must do to get healthy again.

Astrocytoma

1. The allopathic definition:
Brain tumors that consist of astrocytes, the so-called ensheathing cells of the CNS (Central Nervous System).

2. How frequently does this type of cancer occur (incidence rate) in Germany (USA appr. x 3)?
In Germany 1-2 people out of 100,000 get astrocytoma annually.

3. Subdivisions:
Astrocytomas belong to the subgroup of so-called astrocytic brain tumors, and here the differentiation is, pilocytic tumors, (level 1), astrocytomas with low-grade malignancy (grade 2) , anaplastic astrocytomas (malignancy-grade 3) and then the glioblastoma (malignancy level 4).

There is also a different division in which all grade 1 and grade 2 tumors are designated as low-malignancy and all grade 3 and grade 4 tumors are designated as highly-malignant.

4. How is this type of cancer diagnosed by allopathic practitioners?
Children often have vision disorders, endocrinological disorders, or also field of vision failures. Less frequently seizures, and cranial pressure symptoms (nausea/vomitting) occur. In many text books there is also discussion of developmental delays or personality disorders. However this is fruitful field for speculation and ensures more hysteria than illumination.

In addition to the neurological examinations, imaging processes are used, primarily due to the many differential diagnoses: Electroencephalogram (EEG), evoked potentials (acoustically evoked potentials AEP, visually evoked potentials or VEP, sensory evoked potentials SEP), computertomogram (CT), blood tests (e.g. tumor markers), magnetic resonance tomography (MRT), angiography, positron emission tomography (PET), and naturally biopsies.

What are the allopathic therapy concepts?

Basically the astrocytoma is considered treatable from the allopathic perspective, as there are studies in which more than half of the children have lived for more than 5-years through operation, chemotherapy, and irradiation. Unfortunately these numbers also mean that approximately one in two children dies and nobody dares to ask the three questions that are crucial for parents:

1.   Do 50% of the children survive because of the toxic therapies or in spite of the toxic therapies?

2.   Do many children die because of the therapies perhaps, and not because of the tumor?

3.   Are there actually other successful therapies for astrocytomas?

Nobody can answer the first question, not even allopathic practitioners. The second question must certainly be answered with yes, unfortunately we do not know today how high this percentage is. The third question I can also answer with a clear yes, see for example the antineoplaston therapy from Dr. Burzynski, even if many doctors firmly deny this. Here the main argument is always: "These therapies are not recognized scientifically". The fact that this is not even possible, as I have described in this book, however is not discussed.

Surgery

Allopathy usually assumes that fundamentally removal of the entire tumor or reduction of the tumor mass should be undertaken if at all possible from the operation/technical perspective. I fundamentally disagree with this argument, because my personal experiences with patients, who have conquered their brain tumor without operation, offer compelling reasons against it. Moreover, do not forget the high relapse rate after brain operations, as well as the additional operation risk.

Of course I am aware of the meaning of the statement of the above section, I have long reflected intensively as to whether I as parent can do this. However I have reached the conviction that there is no use in beating around the bush in this matter, but rather I must give parents the chance to reflect about the disease of their child from different perspectives. Naturally I am not referring to children with cerebral spinal fluid circulation disorders, in which a primary resection can represent a life-saving operation. Since complete removal of the tumor frequently is not possible, parents are often recommended to undergo a second operation, after irradiation and/or chemotherapy. In this regard however the damages to the brain (particularly for children under three years of age) must be taken into account; and these damages can be severe. This concern is frequently dismissed with statements like: "We have the most modern irradiation devices", or "we know exactly how we must dose chemotherapy", etc. Unfortunately daily experience in the practice paints a different picture.

Basically parents must know that allopathic practitioners proceed from the assumption that the tumor in the brain = cancer, and when this tumor is destroyed, the cancer is gone as well. Consequently they are happy to "automatically" fall back on other tumor-destroying therapies like irradiation or chemotherapy, even if these first, are cancer causing themselves, and second, have side effects which can affect a child for the rest of his life.

Chemotherapy

Astrocytomas are viewed as tumors that are moderately sensitive to chemotherapy. Consequently the toxins are often given to children in high doses. Since children in general are much healthier than adults, physicians assume that they will survive this procedure.

Basically chemotherapies are not easy to use for children because due to the irradiation which is usually previously administered, even greater damage has been done to the bone marrow. Earlier studies with carboplatin, vincristin or antinomycin D are also not very promising, and when read carefully they are anything but convincing. This is primarily because (again) only chemotherapies were compared and a lot is said about positive response rates or remission rates, but no significant life extensions could be proven. Parents here should not allow themselves to be deceived. Destroying the tumor is not the same as a longer life. High-dose chemotherapies clearly belong in the area of research and study. Here there are no meaningful data. Be careful if you are pressed to put your child in such a study.

Irradiation

For low-malignancy astrocytomas usually irradiation is only employed if the tumor continues to grow. With highly-malignant tumors irradiation is always employed with a very high quantity of 54-60 Gy. But regardless of which type of irradiation is used you must clearly understand that the rays pass through the head and thus they always destroy more healthy cells than changed cells. Ask any physician who maintains the contrary, to please explain to you how anything else could be possible. Since Hiroshima, Nagasaki and Tschernobyl, we also know that it is these rays in particular that generate cancer many years later.

The combination of operation and irradiation is often viewed as an absolute must in treating highly-malignant astrocytomas. As previously mentioned, this is due to the perspective that healing will only occur through complete destruction of the tumor. To what extent healing is prevented by this perspective "may not be discussed" without risking the involvement of the state prosecuting attorney.

To avoid misunderstanding: I do not say that you should not let your child undergo radiation therapy. I just allow myself to independently to review the available data in detail, which unfortunately does not support that which is viewed today as standard therapy - not by a long shot. There are no proofs, rather there are only a lot of theories. You can quickly recognize this by they number of different allopathic therapies.

I know that with this statement I do not contribute to a clear policy line that you can follow for your therapy decisions. However I would like to avoid the same mistake that is made by most of allopathic practitioners and maintain that the present data clearly support the current standard therapies – careful study of the available data reveals that this is absolutely not the case.

Additional therapies like hyperthermia, gene therapies etc. see Astrocytomas for adults.

Michael Horwin and his knowledge of brain tumors.

In the following pages I do not want to revisit the issue of who is right and who is wrong. It is important however that you know that there are also other people who have studied the causes of brain tumors, and that today we are far away from knowing what brain tumors are, regardless of who maintains what.

Michael Horwin and Alexander

In 1999 the case of little Alexander Horwin was carried in the press. In 1998 Alexander was diagnosed with a medulla blastoma, and his parents began extensive research to determine which treatment would be the most successful for this disease. They studied the research work of Dr. Percival Bailey and Harvey Cushing, who were the first to report on medulla blastomas. Then they collected all the studies on medulla blastomas and finally decided on the antineoplaston therapy offered by Dr. Burzynski in Houston/Texas.

Unfortunately it was not possible for them to avail themselves of Dr. Burzynski's therapy, because he was only permitted to provide therapy to children, for whom irradiation and chemotherapy had failed. Based on this situation, Alexander was then given a chemotherapy, which he died of a few weeks later. However it is interesting to see what the Horwin family brought to light through their research and that is what I would like to share with you here.

1. Are vaccines carcinogenic?

Mercury, aluminum, and formaldehyde are known carcinogenic substances. A person who would inject even the smallest amount of these products into a baby would be arrested. This is not the case if you are a doctor! Do you know that almost all vaccines contain these three toxins to a greater or lesser degree?

2. Can viruses cause cancer?
This question is answered with a clear yes in the medical literature. Today we know the Eppstein-Barr virus, which is considered to be responsible for Morbus Hodgkin's cancer, or HPV-17 which is frequently cited for skin cancer. Only a few viruses have been tested to determine just how carcinogenic they really are. At the same time children are injected with killed-off bacteria, which almost always contain viruses. Or viruses that have been cultured in animal tissue, which in turn contains its own viral strains are directly injected. The fact is that nobody, not even the manufacturers, know what is really contained in the vaccine.

3. Brain damage after vaccinations
Neurological damages like vaccines, seizures, nerve damage, or Guillan-Barre syndrome (palsy) are cited as "side effects" of vaccines. Unfortunately the observation that tumors spread more easily in areas that have been previously damaged (see also increased liver tumors after hepatitis) fits here.

4. Polio vaccination as cancer cause?
In the 50s and 60s many people were vaccinated against polio with simian virus 40. Only later was it discovered that another cancer-causing virus also nested in the same ape kidneys where the virus was cultured. Upon this discovery the manufacturer changed the species of monkey. Today SV 40 is still found occasionally in children's brain tumors! In 1987, Dr. George Rousch and colleagues published a book which described the relationship between SV 40 virus and medulla blastomas in great detail. Again a study published in 1995 showed that SV 40 viruses were not found in healthy brains, but they were found in brain tumors. A study published in

1999 by H. Huang likewise found SV 40 viruses in all brain tumors.

By the way researchers assume that the child did not even need to be vaccinated himself, but that the virus is transferred from the mother.

5. Vaccination and immune system

Many physicians say that our immune system plays a significant role with cancer. However now we know that vaccines have a negative influence on our T-lymphocytes and that they can strongly suppress them. However when children are less than 1 year, this is very difficult to determine in the blood. At the same time however all pediatricians warn that children with weak immune systems should not be immunized. Thus it would be logical not to vaccinate children in their first year and to test their immune system PRIOR to every vaccination. However this is not practiced in America or in Germany.

This brings up another point. As researchers published in the magazine Science in 2002, many pathogens, such as the worm parasite helminth, stimulate cytoproduction (like interleukin-10). However people who fight infections with vaccines and antibiotics, play down the importance of cytokine production, which could play an important role, particularly for cancer. Thus Professor Kremsner from Tübingen University determined that many people in the civilized world no longer produce interleukin-10 or do not produce it in adequate quantity.

6. DNA and viruses

These days every university teaches that a change in DNA generates cancer. They also teach that viruses cause DNA changes. And they teach that every vaccine contains millions of bacteria or viruses. These are viruses that occur in the growth tissue of the vaccine, and viruses that get in unintentionally. However the universities do not teach that the increasing incidence of cancer could have anything to do with vaccines.

What can I learn from this?
Does vaccination lead to cancer? Certainly, probably, hopefully not. We do not know. But why should vaccines, that can result in meningitis and seizures, that can trigger the Guillan-Barre syndrome, and a lot more, not also be responsible for brain tumors? To what extent do vaccines really disturb the immune systems of our children, which they are actually supposed to build up? Alexander's parents vaccinated their child sixteen times in his first seventeen months. In Germany this is nothing unusual. My son's vaccination records indicate at least fourteen vaccinations and nobody asks the important question:"How many vaccinations can a child bear in the first two years of life?"

Neuroblastomas in children

The allopathic definition of your type of cancer is:
Solid malignoma, that arises from the autonomous nervous system.

2. How frequently does this type of cancer occur (incidence rate) in Germany (USA appr. x 3)?
1 per 100,000 children under 15 years of age (app. 1,400 cases annually). Approximately 35% are diagnosed in the first year of life, and more than 90% are under 6 years of age.

3. Subdivisions:
Neuroblastomas are categorized according to appearance (cell maturation) or malignancy grade under the microscope. Categorization is then made accordingly.

1a =   Diffuse mixture of immature, maturing and mature cell elements (diffuse ganglioneuroblastoma)

1b =   Alternating large areas with non-differentiated Neuroblastoma tissue (Ganglioneuroblastoma of the composition type)

2   =   Mixture of non-differentiated cells and the presence of a few with partial differentiation in ganglia cells

3   =   Non-differentiated, small-cell and round-cell tumor tissue

4 =   Stage 4 is called anaplasia. An anaplasia is nothing
       more than a transition of higher differentiated
       cells into less differentiated cells. In this process there
       are neuroblastoma tissue (1-3) and tumor portions
       without neuroblastoma indicators, which however
       contain large or multinucleated cells.

4. How is this type of cancer diagnosed by allopathic practitioners?
Usually a tumor is detected through imaging processes like CT, MRT, sonography, or x-rays. So-called catecholamine metabolite examinations of the urine or blood are unfortunately very imprecise, as many neuroblastomas do not produce increased catecholamine values. Tumor markers NSE, MIBG determination (noradrenaline derivatives) biopsy of the tumor or the bone marrow. Basically, delimitation to other embryonic tumors is very difficult.

What are the allopathic therapy concepts?
Interestingly enough in stage 4S no therapy is offered and doctors wait for spontaneous remission which frequently occurs. Naturally any thinking person would immediately ask; "Why not do the same in other stages"? Why not compare other stages with no treatment at all or compare a non-conventional treatment with chemotherapy and irradiation? Why doesn't anyone ask how many children die of the therapy? Naturally insiders know the answers to these questions, but does this help all the children?

Certainly not and here I can only appeal to the conscience of every single physician, that they finally commit themselves to making changes in this area. In the interest of every single child with this diagnosis.

Surgery
Basically an operation to remove the tumor is the objective.

Since the patients are still quite young, the risk of an operation should be considered very carefully. Particularly for larger tumors, many oncologists tend to first use chemotherapy to reduce the size of the tumor and then to operate.

Naturally this carries the risk that the tumor will continue to grow faster, in spite of, or because of the therapy, and that the patient will then be too weak for an operation. Please speak with your oncologist, since many people assume that tumors always become smaller during chemotherapy.

Chemotherapy:

Other than in stage 1 or 4S chemotherapy is the first choice. Here the following substances are employed: Cylophosphamide, vincristin, cisplatin, vindesine, ifosfamide, dacarbazin, adriamycin.

Doubtless all preparations can contribute to the destruction of cells and improve the blood values. But will your child live any longer through this measure? Since there are only comparative studies involving different branches of chemotherapy, this question unfortunately remains unanswered, and as long as it remains unanswered it is hard for me to go over to the side of conventional therapies, even if there are statistics, that (could) speak positively for chemotherapy for neuroblastomas.

Bone marrow therapies (BMT)

A. Allogenic bone marrow transplant / stem cell transplant:

Here the patient receives stem cells from a donor. First, high doses of chemotherapy are administered with or without supplemental irradiation, in order to destroy all the bone marrow in the body. Then healthy bone marrow is taken from a different donor. The healthy bone marrow of the donor is then injected into the patient, and this then replaces the destroyed bone marrow of the patient.

A. Autologic bone marrow transplant / stem cell transplant:

With this therapy bone marrow/stem cells are removed from the patient and after administering a high-dose chemotherapy are re-administered. This means that bone marrow is removed from the patient and treated with medication to kill all cancer cells. The bone marrow is frozen for storage. The patient then receives a high-dose chemotherapy with or without supplemental radiation therapy to destroy all the remaining bone marrow. The stored, frozen bone marrow is thawed and then injected back into the patient.

Naturally one should not forget that bone marrow transplant involves a high risk of the patient dying due to the therapy. Neither of these therapies is without controversy, even among allopathic practitioners. For this reason think twice before deciding whether or not you would like to subject your child to this. Moreover studies speak against both forms of therapy because out-patient therapies with chemotherapies (over a year) resulted in the same good/bad results.

Irradiation:

The use of irradiation still plays a major role in treating neuroblastomas. Here the belief is that possibly present cancer cells will be killed off through strong irradiation. For better understanding: No doctor knows whether this is so. This is pure theory and due to this theory children are exposed to cancer-generating irradiation. Thus studies (Mattay 1989) have shown that children do not live longer through irradiation, and also the use of whole-body irradiation as better "preparation" for a bone marrow transplant showed no survival advantages (Ladenstein 1994). Also the use of 131iodine MIBG to this date has not produced the positive results that were expected of it. But considering the generous use of radiation for children with neuroblastomas, often we must assume that oncologists do not read these studies.

Is it not paradoxical that the type of radiation used as therapy for neuroblastomas, is precisely that type, which could possibly be the cause of the disease according to allopathic opinion? Here parents have a particular responsibility, as physicians often generously trivialize all the side-effects of irradiation. I have personally witnessed many times how doctors told their patients that the irradiation only kills the diseased cells.

Consider very carefully why your child will be irradiated and what risks are involved.

Additional therapies like hormones, antibodies, etc.

Cytokines
Although there are approaches with interleukin 2 or LAK cells (lymphokin-activated killer cells) these therapies, as well as monoclonal antibodies, do not play a major role, or they have been discontinued due to lack of success.

General
If you have read the lines above about the treatment of neuroblastomas, and know that there are many children who are between the ages of two and four when they get this therapy, then sooner or later you might ask the following question:

Assuming that over two years a healthy child regularly gets 6-10 different chemotherapies, a high-dosed irradiation, and that the child must stay in a hospital with all the bacteria, viruses and the poor food, and in addition must survive a bone marrow transplant = how many healthy children would die of this therapy?

Certainly a few, would most likely be your response. For this reason I permit myself to point out again and again, that we do not know whether children die because of, or in spite of, these therapies. I am very much aware some parents and

402

many oncologists in particular must find this question shocking, on the other hand it does not help to act as if we knew the answer to it. Nobody knows the answer and whoever maintains the contrary is lying.

Physicians often say that if neuroblastomas were not treated with chemotherapies then the children would have to die. However I would like to contradict this statement for several reasons:

1. I have personally documented cases in which children with neuroblastomas did not die, because they did not get chemotherapy, or although they did not get chemotherapy.

2. Not to undergo chemotherapy is not the same thing as doing nothing and waiting. Also children especially should go through a detoxification process and stay on the oil protein diet, for example.

3. Almost all children in Germany with stage 2, 3, + 4 get chemotherapy. How do all the doctors know that children will die without chemotherapy, as it is known that there are no comparative studies, and there never were.

4. How many children do the doctors in Germany know, who have survived neuroblastomas without chemotherapy? None, one or two? Probably none, because the child would be immediately taken from its parents if the parents did not allow their child to undergo mandatory chemotherapies. The legal point unfortunately is a very serious one. As parents we know that the authorization to bring up a child can be withdrawn, or is almost always withdrawn if the parent desires to have the child treated holistically. This why there is hardly a physician in Germany who would dare treat children without chemotherapy.

CAUTION: Here as well I would like to avoid any misunderstanding: I do not recommend that your child not be treated, regardless of whether in accordance with Dr. Hamer or allopathically. Also Dr. Hamer's therapy does not just consist of waiting, but rather he explains to his patients, or to their parents in detail what they must do to return to health.

The only thing that I permit myself is to completely question the allopathic approach. I do not say that it is wrong. I would only like to encourage you not to undergo any unconsidered treatments, which are irreversible in their effects.

Other therapists have demonstrably treated neuroblastomas successfully with non-conventional preparations. Thus Dr. Aschhoff in Germany published a small study with 5 neuroblastomas, of which 4 were healed, one case was brought to standstill, and 1 case was without positive result. All children were given Ukrain (see under Ukrain). These results are all "unscientifically documented", but this was not important to the patients and the parents, because Dr. Aschhoff's success was evident.

Medulloblastomas in children

1. The allopathic definition:
Brain tumors that emanate from the cerebellum vermis (the middle part of the cerebellum), the posterior cranial fossa, and from the 4th ventricle.

2. How frequently does this type of cancer occur (incidence rate) in Germany (USA appr. x 3)?
App. 20% of all brain tumors in children (2 per 100,000) are medulloblastomas.

3. Subdivisions:
Under the microscope, medulloblastomas are very small and dense tumor cells with little cytoplasm. They divide relatively quickly and the cell nuclei are hyperchromatic and have very different appearances. Thus they are easy to distinguish from the normal round granular cells of the cerebellum.

4. How is this type of cancer diagnosed by allopathic practitioners?
In addition to the neurological examinations, imaging processes are used, primarily due to the many differential diagnoses: Electroencephalogram (EEG), evoked potentials (acoustically evoked potentials AEP, visually evoked potentials or VEP, sensory evoked potentials SEP), computertomogram (CT), blood tests (e.g. tumor markers), magnetic resonance tomography (MRT), angiography, positron emission tomography (PET), and naturally biopsies.

In addition symptoms like severe vomitting and a papilloedema (changes of the eyeground) play a major role, which can occur due to an increased intracranial pressure through water retention.

Primarily tumors of the cerebellar vermis, which strong contrast agents enrich, are frequently viewed initially as medulloblastomas. Differential diagnostically however one must also think of astrocytomas or Lindau tumors (haemangioblastomas).

What are the allopathic therapy concepts?

Surgery
Info: Please see Astrocytomas for children

Chemotherapy
Medulloblastomas are viewed as tumors that are moderately sensitive to chemotherapy. This naturally depends on the age structure and the possibility, of being able to give high doses of toxins to children, as children in general are much healthier. Basically chemotherapies are not easy to use for children because due to the irradiation which is usually previously administered, even greater damage has been done to the bone marrow. Although there are many studies with CCNU, MOPP, vincristin and cyclophosphamide, their results are not particularly promising (Evans 1990, Tait 1990, Levin/DeVita, Gutin). Also the highly-praised HIT studies, in which cisplatin, ifosfamide and methotrexate were used, when reviewed carefully are anything but convincing. This is primarily because (again) only chemotherapies were compared and a lot is said about positive response rates or remission rates, but no significant life extensions could be proven. Parents here should not allow themselves to be deceived. Destroying the tumor is not the same as a longer life.

High-dose chemotherapies such as busulfan and melphalan clearly belong in the area of research and study. Here there are no meaningful data. Be careful if you are pressed to put your child in such a study.

Irradiation
"Due to infiltrative growth, healing is not possible without follow-up irradiation". Most allopathic practitioners agree with this statement, with the exception for children under 3 years of age. Since the assumption is made of metastases via the spinal fluid cannels, cranial spinal irradiation of the entire cerebral spinal fluid area is attempted.

In this process enormous amounts of radiation in the range of 54 GY are recommended (Kortmann et al. 1999). But regardless of which type of irradiation is used you must clearly understand that the rays pass through the head and thus always destroy more healthy cells than changed cells. Ask any physician who maintains the contrary, to please explain to you how anything else could be possible. Since Hiroshima, Nagasaki and Tschernobyl, we also know that it is these rays in particular that generate cancer many years later.

Additional therapies like hyperthermia, gene therapies, etc.
Please read the section on astrocytomas.

Soft tissue sarcoma

Info: Definition and division, see Soft-tissue sarcoma for adults.

What are the allopathic therapy concepts?

Surgery
See under soft-tissue sarcoma for adults.

Chemotherapy
Fundamentally children have vital functions which are totally different than those of adults, and consequently they survive chemotherapy much better than do adults. Unfortunately this knowledge is generously exploited, particularly in the case of soft-tissue sarcomas. For this reason, chemotherapy is part of the basic concept for treating soft-tissue sarcomas in children.

In this case oncologists differentiate soft-tissue sarcomas that are sensitive to chemotherapy and soft-tissue sarcomas that are resistant to chemotherapy. Primarily all rhabdomyosarcomas, but also extraossary Ewing sarcomas and malignant peripheral neuroectodermal tumors are considered to be sensitive to chemotherapy. Fibrocarcinomas and malignant schwannoma however are considered to be resistant to chemotherapies. Leiomyosarcomas, malignant rhabdoid tumors, malignant fibrous histiocytoma and liposarcomas are considered to be moderately-sensitive to low-sensitive.

Today primarily cyclophosphamide, ifosfamide, adriamycin, vincristin, actinomysin and etoposide are used, which however is not undisputed, even among allopathic practitioners, due to the increased risk of leukemia. The view of most oncologists however is still, the stronger the better. This cost however is often significant physical and psychological dam-

ages. One should not forget that according to official statistics (CWS studies 81 and 86) every 33rd to 50th child dies of the treatment!
Please consider the last sentence seriously. Many children die quickly directly because of the therapy or indirectly through the generation of new tumors through the allopathic treatment.

Irradiation
To summarize my research relative to irradiation of soft-tissue sarcomas for children, I must say that I could not find any meaningful studies that prove children lived longer because they had these treatments. There are indeed many studies in all possible combinations with chemotherapies, but these say little about the extent to which additional irradiation will really help children live longer.

It sounds logical that tumors will become smaller or even disappear under irradiation. Unfortunately there are still no clear studies that prove that children will also live longer through this measure.

Also allopathic practitioners are not clear about the quantities that should be applied, or when irradiation should be applied. Many oncologists say that irradiation should be used early and over a large surface to avoid relapses. Others in-turn say that particularly this should not be done, but rather irradiation should only be applied, if there are local relapses. This "dispute" alone indicates how "certain" oncologists are relative to irradiation of soft-tissue sarcomas.

However what is usually not said is that it is precisely these rays, that allow a new tumor to grow. You should not forget that the recommended amount of radiation (30-60 Gy) is very high and nobody can correctly estimate the damages.

Additional therapies like hormones, antibodies, etc.
Approaches like monoclonal antibodies or cytokine therapies

play virtually no role at all in the allopathic therapy of sarcomas.

Fever therapies

My previous researches clearly show that fever therapies (see also Coley's toxin) bring good results with sarcomas, and it is imperative that they are included in the therapy consideration. To my knowledge, the use of fever-generated bacteria and/or hyperthermia (exogen generated fever) in particular is a successful alternative. For small children this therapy is usually not possible, however it is possible for teenagers.

Chemotherapy,
irradiation and 3E

Even if there are few hard facts today that prove chemotherapies help in the case of solid tumors, I am naturally enough of a realist to correctly assess the political landscape and the medical establishment and its immense powers of persuasion. In other words regardless of what I write here, and regardless of how many studies will also fail in the future, there are still too many patients who decide for chemotherapy or irradiation. This is because, on one hand it is very difficult for a patient, under time pressure, to correctly determine which path is correct for him, and on the other hand, patients are still frighteningly subservient to "authority" where health is concerned. For the reasons stated I would like to discuss how you can use the 3E program, even if you undergo chemotherapy or irradiation.

Basically all aspects of the 3E program still apply if you undergo conventional therapy. There are a few points that I would like emphasize particularly. Since most conventional physicians do not care what you do during or prior to conventional therapies, (they argue that it won't help anyway), use this chance. Prepare yourself with the following plan, if it is not interesting to your doctor.

8 days prior to the therapy

· Antioxidants (primarily selenium and vitamin C). If you can afford it, in addition take reduced L-glutathione, L-cystein and ubiquinone (CoQ10).

· Visualize the success of the therapy three times a day.

· Ensure that you drink at least 2-3 liters a day.

· Start drinking fresh-pressed juices 2-4 times a day.

· Organize now who will be bringing you food and freshpressed juices in the hospital. Under no circumstances should you rely on what you will get in the hospital! Just think that so-called nutritionists work in almost every hospital and then think about what is served.

· Find out if you can do the chemotherapy at home or with your family doctor. It is very dangerous to go to a place where the most germs are located, - a hospital, when your immune system is so weak.

During your hospital stay

- Have someone bring your food to you in the hospital. Do not worry what doctors or nurses say and have the courage to be laughed at. If this is hard then think-up an excuse like I am allergic to this or that.

- Continue taking the antioxidants as described above.

- Visualize many times during the day. You have the time to do this.

- Return to your home as quickly as possible. Nobody can recover in the day-to-day hospital environment. Please consider in this regard that the hospital director prefers to see you in the hospital when you are no longer so sick, as you then cause fewer costs. Discuss with your doctor which therapies are planned in the next days and decide whether these therapies are also possible at home.

- Never forget that the purpose of a hospital stay is to get better again as quickly as possible and return home. It is not your job to be voted the most popular patient in the ward.

Pain control

I personally did night duty in the hospital. I went through the rooms and asked patients if they wanted a sleeping pill or pain pill. As I experience frequently, not much changed in the last 20 years in this area. But be very careful, when you are offered "preventative" antibiotics, tranquilizers, or sleeping pills. It is your mucous membranes that will suffer and your cell respiration that will thus be weakened. Be aware that every nurse and every doctor will have their own opinion on this issue and consequently you must form your own. I know that it is not easy to be "unpopular" in the hospital, just because you do not accept what other patients accept – just keep your recovery and the health of your family in mind.

First, pain is something positive, because it makes you aware of certain points in your body. I mention this because I have the impression that today pain is usually viewed as something which is only negative, and every physical and psychological pain is covered over with chemicals. This does not mean that I pillory pain medication, rather I would like to help you better deal with your pain.

Pain analysis is absolutely necessary to get a handle on pain. If you know why you have pain, then you should first consider which medication is available to control the pain. Let me explain this to you with an example. During my week-long visit in a cancer clinic in Mexico, a young cancer patient came to the clinic with extreme pain, he had been receiving morphine several times a day for weeks. Clinic personnel showed the young man relaxation techniques, performed coffee enemas several times a day, and replaced the morphine with paracetomol which is a significantly weaker pain medication. By the time I left the clinic the patient did not require morphine a single time. Almost every doctor will tell you that this is not possible, but at the same time I have experienced precisely this system (relaxation techniques, enemas, and permanent lessening of the dose, or immediate replacement with weaker pain medication) in many clinics, and the physicians and patients were often enthusiastic about it. Before reaching for a pill, determine for yourself, how long, or whether you can withstand the pain without chemicals, or whether the following alternatives might be something for you.

1. Whenever you have pain go into your house on the right bank (see the chapter on mental energy) and go into the relaxation room that you previously create. In this room lay yourself down on a comfortable couch, breathe oxygen through a mask and smell your favorite fragrance. Stay in the room until you feel completely relaxed.

2. Listen to relaxation music or classic music.

3. If it is possible, have sex or masturbate, if your personal religious attitude allows this (this suggestion is serious!).

4. Drink as much as possible.

5. Have a massage.

6. Take a relaxation bath.

7. Have acupuncture or learn acupressure.

8. Divert yourself with an activity that is fun for you.

9. Do something that makes you laugh.

10. Clinics often have the possibility of better controlling pain with biofeedback or TENS devices. Ask your doctor about this and use these possibilities. For cancer patients there is no pain medication with "few" side effects, as all pain medications (even aspirin) can have effects on cell respiration and can stress your mucous membranes, not to mention the additional workload they place on your liver.

11. Consider a build-up program for your intestine with intestinal bacteria or a cure according to Gray.

12. Deacidify yourself, in any case, intensively with baths or with energy drinks (see chapter: Detoxification).

13. And do not forget: Coffee enemas can be an extremely positive influence on pain (see Detoxification).

After the hospital
There is one advertising slogan that says: You've earned it". When you return from the hospital then you have also earned something. I cannot tell you what this is. But you should "allow yourself something", as there is nothing better than getting your immune system up again. Do not delay this point, rather allow yourself something.

Attention: This program can make a significant contribution to your recovery, and most of all to rapid regeneration of your intestine.

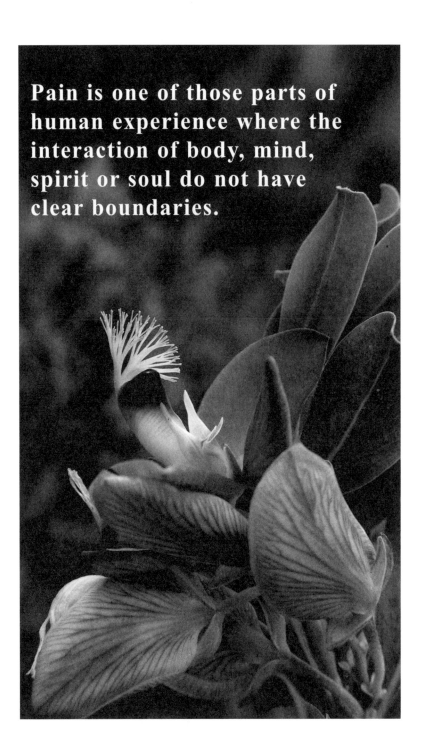

Pain is one of those parts of
human experience where the
interaction of body, mind,
spirit or soul do not have
clear boundaries.

6

The
3E Program

How have final-stage cancer patients
managed not only to survive,
but also to obtain a higher quality of life
for themselves than they had before?

The first E

Eat healthy

Nobody really knows exactly which diet is best for us. This is precisely why thousands of journalists take the liberty of describing totally contradictory guidelines on a daily basis. How long has it been since you participated in a discussion about nutrition, or since you thought about your diet. Most likely it was not that long ago.

The biggest problem with our diet today is that we eat dead food, i.e. processed food. Naturally everyone understands that bread, whose seed has been dressed, washed, polished, sterilized, etc. with chemical agents, in order to then be "treated" with nitrogen oxides, chlorine, persulfates, bromates, arsenic derivatives, etc., does not promote our health. However this does not prevent millions of people in Germany from eating precisely this type of bread, just because it is labeled biologic whole-grain bread, or labeled with some other deceptive name. The same applies for sugar or trans fatty acids (hydrogenated fat), and yet this does not prevent us from consuming these substances on an almost daily basis. Let's take another, more precise look at the masterpiece of creation, the human body, in order to better understand just how important our diet is.

Certainly you know that our body is made up of billions of cells. In turn, each individual cell itself contains millions of minute components. Regardless of what we hear over and over, nobody is even close to understanding how an individual cell manages to produce billions of cells in nine months from two cells, and particularly how it manages to produce different cell groups like nerves or liver cells. Many experts believe they understand that this all has something to do with our DNA; with genes. However the truth is that while they indeed know what occurs in an individual cell under very specific laboratory conditions, they know absolutely nothing about how this cell behaves in the united cell structure of a human being, here we know absolutely nothing – but it is precisely this area that is so important for us. It is not individual cells that can become healthy, but rather an entire human being, along with everything that this entails.

We will only be able to understand what health is, and what disease is, when we are able to understand united structures consisting of billions of individual parts. Since we are still light years away from this knowledge, we cannot simply shut down our understanding and act as if we can draw conclusions about total cell organization from individual cells. When scientists do this, they do it for one reason only, and that is because the other way, the more objective way, is simply not yet possible. Thus when doctors tell us what is going wrong in our bodies, we must never forget, that these words represent nothing more than an assessment. Please do not misunderstand me, I do not mean that we should now forget all diagnostic processes, but rather I simply mean that we must never forget that diagnoses always represent just a piece of a large puzzle, they are not the whole picture.

You must understand this in order to ask yourself the most important question of all, if you have cancer: "What can I do so that these tumor cells once again divide normally". I would like to emphasize this again because it is so important. The question is not, "What can my doctor do, so that I get better, but rather, what can I do?". This book will provide you with possibilities. But if you have cancer, or if you treat people who have cancer, then you must understand that each individual must find his own path to healing. Almost all the cells in our body renew themselves within a period of a few weeks. This means that we are not the same today as we were a few days ago. Imagine a multi-story building from which thousands of bricks are removed everyday and replaced with others, and then imagine that the old, "good" bricks, are increasingly replaced with old, decaying, and crumbling bricks. It is not hard to imagine that this building will collapse sooner or later.

Funnily enough this same perspective has not yet been applied to human beings and the renewal of their cells. Every cell membrane is composed of fatty acids. Logically these are also replaced by new fatty acids on a constant basis. But what actually happens if over years we no longer consume the requisite good fatty acids in sufficient quantity? Do you really believe that your liver can form outstanding brick with which to build the "multi-story building (human being)", from low-quality, crumbling brick? Every doctor answers this question with a definitive no; but at the same time most doctors still believe that nutrition, or as in our example the fatty acids, are not as important as some chemical substance that is mixed together in the laboratory. We constantly talk about hormones, vitamins, and enzymes, and in the process we forget what they actually consist of. Next to water we are primarily made up of proteins and fat. Since this is the case, then wouldn't it be illuminating to discuss which fatty acids we should eat or not eat, for example? Instead, certain interest groups have succeeded in bringing us to a situation, where we daily think about how much vitamin C we should be consuming.

If you ask your doctor if there is a cancer diet, he will certainly deny that any such thing exists. It's possible that he will start out by saying that it is important to eat healthy food, and he will probably say that you should eat whole foods, more vegetables etc. However the fact that this discussion between doctors and patients takes place hundreds of times everyday in hospitals around the world, is also due to the wrong question. The correct question would be: "How many patients do you know who have been successful in getting rid of their tumors thanks to an intensive change in diet?"

Most doctors would then simply respond with: "I don't know of any", or "naturally I don't know any, because there is no such thing as a cancer diet", and patients would then know that while this doctor may be a very good doctor, he has had no previous experience with cancer diets. What would be wrong with this? Should we expect an oncologist to know everything – in this day of specialization? Of course not. But with few exceptions these discussions do not take place, because many patients are not confident in posing "such" questions to a doctor, even though their life is at stake.

I have been reading books about nutrition for more than 25 years, and before I studied cancer intensively I thought that I was quite knowledgeable in this area. However to my utter dismay, I had to admit that in reality I knew little, and that I had to go back to school in this regard. My most important "teacher" was Dr. Johanna Budwig, certainly one of the greatest experts in the field of cancer and nutrition. No reference is made to the "flaxseed lady" from Freudenstadt (as she is called in America), that does not include superlatives. Nominated several times for the Nobel Prize, author of many books and countless scientific articles, hated by her opponents, and loved by thousands of patients who are alive thanks to her therapy. I have spent a lot of time with Dr. Budwig and have traveled several times to the Black Forest to interview Dr. Budwig, and to investigate the documentation that was made available to me. Anyone who has personally become acquainted with Dr. Budwig and/or who has studied the theory and practice of the oil protein diet, can imagine how difficult this work was. However I know today that the effort has been 100% worthwhile, and in all my travels I have never learned more about nutrition than I did from Dr. Budwig. In the meantime I have become acquainted with many therapists and patients who have confirmed what I have learned from her. There is not a month that goes by that I do not meet somebody who enthusiastically reports to me about the successes of the oil protein diet. Recently I have been doing more and more research into the physical aspects of the oil protein diet, and I always discover something new in conjunction with energy work.

Unfortunately I also see many "helpers" who believe that they understand the oil protein diet, and who reduce Dr. Budwig's therapy to nutrition. This would be too easy. Dr. Budwig's therapy includes knowledge of electromagnetic stresses, proper daily planning, the psychological component, and naturally the correct use of ELDI (electron differentiation) oils and alcohol. In our discussions Dr. Budwig warned me countless times of how dangerous "wrong" combinations can be, and how important it is that patients do not undergo a different therapy at the same time. I consider the oil protein diet to be an inexpensive therapy, which almost anybody can follow on their own after consulting with somebody who has studied the oil protein diet, or after studying the theory intensively. For me this therapy takes the absolute no. 1 ranking of all nutrition therapies, and you can be sure that I have carefully considered what this statement means before writing it in this book.

The oil protein diet

As a qualified pharmacist, a chemist with a doctorate in chemistry and physics, who later studied medicine, Dr. Budwig was senior expert for medication and fats in the German Federal Institute for Research on Grain, Potatoes, and Fat. In 1949 she published "New methods of fat analysis", jointly with Professor Kaufmann, which really marked the birth of paper chromatography in the area of fat research. In 1952 she wrote in the work: "Zur Biologie der Fette V. Die Papierchromatographie der Blutlipoide, Geschwulstproblem und Fettforschung" ("About the biology of Fats V. Paper chromatography of the blood lipoid, tumor problem and fat research"), which must be considered to have proven that the highly unsaturated fatty acids are the decisive sought-for factor in the function of respiration ferments , i.e. the second pair, which the Nobel prize winner Otto Warburg was not able to find. What sounds so unimpressive to lay people was in reality perhaps one of the greatest breakthroughs in medicine.

At this point for the first time it was understood that polyunsaturated fatty acid is the decisive factor for achieving the desired effect of stimulating respiration. In interplay with sulfurous protein it plays a role, if not the decisive role, e.g. in building bridges between fat and protein for oxygen absorption and utilization, for all growth processes, for blood formation etc.

With this theory Dr. Budwig was not only able to help many cancer patients, by returning cancer cells to a situation where they could "breathe" though the oil protein diet she developed, but other physicians, like Dr. Dan C. Roehm in Florida, Dr. Robert E. Willner in Miami, and many others in Europe and Asia were also able to help patients.

Dr. Jan Roehm wrote in a 1990 article, that although he was very skeptical initially, he became convinced that cancer can be healed through the oil protein diet. Never forget that we are all heliotropes (beings of light) and that we need light with its electrons (photons). Human tissue is thus unique because it is capable of storing precisely these electrons and giving them off as needed. The absorption occurs via so-called resonance which means that our tissue must vibrate in the same bandwidth as the incoming rays. You can compare this with a television antenna, which must be adjusted.

For this to happen our cells require certain unsaturated fatty acids like linoleic acids or linolen acids. Together with sulfurous proteins these fatty acids form a compound whose dipolarity and inherent resonance allows|the human body to absorb electrons, to store them, and to emit them as needed. It is also this "force", which ensures that we "live" and it controls all vital functions, like our pH level, protein build-up, etc. At the end of the 1920s the Nobel Prize winner Otto Warburg discovered how important this dipolarity was at the conception of human life. What is interesting in this regard is his discovery that oxygen absorption of a fertilized egg cell increases by 2200%.

But let's consider Otto Warburg's work from the very beginning. Warburg attempted to stimulate the idle cellular respiration of cancer cells by experimenting with butyric acid. This failed because at the time there was no detailed information about saturated and polyunsaturated fatty acids. The honor of discovering the factor which was capable of bringing oxygen into the anaerobic living cancer cell is accorded to the scientist Dr. Johanna Budwig. She was the first to publish these important findings.

Dr. Budwig sees the human body as an antenna which is capable of receiving these vital and healing electrons, if the two antenna, called sulfhydyrl, and polyunsaturated fatty acids "are correctly adjusted". In the sulfhydryl group they are

425

on the safe side with cystein and methionine, which occur in dairy products, and for fatty acids they are on the safe side with linoleic acid and linolenic acid. But be careful. The real "secret" lies in knowing where these fatty acids are still present in an intact state. Theoretically there are also large amounts of linoleic acids in margarine. But these are present in the "trans form" and not in the "cis form". In the trans form the atoms are opposed to each other and not parallel to each other, like in the cis form (see the diagram below)

```
   H  H                          H
   |  |                          |
  -C=C-                        -C=C-
                                   |
                                   H
```

cis form   trans form

This small difference naturally is not listed on the lid of the margarine package, nor is it on the label of the sunflower oil that you can buy at any grocery store. However the problem with this trans form is that no electron absorption can take place and thus a vicious circle starts.

How do we get sick? By consuming too many of these "electron stealers", or in other words, by consuming food and toxins which block cellular respiration. Margarine, animal fat, butter, nitrates, radiation, and cytostatic agents (chemotherapies) are known electron stealers. They all prevent absorption of electrons. Interestingly enough antioxidants like vitamins (in certain quantities) are also included here. Consequently do not take high doses of vitamins or enzymes just because you read about this in a book (naturally, nutritional therapies like that of Dr. Gonzales, which have been especially worked out,

426

are something totally different). By the way Professor Linus Pauling, who personally requested Dr. Budwig's work, was aware of this as well. If you read the previous sentences carefully then you will also easily understand why Dr. Budwig's work could not be made known to the "broad masses" under any circumstances. Whole branches of industry would have to change their production equipment and people would probably not purchase the majority of goods offered in supermarkets. In addition:

* The margarine industry could no longer tell us that the polyunsaturated fatty acids in its products are essential, or that they do not have network-like compounds in their carbon members of the fatty acids, and thus nobody would eat any margarine.

* Saturated fats and the wrong polyunsaturated fats as present in products like sauces, in almost all the world's candy, and in most baked goods, would have to be taken off the market, or production of these products would have to be transformed in a manner that would enable production with genuine polyunsaturated fats.

* Denatured products, which comprise the majority of the goods on supermarket shelves, would no longer be produced, either because nobody would want to buy them, or because they would be legally prohibited from being sold.

* Status quo party financing would be done away with. No government could state that they were interested in the health of their citizens and at the same time allow illness-causing fats.

You can easily figure out for yourself that we are not talking about millions here, we are talking about billions, and that we are talking about a revolution in health that would be unique in the history of mankind. But we would also have to look ourselves in the mirror; I mean, haven't we all become so comfortable that we are only too happy to believe the lies put forth by advertising? We no longer take time to check uncomfortable statements; instead we just hope that everything will not turn out to be all that bad.

The following information is provided to acquaint you with the practical application of the oil protein diet. I understand that the food items described here can only be as good as the producers allow them to be. Thus be careful where you buy your food. This point is vital, because nutrition therapy cannot function with food purchased from the supermarket.

Info:

Dr. Budwig died on May 19th 2003, at the age of 94 in Freudenstadt Germany. Unfortunately there is no official successor. I can only promise, that in the future I will tell all that I was privileged to learn from her to as many people as possible. I do this in the hope that generations will yet profit from the oil protein diet.

Nutrition guideline

For the first four weeks, to start the oil protein diet
(Excerpt from the book: <u>The Oil Protein Diet Cookbook</u> published by Sensei)

The essential aspect of the oil protein diet is to exclude fats that are hard to digest. In their place, easily-digestible, easily combustible fats that supply energy and resilience – in other words, good fats, should make up the major share of the diet. Moreover, the diet is so carefully structured that all preservatives, which act like respiration toxins, are excluded. On the other hand, fresh and non-cooked food is rich in those proportions which support the organism's automatic oxygen uptake. This form of nutrition is a whole food diet, a build-up diet. It should not be confused with a "diet" that is just light and bland. Many types of fresh vegetables are used raw. Only fresh vegetables should be used for preparing the steamed vegetable dishes. Canned vegetables or pickled vegetables are avoided. Raw prepared food should be included in some way for each meal. Either as a raw vegetable platter, or prepared raw in conjunction with the warm meal. Fat is used abundantly, however it is always used in proper harmony with protein, for instance quark with flaxseed oil in many variations forms an essential part of this energy-rich and revitalizing diet.

The transition

On transition day nothing should be eaten except 250 g of Linomel (flaxseed honey granulate or flax seed meal as an alternative). In addition you should only drink fresh juices, this means fresh-squeezed/pressed fruit juices, or absolutely pure juices (without added sugar). Fresh-squeezed/pressed vegetable juices, like carrot juice, celery juice, with apple juice, and red beet juice with apple juice, are also recommended. Ensure that you drink a hot drink such as herbal tee, peppermint tea, rose hip tea, or hibiscus tee, at least three times a day. Sweeten it only with honey. Sugar in any form is prohibited. Grape sugar is permitted, also fresh juices may be used for sweetening, if needed black tea is permitted in the morning. For those who are seriously ill a champagne breakfast consisting of champagne and Linomel (flax seed meal) can be taken. This transition day is urgently recommended for seriously ill patients, and they do well with it.

Daily schedule
Drink a glass of sauerkraut juice or sour milk before breakfast. (Author's note: This is very important and may not be skipped!)

For breakfast
eat muesli regularly, which is prepared as follows:
Put 2 tablespoons of Linomel (or fresh ground flaxseeds as an alternative) in a glass bowl. Cover this with fresh fruit; depending on the season, berries, cherries, apricots, peaches, grated apple. Then prepare a mixture of quark and flaxseed oil. Add 3 tablespoons of flaxseed oil to 100 to 125 grams of quark, mix intensively, adding some milk, (2 tablespoons) so that the flaxseed oil is completely stirred in. Then add 1 tablespoon honey. To change the flavor you can vary the quark-flaxseed oil mixture with chopped rose hips, sea buckthorn juice, with other fruit juices, or with ground nuts. Butter is not recommended. Only herbal teas should be taken as beverages, a cup of black tea is also allowed, if needed.

At 10:00 in the morning have a glass of fresh-pressed carrot juice, or fresh-pressed celery and apple juice , or red beet juice with apple juice.

Mid-day meal
a) Cabbage fruit salad as appetizer

Make a quark-flaxseed mixture as mayonnaise by mixing 2 tablespoons flaxseed oil, and 2 tablespoons milk in the mixer, with two tablespoons of quark, then add 2 tablespoons lemon juice or apple cider vinegar, and flavor with 1 teaspoon of mustard and herbs. You can also use marjoram, dill, parsley, etc. adding 2-3 gherkins is also recommended. Use herbal salt. The quark-flaxseed oil mixture combined with a lot of mustard and a little banana is an excellent salad dip. As part of this oil protein diet the quark-flaxseed oil increases the value of the raw vegetables; in terms of taste, you can always come up with new surprises by using seasoning herbs. It makes the raw vegetables even better. The only oil you should use is flaxseed oil. In addition to green lettuces, grated root vegetables like carrots, kohlrabi (cabbage turnip), radishes, sauerkraut, black salsify, pureed or finely-grated cauliflower, are also suitable. Horseradish, chives, and parsley are also recommended.

b) Cooked dish
In addition to steamed vegetables, potatoes, rice in particular, buckwheat or millet, are also part of the diet. Only use Oleolox * (the recipe is in Dr. Budwig's book) as oil. It tastes better with vegetables than does flaxseed oil. Preparation simply involves boiling the vegetables in some water and mixing them with some Oleolox and spices before serving. Soy sauce comes in handy.

The quark-flaxseed oil mixture can also be served with the potato dish and flavored with caraway, chives, parsley, or with other herbs. If you are using the quark/flax seed oil mixture with potatoes then you can add more flaxseed oil.

c) Desert
You can serve a quark-flaxseed oil mixture which can be varied with fruit, similar to breakfast. Quark-flaxseed oil combinations like lemon cream, wine cream, banana cream, or

vanilla cream, are quite popular as a sweet variation. Combining the quark-flax seed oil mixture with fresh fruit always works well.

d) Afternoon

At about 3:00 and at 4:00 for the patient a small glass of pure wine or champagne or also pure juice is recommended, however it should always be taken together with 1-2 tablespoons of Linomel (flax seed meal).

e) Evening

The meal should be eaten early in the evening (about 6:00 pm), and it should be light. You can prepare a warm meal of rice, buckwheat or oatmeal, soy flakes, or similar flakes from a health food shop. The preparations with buckwheat grits are very good and they are the easiest to digest. The preparations can be made as soups, or in a more solid form they can also be combined with hearty sauces. Use a lot of Oleolox for sweet soups and sauces. This gives them more nutrients and they are richer in energy. Use honey to sweeten, all sugar is prohibited. I do not recommend wheat-germ preparations. Wheat germ oil (one teaspoon, twice a day) can be taken to support the cure.

All animal fats, margarines, "salad dressings", and butter are strictly prohibited. Moreover all meat products are prohibited, because harmful conservatives are almost always added to their preparations. Canned meats are strictly prohibited. Sausage must be avoided completely. Only "pure juices" should be purchased as fruit juice, because the way these juices are prepared is important. Juices that contain preservatives are less effective than juices that are completely natural.

Bakery goods, particularly the so-called "little piece" are also strictly prohibited, as frequently these are prepared with harmful fats which are biologically useless.

Drinking sauerkraut juice in the morning on an empty stomach is particularly recommended, but also eating raw carrots, radishes, green peppers and red peppers, raw asparagus, raw cauliflower, kohlrabi, as well as other vegetables that can be eaten raw as a salad plate (if possible vegetables should be grown with biological fertilizers). Likewise nuts, particularly walnuts, and brazil nuts, should not just be used as a snack but as an essential part of the nutritional regime. You should also use nuts abundantly for desserts.

Children should be given nuts instead of candy and suckers. For instance nuts together with dates, figs, or raisins. Hearty seasoning with natural fresh herbs, or dried herbs in winter, is permitted and desired. If you like flaxseed oil you need not fear spices.

A note on milk
These days many people condemn milk as a dangerous product. To some extent this is correct, because of all the harmful substances in milk and due to the allergies that these substances cause. On the other hand, I have known people, with so-called lactose intolerance, who, after three transition days with flaxseed oil, were able to eat the oil protein diet without any problem. Here we must make a distinction between milk as a raw product and quark which is mixed with polyunsaturated fatty acids and consumed as lipoprotein. If you are absolutely opposed to cow milk, then I recommend goat quark.

The Linomel (flaxseed meal) muesli for breakfast is a corner-stone of the oil protein diet:

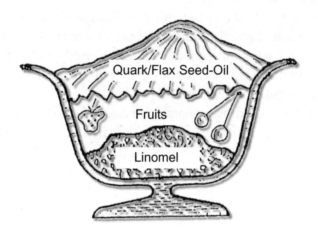

Preparation:
Put 2 tablespoons of Linomel (flax seed meal) in small bowl. Then add a layer of fruit in season as you desire, (see illustration). You can mix the fruit as you would for a fruit salad, or you can just use one type of berry. Coarsely grated apple can be used in many ways in winter, by added cherry, blueberry, and quince juice, or by adding raisins or apricots that have been softened in apple juice.

Quark-flaxseed oil cream
Mix honey, milk, and flaxseed together in a blender, if possible. Then add quark, a little at a time. Mix it all together until it is a smooth cream. You should not see any more oil. You can add some milk if necessary.

This mixture can be varied by adding nuts or bananas, lemon juice, orange or lemon juice in a ratio of two to one, chocolate powder, coconut, fruit juices (which should be added last); vanilla, cinnamon, pineapple or similar items. Cover the layer of fruit with the quark-flaxseed oil cream, and then garnish with nuts or fruit.

Nutrition must be inhaled. Fresh air is important for the sick person. Movement in fresh air is urgently required in accordance with capacity. Rest for balance and recovery is also important for the sick person. Often the bed-ridden patient lacks both proper rhythm of rest and relaxation, and exercise in accordance with available capacity, which is helpful.

Caution

In recent years I have experienced extraordinary successes with the oil protein diet, and many people have integrated it into their daily lives. But all too often I find that people in an acute phase (with tumors), only follow some of the prescribed diet, for example they leave out the important sauerkraut juice and "sin" once in a while.

My experience shows that it is crucial for cancer patients with tumors to precisely follow the instructions in this book.

Nutrition summary:
I have no question whatsoever that there are successful nutrition therapies for cancer patients. Anybody who maintains the contrary should expend the effort required to find out why all the patients of Dr. Budwig, or Dr. Gerson have returned to health, if it was not primarily due to their nutritional concepts. What have you got to lose by following the oil protein diet for 8 weeks. It doesn't cost any more than what you are eating now, and I promise you that you will feel the effects after just a few days. Why do so many doctors fight against cancer nutrition therapies, which demonstrably have helped other people? What kind of fear on the part of a physician would compel him to so vehemently resist changing his view of cancer nutrition therapies.

Since allopathic practitioners always follow the gold standards (usual medical treatment) and because thousands of others are doing the same thing at the same time, in their opinion they could never be considered quacks. Just because many people make the same error, an error still remains an error. Naturally this applies to non-conventional therapists, and if these practitioners intentionally treat patients incorrectly, then they also belong in prison. However there is a difference. If a homeopathic practitioner treats you for 3 months then the damage is significantly less than it would be if you were treated for three months with radiation, or with chemotherapy.

But this means that I can't eat my favorite kind of cake anymore!

"Does this mean that I will never be able to drink a cup of coffee?", or "How long do I have to stay on the oil protein diet?" I hear these sentences or ones like them all the time from patients who start to eat more nutritiously. There are three primary points that need consideration in this regard:

1. What kind of life are you leading that makes a cup of coffee so important to you? Of course I know that this question is provocative, on the other hand it contains a very important element, namely how satisfied are you with your life, or what makes your life worth living? Only if you confront this material you can find a "replacement" for a cup of coffee, or for another "unhealthy", but favored, dietary habit.

2. I consistently experience in our cultural circles that even the slightest changes in lifestyle are viewed as impossible, or that they have too great an impact on the quality of life. However these same people have often been through the Second World War, endured chemotherapies, or experienced days that are much more drastic in their impact. But when some people are asked to eat differently then they forget that the majority of mankind would be happy if they were given a chance to eat such a diet. I do not want to label anyone a "wimp" with these words, rather I would just like to communicate to you that I do not understand why people are so little prepared to do more for their health.

3. If you have been following a healthy diet for a time, and if you have more energy, then naturally there is no question of "going back" to the old diet. Automatically you will prefer biological food instead and fresh-pressed juices over any other homogenized juice, regardless of how it is advertised. Once you have experienced this then drinking a cup of coffee on occasion will not be that important.

Is there a common element that links all nutrition therapies?

No doubt there are widely-varying views as to just what a healthy diet should include. The Ayurveda frowns on too much raw food, and Dr. Gerson says that raw food is essential.

However both theories have demonstrated successes, and both prove to us anew how little we actually know about the significance of nutrition, not about the foodstuff. If we set the Ayurvedic guidelines aside, then there are certainly shared elements:

* Polyunsaturated fatty acids

* Biological food, i.e. as natural and fresh as possible

* A lot of raw food

* Little (no) meat

* Fresh-pressed juices

If you expected a longer list, then I am afraid I must disappoint you. These are the main characteristics that you can find in the work of all those who have intensively studied the issue of cancer and nutrition. Most of the other information clearly differs relative to diet composition. There is no consensus at all relative to how much fat, protein, and carbohydrates you should eat. It gets really "complicated" when you read the opinions about individual food items. Some recommend tomatoes, the anthroposophists say cancer patients should avoid all plants in the nightshade family. Some recommend sourdough bread, others say that you shouldn't eat any bread. Some recommend a little fat, others recommend a lot of fat etc.

As far as nutrition and cancer are concerned, science leaves you on your own; or do you know how much vitamin C you need? You cannot rely on some books by "nutrition scientists" and "professors", rather you must rely exclusively on the combination of science and empiricism (what experience teaches). Here I emphasize the word, **and**. I consider it to be a serious error to neglect either one of these two areas. First we need a theory of nutrition which has demonstrated that it can help people, and once we have that, then we need the science. I know that the path today is just the opposite, and this is precisely the reason why so many therapies fail. The way out of the laboratory does not function if we do not concurrently include all the experiences of the "users".

Nutrition in the 3rd millennium

Despite all the successes achieved by nutrition therapies, we should not forget that it is becoming even more difficult to live a healthy life and to purchase biological foodstuffs. Consequently you must place the utmost priority on this point. It makes a significant difference whether you use quark for the oil protein diet that contains hormones and antibiotics, or quark made from cows whose milk is free of these substances. This point determines whether the whole therapy will work or not, and cannot be over-emphasized. I consider this point to be even more important for the Gerson therapy than it is for the oil protein diet. Don't be intimidated by these "negative" statements, like "biological products are just more expensive". There are huge differences between the individual food products. Even if there are no guarantees, at least buy quality natural products, or even better get to know the farmer personally from whom you get the product. Never forget that your life is at stake, and that you are bound to confront these issues sooner or later.

If you are still undecided as to whether a cancer diet is right for you or not, then I would like to offer the following for your consideration to conclude this chapter: There is only one way to determine whether a cancer diet therapy can help you or not: and that is by trying it. Please do not forget that if I am right, then perhaps this decision can save your life, and if I am wrong, then the worst that can happen to you is that you will have eaten a healthy diet for a few weeks.

439

The somatic-psycho influence of a healthy diet

Have you ever run into the term somatic-psycho? (Soma = body). Probably not. Although we read over and over how important the body-spirit unit is, few scientists have studied it. Specialization on a different, specific area, significantly increases the chances of winning a Nobel Prize.

Over the last few years however there are also various currents which increasingly deal with this aspect of the statement: "A healthy spirit can only dwell in a healthy body". There is increased activity in this area on the part of researchers studying aging, genetic engineers, and neurosurgeons. I share the opinion that there has been far too little research in this area. An example: Have you ever considered how decisions are made? Are they made on the basis of experience alone?

Let's assume that you are sitting down and thinking about whether you want to go to the mountains or to the sea for your next vacation. Finally you decide to go to the sea. Why the sea? Did the decision come from a feeling? What is a feeling? An increased secretion of hormones, and why did your body secrete them at precisely this moment? Now there is a totally different way, which is being confirmed scientifically through ever more research.

While you are sitting there consciously considering the relative advantages and disadvantages, thousands of bodily reactions are taking place. When thinking about the sea, for instance, your body temperature climbs from 37.258 degrees to 37.345. On the other hand when thinking about the mountains, your temperature decreases from 37.258 to 37.155. Even if this temperature difference does not reach your consciousness, it is present nonetheless. However perhaps your adrenaline level climbs by 0.01 percent when you think of the deep blue sea. What is certain is that while you are thinking of your vacation, many different processes take place in your body. Your body analyzes these reactions and evaluates them.

Finally after it has placed all its reactions in the balance, your body tells you that it is probably best to go to the sea.

There is an infinite number of examples from daily life that demonstrate how strongly our body influences our psyche or our thought process. Just think about those times when you have a full bladder in the morning and you start to dream that you are going to the bathroom. (By the way the physician Hippocrates described this phenomenon as early as 500 years BC).

Or just try to maintain a rigorous physical training program for several weeks and eat a poor diet like hamburgers, at the same time. Again this is almost impossible, because your body will tell you what foods it wants and it will automatically set desires for healthy nutrition. Or who has not heard the statement: "Just leave her alone, she is having her time and she is irritable." This means nothing more than women are more often sensitive, more easily provoked, and more aggressive during menstruation. The same holds true for athletes who take anabolic steroids. These athletes are also more easily provoked and more aggressive. But what is actually happening here? How can hormones make men and women more aggressive or more gentle? If hormones are capable of making us all more aggressive, then are they also perhaps responsible for other feelings like, friendship, depression, hate, and love? Or do they just amplify whatever is already there? Are they perhaps responsible for whether I just insult a person with words, or whether I inflict bodily harm on that person?

I have been involved in sports since I was six years old, and I have been involved in martial arts for more than 30 years. Intensive involvement with psychology on one hand, and with my body on the other hand have allowed me to develop a high degree of sensitivity for processes in my body. In addition, in recent years I have often spent time with top athletes and people who are seriously ill and from them I have been able to learn a lot about which processes a person can be aware of within his body. The basic prerequisite for a satisfied life is only possible in unity with a healthy and active body.

This interplay of multiple processes (hormones, enzymes, various cycles etc.) changes when you are sick, consequently other disappointments also occur. It is a scientific fact that underweight people have a limited thinking capacity and that they are not capable of making vital decisions on their own, e.g. this has been observed in anorexics, prisoners of war, or undernourished inmates.

All these observations naturally cast the importance of a healthy diet for cancer in a totally different light. Even if nutrition therapies cannot make "direct" tumors disappear, this could be possible via the psychosomatic route, and it is primarily for this reason that you should be concerned about diet therapy.

Thus the starting point for a change is, first a healthy body - regardless of tumors or other changed cells – and this requires the best nutrition that you can find.

The second E

Eliminate toxins

Whether we like it or not, we are exposed to countless toxins on a daily basis, or we introduce them ourselves into our body through our diet. Unfortunately the likelihood that we will one day regain control of these toxins is remote. Consequently we are compelled to learn how we can avoid these toxins and how we can get those that are stored in the body out of our body. Detoxification plays a central role for cancer patients.

Many people still believe that all of our cells are directly connected to our circulation system and thus they obtain an optimal supply of nutrients. This is not the case. Let's consider a typical tissue situation in more detail.

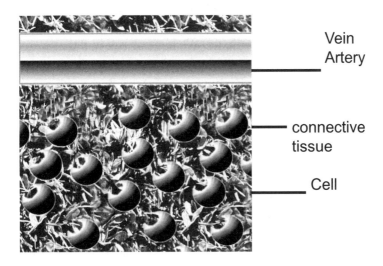

Vein
Artery

connective tissue

Cell

As you can see, only a few cells are directly connected to the circulatory system, and the others must rely on whatever gets to them through the interstitial tissue. Here it is easy to understand that the permeability of this tissue (mesenchyme) is very important. Great authors like Hauss, Pischinger, or Heine, have long referred to the importance of interstitial tissue for the occurrence of disease and healing of diseases. Since all organs are surrounded by this type of tissue, naturally "communication disorders" can occur quickly if the tissue protecting these organs is full of toxins and deposits. Doctors call this a basic regulation disorder.

Often for cancer patients detoxification and future avoidance of toxins is a question of life or death, and cannot be overemphasized. When you read books dealing with the history of medicine, you will quickly notice the significance role that detoxification measures have played in all civilized cultures, and you will realize what a disgrace it is that "modern" medicine apparently has completely forgotten the knowledge which has been collected over millennia. Not to mention the fact that physicians prescribe even more chemicals to their already-contaminated patients without initiating a detoxification program at the same time.

5,000 years ago Mesopotamian medicine described detoxification therapies in the Ashipu handbook just as they were described in Egyptian medicine. We have also found that what was known to American shamans, Aztecs, and Mayas, was previously known by the Romans and Greeks. Just think of all the baths from England to Asia that were built by these high cultures. Detoxification therapies played central role there and they still do.

An increasing number of doctors around the world are learning about the positive influence a detoxification therapy exerts on our body, and they are learning this from aborigines, African healers, and naturally from traditional Chinese medicine and the Indian "Science of Life" (Ayurveda). In later cen-

444

turies great teachers like Paracelsus, Bircher, and particularly Pastor Kneipp have taught us why we should not forget this ancient wisdom. But when cancer (a "model disease" for toxins) is involved, (just think of the thousands of studies listing new carcinogenic substances) then apparently the word detoxification appears to be a foreign term.

Unfortunately you can expect little support and instruction in this area from most physicians, and as a consequence you cannot avoid either looking for a capable therapist, or gathering the necessary information yourself. However there is one thing that you should not do under any circumstances: And that is believe that you can get by without detoxification! If you have cancer then your cells have a communication problem, and this is almost always associated with toxins. Do not take the information in this chapter lightly, and please do not think that some kind of pill would be more important than detoxification therapies, since most pills cannot work effectively in impermeable tissue anyway.

Eliminating toxins
First it is naturally important to get the toxins that have accumulated in the body, out of the body. In this regard you can have a doctor determine which heavy metals or other toxins have accumulated in your body, in order to better determine the degree of therapy. On the other hand this is not necessary as you should undergo an intensive detoxification processes anyway.

Teeth
If you are a cancer patient, then it is 100% certain that you cannot avoid this issue. I have seen miracles just through removing amalgam fillings, and the more I study amalgam fillings, the more logical this becomes to me. For years dentists and insurance companies have been telling us that amalgam fillings and root canals (dead teeth) are not dangerous. I

could fill the following pages with studies proving the contrary, however I unfortunately know that studies will not motivate people to go to their dentist, consequently I will spare you all of this and appeal instead to your reason. Do you really believe that highly-toxic substances like mercury cannot harm you? If this were so then why do we find high concentrations of these substances in the blood? Do you really believe that root canals (dead teeth) cannot harm you through production of countless siphanospora germs? Do you really believe that a permanent high voltage caused by different metals in your mouth cannot harm the organs and your brain, which are only a few centimeters above these metals.

Today we know, primarily through TCM (Traditional Chinese Medicine), that all teeth are connected with certain organs via meridians. The siphanospora bacteria (also referred to as cadaveric poison) because they are found in all decomposing matter, play a significant role, particularly for cancer patients. These bacteria have a toxic effect in your body. Furthermore parts of the fillings are absorbed by the body and stress your nervous system and immune system. But this is not all. Different metals represent counter electrodes, e.g. to amalgam, and consequently you have a permanent battery in your mouth. These galvanic currents are an irritation to the entire body system 24-hours a day, and they impose major stress. An increasing number of holistic oncologists even go so far that they will stop treating cancer patients who do not have their dead teeth removed.

But other disturbances like old oral dental infections or dispersed amalgam particles are every bit as important as removal of your amalgam fillings. Please do not simply go and tell your dentist that you want to have all your amalgam fillings removed, rather you should follow a removal plan as published by different organizations or dentists. On the following pages I would like to suggest a plan to you which contains the absolute minimum program.

446

Amalgam removal program

1. What the dentist must know:

* Only remove one filling per session

* Low RPM drilling

* Constant suction

* Take the amalgam home with you for possible homeopathic treatments.

2. What you should do in addition

* Take DMSA (Chemet) and DMPS (Dimaval) capsules in alternation.

* Take sodium selenite (selanase).

* Bear's garlic (also called ramson or wood garlic) and coriander drops

* Algae preparations

Fluorine is also an issue. There are numerous studies which prove that this strong cell toxin, (which fluorine actually is), harms you daily. Unfortunately there is an immense financial interest in selling fluorine. I intentionally do not discuss this subject in detail, but I would simply ask you to answer the following questions on your own: Do you really believe that such a strong toxin will do your body any good? I can only advise you to stop using toothpaste that contains fluorine and read books about fluorine and then decide for yourself whether you need fluorine for your teeth.

Colon

Cleansing your colon is every bit as important as removing amalgam fillings. Until the earlier parts of this century colon cleanses were part of every practitioner's standard program and physicians realized that "death is in the colon". Official documents show that 700,000 colon cleanses were performed between 1910-1954 just in the city of Karlsbad alone. If we extrapolate this number over all health resorts, then we quickly arrive at a number representing millions of colon cleanses.

This is even more astounding considering that earlier the colon region was associated with far greater shame than it is today, particularly in Christian countries, and yet patients overcame this problem, because they were aware of the importance of this therapy. There is a wide variety of therapies for the colon and I can only introduce the most important ones below. But each of these therapies is concerned with establishing a symbiosis (healthy co-existence) with bacteria and eliminating toxic deposits (particularly heavy metals).

There are many colon cleansing programs such as the colon cures developed by Gray, Ejuva, F.X. Mayr, R. Anderson, and many more. But each colon cure should start with a cleaning "from below" and not with oral preparations.

Colon-hydro therapy

A gentle rinsing of the colon is undertaken with purified water. Through a special hose system rinse water and colon content are rinsed out at the same time – it is almost absolutely clean and odor-free. After repeated treatment intervals the constant alternation of water introduction and discharge loosens even stubborn deposits and adhesions in the colon. The colon is massaged from inside and cleaned from inside. If you have never had an enema then this certainly represents a first option. I consider this to be extremely important, it is not just for cancer patients, and cannot emphasize this therapy enough.

Coffee enemas
See Diet/Gerson. A few words about execution: Make coffee with about 800-1000 ml water (according to Dr. Gerson you should use distilled water) and 3-5 tablespoons of biological coffee with caffeine, in the usual manner. Wait until the coffee has cooled to body temperature and then introduce it into the colon. It is best to use an irrigator (bucket/tube system, app. 10 ≠) from the pharmacy and some Vaseline. First let out a few drops to ensure that no air is in the system and then introduce the rest.

The coffee should remain in the colon for app. 10-15 minutes to ensure that all the caffeine is absorbed. Do not be alarmed if the colon completely resorbs everything, and nothing comes out after 10 minutes, this is entirely possible.

ELDI enemas
ELDI stands for electron differentiation and is a collective term for ELDI oils according to Dr. Johanna Budwig. Among other things these oils introduce energy into your body as quickly as possible. Particularly in cases of the most serious illness this represents an important option. Ideally it is introduced with a large syringe. The first option is the ELDI-R oil.

Attention: Enemas do not replace the necessary daily rubbing-in of ELDI oils, but rather represent a special instrument for low energy situations.

Enemas in general
Naturally in Ayurvedic medicine and in German alternative medicine there are many other possibilities of combining enemas with a wide variety of herbs or oils. Study enemas intensively – it's worth it!

Bacteria

The word "bacteria", usually has a negative connotation. Many people simply forget that evolution has not just found a way for us to coexist with bacteria, they forget that without bacteria we would quickly be dead. We have billions of helpful bacteria just in our colon alone, and without their help we would not be able to digest a single meal. Cancer patients are not the only people who have had their intestinal flora destroyed and for whom it is imperative that the intestinal flora be built-up again.   It is a fact that intestinal flora are seriously damaged after chemotherapies, or after using antibiotics, and that they should be restored using biological dairy products, juices (sauerkraut juice) or capsules with bacteria like lactobacillus acidophilus and particularly bifidobacteria.

Sweating

Sweating is one of the most simple and most effective possibilities that our body has of transporting toxins out of the body. If you have ever fasted, or if you have undertaken an intensive diet therapy, then you know what I am talking about. The odors that occur and the substances which you can find on the skin are often unbelievable. Our skin always mirrors our health, and for good reason.

Sport

Usually we sweat through physical activity, either sport or hard work. Cancer patients should avoid these activities as long as they still have a tumor in the body.   In addition to all its advantages aerobic sport has three major disadvantages:

1. Production of free radicals

When we are involved in aerobic exercise, we require increased oxygen. These oxygen molecules mean more free radicals, which attack our cells, and these free radicals must be neutralized, e.g. with additional vitamins. Naturally you can then hope that your cells will produce enough enzymes. Unfortunately you will only be able to determine that this is not the case, after you have sustained irreparable damage. Please be aware of this point regardless of which aerobic sport you are involved with.

The European Journal for Applied Physiology reported in 1995 that even one hour of jogging or riding a bicycle causes a dramatic increase of free radicals in your red blood cells. Researchers at the University of Utah and the US Army Research Center discovered something else. Free radicals occur in increasing amounts when you exercise aerobically, in the mountains, when it is hot, and when it is cold, and some athletes do this. As improbable as this may sound, it is better to refrain from jogging to work everyday, or riding a bike for several kilometers, in any kind of weather. The same applies for high-altitude training. Unless you are preparing for the Olympics and require a lot of red blood cells, then do not subject your health to this.

2. Increased absorption of ozone
In 1840 the chemist Friedrich Schönbein discovered the gas ozone. But it was not until 1913 that French scientists recognized that ozone forms in a high layer of the atmosphere, and it is formed through solar radiation. In 1985 J.C. Farmann discovered that apparently there is hole in this ozone layer over Antarctica, and this is when we all became aware of ozone, that it is a toxin, and that it is particularly damaging to our lungs.

By the way, in recent years jogging through the forest in the evening was considered to be the healthiest thing that you could do for your body. However this is no longer the case. It is much healthier for your lungs to run through the forest early in the morning when the ozone levels are not so high. Unfortunately it is no longer a rare occurrence to find damaging ozone concentrations of 180 micrograms per cubic meter of air, in the forest in the evening. When ozone reaches this level of concentration there are usually warnings on the radio against athletic activity. But even at much lower concentration levels there is a risk that you will get headaches, become tired, and that your respiratory tract and eyes will get irritated. Irreversible lung damage is possible at concentration levels greater than 350 micrograms.

At first it seems odd that ozone concentration in the evening would be highest where there is the least air pollution, in other words in areas where there is no automobile traffic and no industrial emissions. This is due to the fact that ozone occurs primarily because nitrogen dioxide gives off an oxygen atom through solar irradiation and combines with our air to form ozone. Then the wind carries this ozone into forests near the city where decomposition is difficult. In the city, on the other hand, ozone can more easily bind with nitrogen atoms and thus ozone content in the evening is lower in the city than it is in the forest. Thus if you can choose to run either in the morning or in the evening, then run in the morning. If it really hot outside, then you should take particular care to avoid anything that will increase your pulse rate. Increasing your pulse rate under these conditions causes much greater damage to your body than you might think.

Hot baths
A hot bath is certainly the most simple, and the best-known detoxification therapy. The hot water increases blood circulation and extends capillary vessels, which results in better elimination of toxins. Never forget that baths are real therapies and that they require a lot of energy. Thus they are not suitable for every person. Before you bathe you should wash your entire body and lightly rub the skin with a brush.

There are two different theories relative to water temperature. The first says that the temperature should be app. 42/43°

C, (very hot), so that the pores open wide. The second theory states that the temperature should be app. 37° C (body temperature) for more than an hour. There are pros and cons for both theories.

Likewise, the amount of time you spend in the water depends on your constitution, and there are no rules in this regard. You must shower before leaving the tub. In any case you should stay in the well-heated bathroom for 15-20 minutes after the bath.

Different baths

Epsom salt (magnesium sulfate) baths are known for better elimination of toxins as they change the pH value of the skin. **Sodium bicarbonate (baking soda) baths are used to positively influence the acid/base balance.** With each of these baths the idea is to have bath water with a pH value of approximately 8.5.

Baths with clay/healing clay also balance the acid/base balance positively. Depending the objective associated with the additive, applications with formic acid, valerian, oak bark, fir needles, camilla, rosemary, melissa, or mustard are also employed.

Naturally clinics have the advantage that they can also offer you a totally different selection of baths like moss, partial baths, hydroelectric baths, (with electric current), Schiele foot baths and particularly the permanent shower. In terms of a detoxification instrument I consider the permanent shower to be an outstanding therapy, which is used much too infrequently. (In a permanent shower, you lay on a framework in a preheated room and a shower head constantly moves over you, at a height of app. 150-200 cm.

Do not use any chemicals in the water. Read the label carefully. If you are not sure, then opt for a bath without additives, instead of using bath additives that contain substances that you are not sure of.

Sauna

For centuries sweating in a sauna has been considered one of the preferred methods of detoxification. Anyone who regularly takes a sauna recognizes the benefits of this therapy. There is a distinction between dry saunas and steam saunas. In a steam sauna, as the word indicates, steam is generated, often with herbs. Today there are a wide variety of saunas and the type of application depends on your constitution. Regardless of how the individual areas of application may be described, and regardless of whether dry sauna or a steam sauna, in the final analysis the important thing is healthy sweating. This eliminates toxins and causes the blood to be saturated with oxygen, and healthy sweating usually has positive effects on your emotional situation as well.

Often cancer patients are recommended not to take a sauna. I do not agree with this opinion, (unless there are reasons to the contrary). But a tumor is no reason not to take a sauna.

Compresses

Long before the name of Sebastien Kneipp was recorded in history, a man by the name of Vinzenz Prießnitz (1799-1851) described various healing applications of water. Prießnitz was known through the compress named for him, and he treated thousands of patients in Gräfenberg.

Compresses can be used to attract heat (as with the well-known fever compress), dissipate heat, to detoxify, and they can be used to treat a skin irritation. Since cancer patients often have other illnesses as well, the use of compresses is frequently indicated. I will only discuss two compresses in this report:

1. Liver compress

Professor Hackethal's patients were not the only ones who have been treated with a hay compress applied on the abdomen 30 minutes before the mid-day meal, to stimulate gastrointestinal activity, and for better blood circulation in the liver. This should not be viewed as a real alternative to coffee enemas, but many people cannot have an enema after an operation, and in these cases promoting blood circulation in the liver is a sensible alternative.

2. Wet pack with ELDI (electron differentiation) oils

The ELDI oils developed by Dr. Budwig are capable of giving off energy at the "event location". ELDI compresses are particularly prescribed for liver tumors or for lung cancer. Here you soak a cloth/cotton batting with the respective ELDI oil and place it on the skin. And you then place another cloth over the first and leave this combination on the body for a period ranging from 1-8 hours, depending on the indication.

Homeopathy

Adherents of Samuel Hahnemann also have quite a bit to say about detoxification. However considering the countless mixtures available, you should look for an experienced homeopathic practitioner who is capable of testing out the correct mixture for you.

Trampoline

Jumping on a trampoline is a simple but effective way to increase your lymph circulation. Try it with light jumps, and without having to breath heavily, for 5-10 minutes a day. Please do not underestimate the pronounced positive effects that jumping on a trampoline can have on your lymphatic system. Even if you do not feel the healing effect immediately, this simple device offers immense support to your detoxification efforts.

Light

Have you ever thought about how we are able to maintain our body temperature at a constant 37° C, even though our environment is usually significantly cooler. In school we learned that the reason for this is that when we generate energy (citric acid cycle) heat is produced as a by-product. But in order for this theory to be correct, nutrient intake would also be necessary, which would mean that our temperature would decrease significantly when we fast! But when we have a fever we usually eat less, not more. How does this fit together? However the fact is that it is not just during those periods when we are fasting or when we have a fever, that our energy balance from food is absolutely out of balance, and it is a fact that we can burn considerable more energy than we take in through our diet.

Most faculties do not like to be asked this question because then they would have to recognize that a human being is a heliotrope (turns to the sun) this means that we need light with its electrons. Human tissue is thus unique since we are capable of storing these electrons and giving them off as needed. Absorption occurs via the so-called resonance which means that our tissue must vibrate in the same bandwidth as the light we receive. You can compare this with an antenna which is adjusted accordingly. Naturally there are many different detoxification measures that contribute to proper realignment of our "antenna". Relaxation exercises also contribute to our ability to absorb the offering of biophotons (light).

One of your assignments during therapy is to you ensure that you absorb sufficient light. Consequently I deem going outside for at least app. 20-30 minutes twice a day to be important therapy. If possible do not wear (sun) glasses, as light is absorbed primarily through our eyes and forwarded to our brain. In addition "show the sun some skin". The following occurs in this process:

* The production of lymphocytes in the skin is stimulated.

* Suppressor cells are activated

* Excessive cortisol is consumed

* Interferon is produced
* Cellular respiration is improved

* Phagocytosis is stimulated (consumption of cellular particles that must be eliminated)

As you see, spending some time in the sunlight on a daily basis can be far more effective than the latest medications. However the most important thing is that your cells "recharge", so to speak. Don't fail to take advantage of this opportunity.

Infusions
Physicians can give you infusions, which, in the first place, can improve the acid/base balance and, in the second place, can bind heavy metals.
1. High-dose vitamin C infusions for detoxification, for binding free radicals, and for a direct attack on tumors.

2. Selenium infusions for binding metal ions.

3. Chelation with EDTA (ethylenediaminetetraacetic acid) for binding heavy metals.

Oil leaching
With oil suction, also referred to as oil leaching, you rinse your mouth out with a teaspoon of oil morning noon and night before eating (usually sunflower oil, alternatively flax seed oil, sesame oil or wheat germ oil). To be more precise, you

leave the oil in the mouth for about 10 minutes and move it back and forth. The theory, as described by G.P. Malachow (among others), is that this procedure activates the saliva glands and acids and toxins are bound. Furthermore the muscles in the head, which play such an important role for an active lymph system, are brought into movement.

Water

I could write an entire book about water, that's how important it is. Consequently do everything you can to obtain additional information in this regard.

According to all that I know about water this substance will play a significant role in future medicine. Primarily water is a carrier substance for information and for energy production. Perhaps one day we will not only drive hydrogen cars, we will also use water as an "inner energy source". This is why just filtering water is ineffective (regardless of whether with charcoal, reverse osmosis etc.), in filtering out chemicals, but you should also delete the information contained therein, e.g. through vortex systems such as those described by Viktor Schauberger. Just using a vortex system, or just using filter system is certainly not enough, you need both! As far as the amount of water to drink daily, personally I still somewhat divided. On one hand there are many reasons why we should drink 2-4 liters of water daily, on the other hand the animal world shows us that other approaches are also possible. The primates, which are right next to us, drink very little.

My opinion however is that during an intensive detoxification therapy we should ensure that we drink 3 liters of water daily, to flood toxins out in sufficient quantity.

Acid-base equalization via alkaline substances

The pH value can also be positively regulated via the gastrointestinal tract. Carbonate mixtures (e.g. with calcium, magnesium, potassium, sodium, manganese etc.) taken as a powder with water can be very helpful here. Check the success by measuring the pH of your urine. The reading from your second urination in the morning should be in the alkaline range (pH greater than 7). Naturally don't do this during detoxification therapy, because increased acid will be eliminated during the detoxification therapy.

Avoiding toxins
The first measure for every cancer patient should be avoidance of toxins. Your body is stressed enough as it is, and what can the best detoxification measures do for you if you introduce toxins at the same time?. Make it a priority to do all you can to create toxin free zones.

Nutrition
Only buy biological products. Forget all the Bessis who want to make you wise, by saying that all foodstuffs are the same. This is not true. Naturally on the market there are poor products which are labeled as biological products – there are criminals everywhere. But do not just stick your head in the sand and say: If you know one you know them all – I consider this to be very dangerous.

Cosmetics and cleaning agents
Our skin absorbs toxins very easily, consequently you must be 100% certain of what you are putting on your skin, on your lips, in your hair, or in your bathtub. Just read what's in your shampoo, and ask yourself how many of these substances you are familiar with. You will be surprised. Particularly avoid fluorine, propyl alcohol, and aluminum. The same applies for laundry detergent and cleaning agents

Microwave
If you have a mortal enemy then give him your microwave – if you do not have a mortal enemy, then dispose of it today.

Nothing else comes close to the damage that a microwave can cause. As a cancer patient you must understand that our cells communicate via light signals and that we cannot survive without this cellular communication capability. Consequently we must protect ourselves from waves that function in such a manner that high frequencies have been "modulated up" on signals with lower intensity, which is the case with microwaves. Whenever you switch on the microwave these waves will compete with the healthy waves of your cells.

But that's not all. Any food that you heat up in a microwave gets a different vibration pattern, (in contrast to normal heating, which occurs via oxidation), and cell walls simply become more permeable. Every foodstuff has its own vibration and this is what we want to particularly preserve when we eat something. In addition "polarization rotation" occurs, i.e. "healthy" right rotation of light polarization is reversed to "sick" left rotation of light polarization. Stay away from microwaves!

Electromagnetic stress
This collective term covers all the devices to which we are exposed on an almost daily basis. Regardless of whether mobile phones, radio alarm clocks, halogen bulbs, heating pads, neon tubes, computers, monitors, and particularly the transmission towers for mobile phones, we cannot completely remove ourselves from the stresses of the 3rd millennium, even if we moved to a remote island. The issue of electro smog has become so significant that you can read thousands of articles about its hazards in any library or on the Internet. I do not want to burden you with all the hazards in this book, and the reasons why our politicians don't do anything about it, rather I would like to offer a brief summary of what you can do so that your cells are not too strongly affected:

1. **Have a demand switch installed.** This is small device (it costs app. 100 Euro) that prevents, electricity from flowing into your bedroom at night. When you switch off the light, power still flows in the wall. Many people lie down with their head just a few centimeters away from the wall in which electricity is flowing. This has various negative effects, primarily on the brain. Thus shut off the power while you sleep.

2. Do not have a radio alarm clock or other electrical devices in the bedroom.

3. Do not have a wireless telephone in the house (especially not a DECT phone).

4. No mobile phones, and if you cannot live without one, then always use an external microphone)
5. Do not have mattresses with springs, or beds with metal these act as antennas).

6. Do not have any chairs with 3 or 5 "feet", such as most office chairs (these also act as antennas). It is better to sit on a wooden chair with 4 legs.

Earth rays
When I studied this subject for the first time, I thought I had gone to the wrong movie, and put the literature aside. But after I had repeatedly encountered illness-causing aspects of this subject I began to deal with it more seriously, and today I regard books that report on the amount of energy that was expended in the past to find the right location for churches, schools and houses, in a totally different light.

I have been to China several times and had studied this topic intensively long before the term Feng Shui was introduced to Europe in the mid 90s. However it is only today that I understand what these Feng Shui masters really do, and the importance of an environment in which energy can flow. Even "serious science" is more and more involved with this topic, as many physicists have recognized just how important our magnetic environment is for us.

What are rays actually? We must make a distinction between our earth's electromagnetic waves and the waves which flow to the earth in the form of elemental particles (protons, neutrons, electrons). Waves can be very short, in the range of nanometers, like x-rays, or they can be kilometers long like radio waves. When waves are between 400 nm and 700 nm long then we call these waves light. If they are shorter, then we refer to UV radiation, just think about your last sunburn. If they are even longer then they extend into the infrared range. We all know that a compass needle always points north and that this "somehow" has something to do with the earth's magnetic field. We also know that there is a magnetic force extending from north to south, and from east to west , and vertical force lines which radiate directly up from inside of the earth can also be measured.

Naturally it makes sense that there can be "circumstances" which prevent these natural rays from emanating normally from the earth, because water is present, or there are unusual displacements or fissures. These circumstances change the magnetic field to which we are accustomed. In past times when there were fewer artificial waves, animals in particular, but also people could feel these "other" waves. To do this today we need the finest measurement devices or extremely sensitive water diviners, who however are finding it increasingly difficult due to the many artificially generated waves. You see, water diviners are not esoteric cranks, they are people who have nothing more or less than the capacity to track these waves.

In the 19th century in England, A. Haviland determined that considerably more incidences of cancer occurred in special areas (limestone and chalk) than occurred in other areas (clay). Other researchers like Watt or Brand, but also Robinet or Rambeau in France, confirmed Havilands research. Then in Germany it was Hager and particularly the famous Baron v. Pohl, who was able to prove in 1932 that 50 people who were officially registered as cancer patients slept on geopathic zones. In the late 60's E. Hartmann confirmed all the findings of previous researchers with his extensive studies. He was also the person who described in detail that the distances between the bands (Hartmann and Curry bands or Hartmann grid) were between 30 cm and 200 cm.

What does this mean for cancer patients? You will not be able to avoid having your bedroom examined. Look for someone in your area or contact a company that is involved in this field.

Textiles
There are many toxins in textiles, particularly in cheap textiles. Impregnating agents and preservatives, pesticides, fungicides, softeners and disinfectants are only a few of the hundreds of toxins that our textiles are exposed to today. In addition grease-dissolving toxins are released when these textiles are worn, and these toxins are reabsorbed via the skin. Thus people are contaminated with toxins like formaldehyde, pentachlorophenol, or pyrethroid. What these toxins have in common is that they all disturb cellular respiration in our mitochondria, or even weaken it. Consequently when purchasing clothing, pay attention to where it was made, and who made it, and invest a few more Euros in healthy clothing.

Polyamides
Although artificial fibers have the "advantage" that they are

usually treated with fewer toxins they have perhaps an even greater disadvantage: They disturb our organism's energy flow by disrupting our body electricity through electrostatic charges. This forces our body to permanently correct this "constant stress" which uses up so much energy, energy, which we know plays the central role in cancer therapy. Consequently wear natural materials like cotton or silk as much as possible. For women it is important to know that in this regard brassieres are very negative, as most brassieres are produced from artificial fibers. As the anthropologists Sydney Ross Singer and Soma Grismaijer have determined, the risk of getting breast cancer is 125 x greater for women who wear a brassiere 24 hours a day, than it is for women who do not wear a brassiere (see also under breast cancer).

Metal jewelry
The permanent wearing of "closed" jewelry on the arms, legs, and neck, can also have very negative effects, because these items hinder the flow of energy. Metal necklaces in particular, can cause problems and consequently you should always have a link made of plastic worked into the necklace or just wear it for a short time.

Laughter
Laughter as therapy? If you think that this is crazy and some-thing to laugh at, then I am happy, because laughter can con-tribute much more to your recovery or to improved detoxifi-cation than you might think. While millions of dollars are spent around the world in laboratories to find out how we can strengthen our immune system, we all have the best means of doing this right inside us. Thanks to the physician Patch Williams we know today that this theoretical knowledge can be implemented in practical application. He proved under clinical conditions, what many scientists only anticipated in their studies. Now this knowledge is used for children, and

there are clowns in many clinics in children's wards. But why just in children's wards? Don't grown-ups need a daily "immune boost" even more than children do? The answer to this question is certainly a definitive yes, but what would you say if your doctor showed up with a red nose? We must start thinking differently and return to the understanding that we did not come into this world to be sick, we came here to accomplish other tasks.

If you believe that you have nothing to laugh about at this time, then change this situation. Ensure that you have something to laugh about, it's certainly possible! Get the excellent book Gesundheit by Patch Adams.

Do not simply dismiss this point by thinking: What nonsense. Laughter will play a major role in the medicine of the next century even if it is not discussed in any "scientific" text book today. The effects of laughter have far greater effects on your immune system than those offered by many medications which have been prescribed for you or which will be prescribed to you.

A small exercise:
Grin every morning for at least 2-3 minutes without interruption. You will quickly notice that you will feel better just by doing this simple exercise.

A lifelong exercise:
The next time have trouble making a decision, because you are not sure what to choose, then immediately start smiling and be happy that you are capable of making a decision at all. Be happy that you can make a decision and that others do not do make them for you. Likewise rejoice that you are part of a privileged majority on this planet who have the good fortune that they can always choose between two or more things. Do this exercise again and again. The results will be rewarding for you and the following things will quickly occur:

- It will become easier for you to make decisions.

- You will be aware that you lead a life that you can determine yourself.

- You will recognize that to be happy deciding for this or that is a secondary consideration.

- It will give you the energy to start something new.

- It will no longer be so important for you, whether you decide for this or for that, rather you will always rejoice anew in the fact that you are able to decide.

The third E

Energy

In this chapter I would like divide the subject of energy into two categories: Mental energy and spiritual energy. Regardless of which type of energy I refer to, I am convinced that if there is really a miracle cure for cancer patients, it is energy therapy. No matter which final stage survivors I spoke to, whether Russian, African, Asian, or American, they all had one thing in common, they all told me how they "built themselves up energetically". Even if each of these patients most likely understood this differently, all of them were again capable of letting their energy flow freely. A free flow of energy always has something to do with (personal) happiness, satisfaction, setting goals and positive thinking. This is why I will explain what you can do to get closer to all of these points, on the pages that follow.

An introductory comment. If you have cancer, or if you want to change something in your life, then don't just read this chapter, bring it to life by filling the empty lines with your thoughts. The only way to reach the point where energies flow freely again is to start thinking about the following points and have no fear of changes. Even if you do not understand why this is so important at this point, I would request in your interest that you not just read these lines but fill them with life.

3E mental training

We have all enjoyed an upbringing which makes us the person we are today. Of course our life as an adult has contributed a lot, but we should not forget that we laid the foundations for our thought structures as children and youth.

Unfortunately we also have "programs" from our parents, teachers, and friends, which we often run unconsciously. Consequently everything that flows into us in the course of our daily life is sorted by these programs and found to be good, bad, optimal, insufficient, satisfactory, etc. When a person is sick it is a great advantage to "reprogram" these programs, or it is even easier to learn new programs. You will learn new visualization techniques (right brain) to do this, and you will also be intellectually challenged (left brain).

If nothing changes, nothing changes!

This statement is very important because your previous life has resulted in the fact that you have cancer. This statement has nothing to do with your assessment of your life, it just describes the status quo. Consequently the introduction of changes takes on major significance for people who have tumors or energetic abnormal cells. But no doctor in the world can tell you which changes are necessary in your life. You are the only one who can find this out, or you can find it out jointly with others. But how does a person actually find out what is good for that person?

How do I found out what is good for me? "But that's really easy", you may think. I can tell you, however, that based on my experience with many people, it is not really easy. Take a look at your circle of acquaintances and you will certainly find a similar situation. There will be people who drink too much alcohol, or who take other intoxicating substances. There will be mothers and fathers who hit their children, or who have even been incarcerated. There will be men who are unbearable machos, irredeemable pashas, or who gratify themselves at the expense of others. Do these people know what is good for them? How come these people show no interest at all in what others are feeling?

The answer is simply: They do not recognize what is good for them over the long-term. They give themselves over to short-term, mood-altering things, which in the case of addicts, or in the case of the unfortunately too well-known pashas, one day gain the upper hand, and then these things can no longer be controlled. Not infrequently this automation ends in death or in serious illnesses. Do we really know why we chose our profession? In your case was it out of self-interest or was it because your technically gifted father bought some experimental kits every few months in the hope that his son would be just as interested in them as he was?

Why do we always fall for the same type of person? Is it because the same values that our parents have taught us are also important to these women or men? Or is it because these women or men are precisely opposite to what our parents would consider to be an optimal daughter-in-law or son-in-law?

Are you often insulted although objectively it has nothing to do with the matter at hand, but rather because your partner does not pay enough attention to you, and by being insulted you get a few strokes? What would you bet that you can answer all of these questions with no? Probably not very much. But even if you are aware of your behavior, this awareness unfortunately does not mean a positive change. Do you believe that alcoholics aren't aware that they drink too much? Or that men who hit their wives do not know that this is wrong? Or that women with eating disorders do not know that vomiting ten times a day is harmful to the health? In all these examples the people involved are very well aware that their behavior does not promote their happiness. Then why aren't we capable of changing the processes of which we are aware? The word fear plays the decisive role here, or to be more precise, fear of the unknown, combined with the fear of changes. Our psyche plays many pranks in this regard, as it knows many ways to prevent us from changing. The first important step toward change is the insight that something should change. Without insight there is no possibility to change, regardless of whether this comes about through force or through analysis.

Perhaps it is the same for you as it is for many other people. On the whole you are actually quite satisfied with your life – if there just wasn't this problem with cancer. You would not change places, or want to change places with anybody else in the world.

Have you ever wondered why almost all people answer the question: "Would you like to change places with anybody?", with a resounding no? How come people only want to be richer, more attractive, healthier, more famous etc., in conjunction with their own experiences and their own past? In order to initiate long-term changes you cannot confront just your understanding, but you must also deal more intensively with the world of your feelings. Regardless of all the bad experiences in the past, we each feel best in our own skin, because we know this situation better than we know any other in the world, and at first that which is familiar generates a positive feeling in us. The opposite situation is represented by new things, which initially invoke negative feelings, regardless of how positive they may turn out to be later. This is why there are so many books about change, and why so many people fail daily in fulfilling their desires, although they have all the prerequisites to fulfill them. If you deny yourself the adventure of

470

the new, then the same thing will happen that has always happened. Only he who is open to something new can have new positive experiences. As soon as it becomes clear that it is OK to be afraid of new things, and that fear is only a feeling, like sadness or joy, you can open yourself to something new and change your life.

An old man was once asked what he would do differently if he was 20 years old, and he answered: "Nothing, absolutely nothing. I would do everything again - only better."

Only better! What would you do better if you were 10, 20, or 50 years younger? Would you still choose the same career, marry the same spouse, and live in the same city? I assume that you can think of a lot of things that you would like to do differently. That is why the first important sentence of the long letter called change is:

I know that something must change.

I have traveled over all the continents on this planet and I have friends throughout the world. Through my work and my former athletic activities, I have become acquainted with a lot of people. My previous experiences and the observations of many professional helpers, clearly show that fundamentally people first avoid changes. Naturally this is mostly done unconsciously, just think of the countless religious fanatics, or people who have experienced something so horrible that their repression mechanism no longer allows truth into their consciousness, as is the case with sexually-abused children. But also people who are aware that changes are necessary in their life, so that either they themselves, or others will have less anxiety, pain, suffering etc, are often incapable of charting the new courses that are necessary. I am sure that you know people personally of whom you often think: "How long will this go on?" or: "What has to happen so that finally…" Unfortunately the knowledge alone that something must change is insufficient. This problem confronts psychoanalysts from the classical school daily. The analysis is clear, the problems are clearly recognized, the repression mechanism is reduced to a healthy measure, and still it is not possible to break through the destructive behavioral structures, or to switch them off.

As cancer patient it is important for you to first understand that any path of change starts with the insight that something must change. Do not close your eyes to changes now. They are necessary for your recovery. Start today and make yourself aware of what must change. In the following pages I will explain to you why we fight changes and how you can defend yourself against these protection mechanisms of your ego.

Why we resist changes

The professor system

Many changes are not made because they are destroyed by your ego in the initial stages. Many people set their goals so high that failure is pre-programmed, so that they do not have to change. This is nothing more than a destructive system which I call the professor system. In this process extremely high goals are set, without having a realistic plan of execution. Naturally the probability of then achieving these goals is quite remote.

A good example would be a man who really wants to become a professor but after he reads 5 books it becomes clear to him that it would be better to choose a different profession because: "Becoming a professor is actually stupid" or: "It's not for me", or: "Professors are all narrow-minded people" or: "They are theoreticians in an ivory tower", etc.

In this case the goals are not the problem. Actually we can't set goals that are high enough. Most people set goals that are too low. No, the problem is the inadequate, (or totally lacking) plan for execution. Very few thoughts are focused on the issue of just how these goals can be realistically achieved. There is no precise definition of intermediate goals, and consequently the person becomes his own victim. Observe your acquaintances closely and you will discover many professors.

There is a well thought-out system behind all of these unachieved goals, which allows you to consciously undertake something without being disappointed in yourself when it does not succeed. Actually it is a good system, since it protects the psyche and it always supplies an excuse for failure when we look in the mirror. However the handicap in the system is that you will never be successful in instigating permanent changes until you break through it. I would like to use an example to explain why we repeatedly use this system. The 90s were characterized by the word Perestroika, in English: Change. The collapse of communism, the abolition of borders, the possibilities for an individual to develop his own possibilities independent of state systems, and parents who are viewed first as friends and then as authority figures. Pure freedom was proclaimed. A few years ago I met with acquaintances from Romania in a restaurant in Istanbul and heard why things got worse in Romania after Ceausescu's death instead of better. The arguments listed by my acquaintances were the same as those which are heard everywhere in the world. Everyone was suddenly on their own (more correct would be= the individual is now independent), there was no cohesion like there was before (more correct would be= now I can find my group on my own), the financial situation was even worse than it was before (more correct would be= now it is possible for me to earn 10 times what I did before) etc.

I certainly do not want to trivialize the precarious situation, and often inhumane living conditions in many Eastern countries, as I have worked for an extended period in Turkey. Nor do I forget the pressure of unemployment in western countries, but I would like to show you why millions of people use the professor system in order to better process personal failures, regardless of the country in which they live.

Unfortunately, knowledge of how a person can develop freely, think constructively, or be artistically active is not given to us in the cradle; we have to learn these things, like we learn reading and math. Please do not mistake artistic development for an aptitude for art. They are two different things. A high value is still not placed on learning how the individual can develop his own potential, even in the western world. Unfortunately our school system still deems it more important that students memorize the citric acid cycle in biology than it is to teach them how they can consciously open themselves to new experiences. This means how an individual can allow himself to become better acquainted with his feelings, his needs, and his desires, and thus to find that which is right for himself among the multiplicity of offerings.

First of all the professor system protects us from deep depression. In other words admitting that I am not capable of handling freedom means I feel that I am a failure. This (incorrect) idea is the first step to depression. We unconsciously implement our professor system in order to protect ourselves from this depression. Unfortunately it prevents us from consciously considering our life and dealing with disappointments, because it uses two powerful weapons, which are generally termed repression and projection.

Without going deeper in the problems associated with these two terms, I would like to use brief examples to explain them to you in a few sentences. To a greater or lesser extent both systems are present in all people, and they are particularly necessary in childhood for healthy development of the personality.

Repression

Let's assume that you have had recurring pain in the lower stomach area. The logical consequence would be a visit to a doctor. Alternatively however you can get by for several more weeks, not noticing, denying, repressing your pains and, indeed you can do this, with logical arguments, such as, "I have often had something like this", "children often have stomach aches", my neighbor with similar symptoms has been to the doctor three times, and the doctor never found anything. This would be repression (of your stomach pains).

In the first place repressions are not negative. They help us to forget, and they protect our soul. They help us to get over psychic pain and they divert us from the fear of new things. Unfortunately repression mechanisms often do their work much too well and they go beyond their objective. As consequence over the years we become world champions when it comes to repression. A few examples:

- Smoking is only slightly harmful.

- What do a few extra pounds matter?

- My husband only hits me occasionally, otherwise he is the dearest man in the world.

- My parents only want the best for me.

Moreover the reason why we do not consider (want to consider) our repressions more, is also due to the little word "desire". Repression provides us with an incredible amount of joy. Or do you think that you could smoke a cigarette if you were aware of what you were doing to your lungs? Or do your think that it would be possible to go out with your neighbor and enjoy sex while you are thinking of your wife and children? Or could you sit down with your parents next Sunday for coffee, knowing full well that your parents did not allow you to go to the university, and that they threw your great love out of the house?

You see, repressions bring their own protective wall, indeed in the form of desire, fun, and joy. Do not get caught in this trap, and please do not believe that there is no desire without repression. The opposite is the case. Conscious desire is the big sister of repressed desire, not its little brother. Conscious sex is the best example of this. Or to consciously decide for a child or a partner.

Until we confront these powerful repressions with all our might, very little will change in our life. Naturally many actions are performed without engaging our consciousness and consequently these actions are not identifiable. But when you want to bring about changes, in order to change your life

476

positively, then you should learn to use the techniques described in this book for a more conscious life.

The more often you use these techniques, the more powerful your weapon against your repression mechanisms will be. It is up to you to undertake something, to become independent from your parents, or to stop falling for the wrong women, men, or counselors.

Projection
Projection is the little brother of repression. Let's stay with the stomach ache example. If you are having a cup of coffee with your friend and you notice that your friend's skin color is somewhat more pale than usual, and that he just eats one piece of cake instead of his usual two, and then you forcefully urge him to see a doctor; this would be a classic case of projection. Projecting your own problems (your fear of visiting a doctor) onto another person.

I would like to offer you a little trick here. The next time you think: "How could he (or she), of all people, say such a thing?", then please realize that your interlocutor is probably projecting at this time. It is usually the apparent things that are projected onto others.

You can experience projections every day:

-   "Don't eat so many unhealthy foods" (while you eat the second portion of French fries).

-   "I think that Ms. Mayer should smoke less because of her poor skin" (while getting a pack of cigarettes from the vending machine).

-   "I think there's something is wrong with the Schmidt's marriage" (although you are upset with your wife and haven't spoken to her for 24 hours).

Projections fulfill purposes that are similar to those that are fulfilled by repressions. They help our ego to avoid facing facts. Instead we can continue to live in the world, even the unreal world that is familiar to us. You see our soul has given us powerful weapons along the way so that we can casually and easily spend an entire lifetime, without ever having to confront the challenge of change. As long as we are leading a happy and fulfilled life, it is not necessary to confront the challenge of change. However my experiences show me that this is only granted to a few people. When analyzing your own life you will quickly recognize that each of us, particularly in puberty, was a little professor.

The professor system is often encountered in conjunction with a different system that I call the dwarf technique. I will use another example to explain this technique. A friend of mine holds seminars in London for Russian bankers. Some of these people come from the most remote areas of Russia, on average they earn approximately 100 $\neq$ to 200 $\neq$ a month, and they live in apartments that are rarely larger than 50 sq. meters. In London they stay in a five-star hotel and are also treated with a lot of deference from attentive hotel staff. It usually takes just a few hours until the dwarf technique becomes manifest in its purest form. The bankers complain, for instance, that their hotel room is not big enough, the swimming pool is not heated properly, the taxi is late, the five-star chef in the restaurant doesn't have a clue about cooking, etc.

Certainly such encounters are not unknown to you. Have you ever considered why these people act (must act) this way? It is nothing more than that they must protect their ego from the knowledge of being a failure, which brings us back to the professor system. These people come from socially underdeveloped areas, they had to push and shove their entire life, they subjugated others, and allowed themselves to be subjugated, in order to reach a respectable position. Within their life system and thought system these people are very well recognized personalities. Suddenly in London they meet giants, i.e. people who to their understanding are richer, more powerful, and more attractive. In order for them not to feel like a dwarf, they suddenly behave as they think an even bigger giant would behave. The result is then, that for this giant, naturally the room is too small, the food is inadequate, etc. Existing objects or people are made out to be small (bad), so that one' own ego appears larger (better). I make the giant into a dwarf, and then I am again the biggest.

I am convinced that you also know some genuine world champions were the dwarf technique is concerned. Almost every soccer team has a player who uses this technique to cover his own incapability. Macho men are masters of the dwarf technique, the know-it-alls who are beloved everywhere, use the dwarf technique in its purest form, and politicians are the true world champions. All it takes is watching a single congressional debate in order to understand exactly what I am talking about. Observing politicians allows you to see that what people believe themselves, is more effective or is what advances a person. Instead of showing others what he/she is capable of achieving, politicians spend 99% of their time playing the dwarf game in order to make others look bad. In the meantime the dwarf game has taken on such dimensions in our society, from politics to the daily mobbing in corporations, that only fundamental pedagological counter-measures could help, to bring about a social change in this area. But in this case we would again need fundamental changes in how we raise our children – and as you know the politicians are the ones who are in charge of this area. Thus you see things are not as easy as they sometimes appear to be. But we have all used the dwarf technique to a greater or lesser extent. The important thing is how often we have used it and how old we are when we use it.

There is a big difference whether a 14-year old on the way to healthy self-confidence uses this technique, or whether a

40-year old man uses it to consciously or unconsciously put other people down. There is also a difference between using the technique twice a year, or using it 10 times a day. By the way the latter makes you a very unloved person.

In this section I have shown you that the most important thing is that you recognize or feel that something should change in your life. The professor system using its assistants, suppression and projection, tries in conjunction with the dwarf technique to prevent changes. This is why you should become acquainted with these inner defense mechanisms.

Just knowing about these mechanisms will help you to recognize them in others first, and then to quickly recognize them in yourself. When you are successful in recognizing defense mechanisms in yourself, then you have taken the greatest step possible toward positive change. So during the next coffee break with your friends or when smoking a cigarette with your colleagues, start listening more closely to what they are telling you. Do not interrupt. Just listen, and try to determine when someone is playing the professor.

I know what I want!

"That is one of my littlest exercises" you might say. I just want to be healthier, richer, thinner, funnier, more successful, and more attractive, and then I will be the happiest person in the world. Question: "Is Bill Gates the happiest man in the world, although he can't take three steps without bodyguards?" Or perhaps Naomi Campbell, who apparently attempted suicide? Both of these people are attractive, rich, and envied (even if the first attribute may not be applicable for Bill Gates).

In the following pages I would like to share different techniques that will help you find out what you really want in order to enjoy a happier life, in a way that is better, easier, and more certain. All of these techniques have one thing in common. They should become constant companions to you, because changes take time. You cannot resolve deep childhood anchoring just by walking over burning coals for 3 seconds, or briefly confronting a different fear. Changes require time, often a lot of time, this is why you should start today and become clear on what you want to change.

Before we deal with the various techniques, I would like to ask you to clearly define what you do not want to change. For example take two minutes at the most and spontaneously write down three things you like about yourself, and three things that other people like about you.

What I like about myself:

1_____

2_____

3_____

What others like about me:

1_____

2_____

3_____

Many years ago I applied for a job at a psychoanalytical hospital in Stuttgart. I still remember my interview very well with Dr. Theodor Seifert, one of the best-known psychoanalysts in Europe and author of many specialized books. Neither my references nor the positive result of my first interview in the clinic (which he did not participate in due to vacation), impressed him. The second question he asked me was, what were my strengths, and why it would be good for him to work together with me? Because I was aware of my strengths, and because I could clearly express them, it was also possible for me to convince him that it would be positive for him to work together with me. I got the job and for three years I had the privilege of working with a man who had a wonderful way of making the people around him feed good.

This is why I want to motivate you to first be aware of your strengths. If you have not spontaneously written down 6 of your strengths, then it is certainly not because you do not possess these strengths, but rather it is because you, like a lot of other people, would prefer to deal with your weaknesses. You believe that if you can just become familiar with these weaknesses then changes will also be possible. However I would like introduce you to your strengths first, because you will thus determine that you have far less to change in order to lead a happier life, than you have previously thought. Please use the following technique to identify these strengths:

The Jefferson technique

According to Thomas Jefferson,
author of the American Declaration of Independence

A simple and successful technique. I would like to invite you to try out the following thoughts of independence. Imagine the following situation:

- You do not have a boss.

- Your parents have been living in Australia for 10 years.

- You are not married, you live alone, and do not have any children.

- Regardless of what you do for work you will always earn 10,000.00 Euros per month.

And now answer the following questions as spontaneously as possible:

What would you do for work?

_____

Would you move to a different country, or live in a different city?

_____

Would you prefer to live alone, with a partner or with children?

_____

What would you buy first?

_____

Would you be capable of falling in love?

_____

And now I would like to show you a way to become better acquainted with your yet unconscious strengths, by using the answers to these questions. The analysis of your answers is quite simple. Regardless of which change you imagine, it will show you how you can better develop yourself if you promote precisely these strengths in the future.

One example. You are a banker and you have answered the questions as follows:

Work:	As an alpine guide and ski instructor
Live:	In the Alps or Austria
Life:	Wife and children
Purchase:	House and garden
Love:	Yes

Now please write down next to Alpine guide/ski instructor, all the attributes that are required for this job, such as:

Alpine guide/ski instructor: Discipline, precise work, enjoy speaking with other people, leading other people, and instructing them, love of nature, excellent physical fitness.

Now consider your present profession. You believe that being an Alpine guide has nothing to do with the job description of a banker. On the contrary. As a bank employee you also require discipline and your work must be precise. To enjoy speaking with other people is even a prerequisite. The ability to lead other people will be required the first time you are promoted. Good physical fitness is likewise recommended, since as an employee you cannot do anything to stay fit during work. Precisely for this reason you should be looking for a physical balance. The only thing on the list that you certainly do not require for your profession is love of nature. In this case you must determine for yourself how important this point is for you. If proximity to nature is important for you, then there are outstanding banks in Oberstdorf or Geneva that are looking for employees like you. Thus you could fulfill your second wish at the same time, namely living in the Alps or in Austria.

You are married and have children. This is precisely what you wrote down under the Life category. Then you are the happiest person in the world. **No?** Then why not? Is it perhaps because you are not always conscious of your good fortune? In the course of my life, I have met many people who objectively lacked for nothing. They had a career, a family, and they were healthy. Nevertheless they did not consider themselves to be the happiest people in the world. Then they were hit with a catastrophe. They became sick with cancer, they lost their wife/child, or they were confronted with some other profoundly negative thing. You can probably guess what happened then. The priorities in their life suddenly shifted by 180 degrees. For a cancer patient the career that was previously so important slipped suddenly from top of the list to position 300. His health suddenly shot to the top of the list, with his family in the number 2 position. This same shift in values also occurs in older people. What is really interesting here are the common denominators.

They are always the same: Health, family, and friends.

We can learn a lot from these people, because usually in our younger years we believe our happiness depends on external circumstances. But we already have everything we need to be happy today. Nobody can stop us from saying that today is the happiest day of our life. If you have a family then that is just one more reason to be the happiest person in the world. Be honest, when was the last time that you sat comfortably in a chair, and looked at your wife/your husband/your children and were aware that this is the greatest happiness that can be given to a person on earth?

Start taking a closer look at what you already have. Striving for more and more obstructs our view of the existing beautiful aspects of our life. You cannot look to the right with one eye and look to the left with the other eye.

An old monk was once asked by his student, how long it would take to learn the monk's teachings if he (the student) studied for 12 hours a day. The monk replied: 10 years. Then the student asked how long it would take if he studied for 16 hours a day. The monk replied: 20 years. Naturally the student was astonished, as he had expected the period to be shorter. But if we forget to look inside ourselves, and if we cannot enjoy the things around us, we will certainly not find them anywhere else, even if we spend 16 hours a day looking for them.

This little story illustrates that striving for more does not automatically mean that we will also get more in return. But let's go back to your answers. Under Purchase you wrote down a house and garden. This is the dream of every Swabian and the dream of a lot of other people as well. But what does this wish tell us? Regardless of whatever wish you wrote down, write down why you want this wish, below it.

- I would like to have my own home so that there is more

  space between me and my current neighbors.

- I would like to be able to impress my friends and enemies.

- I want to see my children play in the garden.

- I want to have a capital asset.

Then write down how you want to satisfy these wishes until they are fulfilled.

- I would like to have my own home so that there is more space between me and my current neighbors. Perhaps I will invite my neighbors over for a cup of coffee?

- I would like to be able to impress my friends and enemies. Be honest, do you really   need to impress your friends and enemies? Is this really all that fun?

- I want to see my children play in the garden. I can play with my children anywhere. Just spending more time with them is much more important to my children, than a nice garden.

- I want to have a capital asset. I am a banker. There are plenty of capital assets.

- _____

You answered the last question, as to whether you could fall in love again, with a clear yes. You did not say probably, perhaps, or even a definitive no. Become aware that you have the capability to acquire the greatest gift humanity has to offer. Love.

Are you in love now? Are you loved? Do you love one task above everything else? The truth in the biblical passage: "It is more blessed to give than to receive", is most manifest in love. Many people know what their partner desires better than they know what they desire. Whatever they would love to do for themselves comes as a secondary consideration. Is it more interesting for you to buy gifts for other people than it is to buy things for yourself? Do you know why? It is because you are spending less time finding out what you yourself love, or what you need for your own happiness. This is one of the high-priority teachings of Christian churches: "It is more blessed to give than to receive." We all grow up with this scripture, it is communicated to us consciously and unconsciously thousands of times.

"Love thy neighbor as thyself", is the biblical response to "It is more blessed to give than to receive". Only he who has come to know himself empathize with other people. This includes identifying your own weaknesses **and** strengths. This is why it is so important to first be conscious of your strengths. Unfortunately many people are more strongly conscious of their weaknesses than they are of their strengths.

Strengthen your strengths and your weaknesses will become weaker.

When you know what you would most like to do in life, then you have taken the first step toward getting to know your strengths. Intensify the Jefferson technique. Do it often and correct your path if necessary. Maybe today you are a secretary but you would rather write books. Or today you manage a trading company but rather would rather be an aid worker in developing countries. Just the fact that you know you would rather be an author than a secretary shows that you enjoy being creative (discovering stories).

To know you would like to help unknown people in a foreign country proves that you are capable of obtaining everything that you require for your life from the joy of others. Would you rather live in a different city or in a different country? What's really preventing you from going there? Are you happy where you are now? When was the last time that you were really conscious of this? So conscious of the fact that you could really get quite happy about it?

The question, of what you would buy first reveals more than just your material desires. The answer can show you much more. Is it something that just makes you happy? Or is it something that also makes other people happy, or is it something to impress other people, such as the coveted Porsche, or the Rolex watch. Is it a luxury item, or is it simply something you need at this time? Your answer will help you not only to identify **what** you desire, but on closer consideration it also will help you to identify **why** you want it. In addition this "why" will strengthen a different capability: Your empathetic intelligence, or in other words, your ability to put yourself in other's shoes.

Our dogmas and how we get rid of them

Dogmas, idiosyncrasies, habits, what we inherited, etc. these are all words for "programs/anchorings" in ourselves that we have taken over from other people, or that we have so embodied for ourselves, because we understood it that way at the time. We all have our own dogmas, and first you should understand that this fact is neither positive nor negative. But when we are seriously ill, we should deal with this subject, as dogmas can really "restrict" us. If you have the opportunity of working with a kinesiologist, then take advantage of it because kinesiology can be effective here.

But how do we determine which dogmas our brain has stored? Which dogmas confine us, and which dogmas help us to lead a happy life? On the following pages I would like offer some possibilities of how you can find this out, so that you can better work on redefining these dogmas. Naturally I am aware that for many people this represents a lot of work, the kind of work that is better undertaken with a trained therapist. On the other hand all too often I experience that people do not always (want to) go to a therapist regardless of the reason. Consequently I consider it better if you at least start to bring about changes, even if the process would be a lot better with a therapist. Please take sufficient time for this, it is well worth the effort.

The Pasttoda exercise
On the following five pages list the 5 most important people in your life. These could be your parents, your grandparents, your brothers and sisters, but also teachers or close friends. Decide who was important for you. Please note that it does not matter how much you loved these people, or how often you were with them, what matters is how significantly they have influenced your life. Then list what was important to these people in their life (career, marriage, sport, hobby etc.) in the

491

individual lines, list their guiding principles ("whoever strives will achieve", "Fortune favors the industrious", "I want you to have what I did not have", etc.) and then write down whether these people remained true to their principles. Many therapists forget this point. But it is very important, because children know at an early stage, whether people live what they profess. If this is not the case then they go into inner opposition and imprint the opposite of what they have heard. Thus it may be that an individual had parents who were very strict, and then he raises his children in an anti-authoritarian manner that is extremely negative. In this case **oppositional** anchoring occurred quite early on and they were lived out by the individual, or they were lived out jointly with the next generation.

I cannot overemphasize the importance of the Pasttoda exercise. It is the beginning of your change and it will help you instigate major changes in a short time. Do not simply skip over the exercise, keep going until all five pages have been filled out.

1. Person: _____

The important things for this person were"

_____

_____

_____

His/her guiding principles were:

_____

_____

_____

The following guiding principles **were not** lived:

_____

_____

2. Person: _____

The important things for this person were"

_____

_____

_____

His/her guiding principles were:

_____

_____

_____

The following guiding principles **were not** lived:

_____

_____

3.Person: _____

The important things for this person were"

_____

_____

_____

His/her guiding principles were:

_____

_____

_____

The following guiding principles **were not** lived:

_____

_____

4. Person: _____

The important things for this person were"

_____

_____

_____

His/her guiding principles were:

_____

_____

_____

The following guiding principles **were not** lived:

_____

_____

5. Person: _____

The important things for this person were"

_____

_____

_____

His/her guiding principles were:

_____

_____

_____

The following guiding principles **were not** lived:

_____

_____

The sandbox exercise

When you relax and think back on your youth, then it is likely that many stories and anecdotes will come to mind. Nevertheless we are all often blocked and either cannot, or do not want to, remember a lot of things. Nevertheless we can decide now and immediately to view the events from our past, which we can still remember, differently than we did previously. In order to do this, we must know how we evaluated our behavior years ago, and the next exercise helps us with this.

Talk to yourself as you were when you were 5, 10, and 15 years old. You will be amazed at what you can still recall. Imagine a situation where you meet yourself. Sit down in the sandbox with the young boy or girl (yourself) and talk seriously about the things that are important for that child (you) or about the challenges that child is facing at the moment. Take enough time for this exercise, and ensure that you are not disturbed while you are doing this.

Directly after the session write down what was important to the child (you) at that time, in key words. Then take time to reflect on the question of whether you view that which was important at that time, from a different perspective. Permit me to illustrate this with two examples from my own evaluation.

1. I remember very well that when I was approximately 10 years old the movie King Kong was being shown on TV at about 10:00 PM. Everybody in my class at school was talking about it and every one of my friends said that he would watch the movie that night. On this same evening my mother was having a voice lesson and returned at about 10:15 PM. For me this meant that my brothers and sisters would let me watch King Kong for 10 minutes and then I would have to go to bed before my mother returned.

What I remember very well were the words of my mother that this kind of movie "is not for children", and I was mad at my mother for days because of this. Today I make the same decisions for my children, and I understand my mother's view very well; naturally I "forgave" her a long time ago for this. This forgiveness is only possible when one reconsiders the "old stories" with a new understanding. This is why it is very important to consistently revisit **what** I decided and **when,** and to ask myself whether this decision still applies today. However for this I must first know what I decided and when, and the exercises in this book will help you.

After working with patients for more than 10 years in psychiatric care facilities and psychoanalytical clinics, I well understand that dogmas often cannot be changed because it is so incredibly difficult to remember them. For example when working with anorexics I experienced more than once that the source of the addiction was serious physical or emotional abuse. For this reason I also tend to bring cancer patients together with professional helpers. But I have stated several times in this book that I am a realist, and naturally I know that far too many cancer patients are not capable of getting professional help, either for personal reasons, or for purely financial reasons.

So use this book as a workbook. As a cancer patient you cannot just read this book. If there is one thing that I know it is this: The great difference between people who survive and those who must die is that the survivors actively work on themselves, and this includes working on their psyche. Because it is so important: This has absolutely nothing to do with cancer patients "not being in order" psychologically. What is involved here is allowing yourself to be helped to become a healthier and a happier person. Please tell me what is not worthwhile here? The Pope and the Dalai Lama take on this task daily. Why can't we do it as well?

5 years

What was important to me then:

How I assess this today:

10 years

What was important to me then:

How I assess this today:

15 years

What was important to me then:

How I assess this today:

After you have done both exercises, please write down the guiding principles that determine your life today, and write down the guiding principles you believe you should change. Later if you make a tumor contract with yourself (see Tumor contract) then you can use everything that you write down now.

The following guiding principles determine my life today:

I will rethink the following guiding principles:

Another thought for all those who believe they do not have to work on their guiding principles.

I have met many alcoholics in the course of my life who told me that alcoholism is the best thing that ever happened to them. The same applies to cancer patients. Many cancer patients have told me that they never would have had the courage or the pressure to change their live positively, without the tumor. I do not want to discuss these sentences in more detail, because there are many pros and cons here. But one point seems important to me. Even if you are quite happy with your life, except for the tumor, what's wrong with working on even greater happiness in life. No matter how you live. The fact is that it is precisely this life, which has contributed to your present confrontation with cancer.

The worse thing that you could do now would be to keep living the way you used to live. It doesn't work without changes. But please do not make the same mistake again and believe that you already know what you must change, without spending some time thinking about it. Perhaps you have climbed a ladder and only realize that it was the wrong ladder, when you reach the top.

Or in other words: Take the necessary time to obtain the awareness of **what** you must change. If not now – then when?

504

The problem with our language

I know what I want also means sharing these desires with other people. However our western upbringing has developed a language over last two thousand years that I call, watch-out language. We have all been confronted with this language thousands of times, and we encounter it every day anew. The mistaken notion associated with watch-out language is that many adults still believe that negative inputs to other people, primarily children, will have the same effect as positive inputs.

The reporting methods in the media offer one example. The more humdrum the material the greater the chance it has of being broadcast. Apparently the view is firmly planted in the heads of those responsible for programming throughout the world that we are all still interested in seeing something curious, unusual and base. In this case as well, a sick person must ask himself, whether he really wants to spend his valuable time in this manner.

Programming directors have also learned to speak in a negative manner from their parents and teachers. One would have thought that educators in particular, would have learned a different, more positive language during their studies. Not by a long shot. My experiences unfortunately have caused me to take a different view. This is not a general attack on educators. It just shows that communicating content is still more important than the manner in which the content is communicated.

Here are a few examples that are probably not unfamiliar to you:

Watch-out language We say:	Positive input It would be better to say:
Don't run so fast!	Please walk slowly.
It will soon be dark and if you don't get into the house right now the boogie man will get you.	I am worried, when you are outside and it gets dark.
Don't come to my house any more	I am mad at you and want to speak with you.
If you don't do your homework then you may not play soccer tomorrow.	If you do your home-work now then we will play soccer tomorrow.
Don't be afraid!	We will walk slowly over the bridge and I will hold you tight.

Most people including me had parents and have parents who often used watch-out language instead of giving their children positive inputs. Don't fall victim to this error and believe there is no difference if I say: "Don't run so fast or whether: I say, "Please walk more slowly". In the first statement your child hears the word run combined with a negative input, and in the second statement the child hears the word slowly combined with a positive input. The following example demonstrates how stubborn negative inputs can be: Let's say I promise you that I already know the lottery numbers for the next drawing, and that I will share these numbers with you under the following conditions:

1.) You must eat an entire strawberry cake on Saturday 15 minutes before the official drawing.

2.) Prior to this you must play monopoly non-stop for 10 hours.

3.) While the lucky numbers are being drawn, you may **not** think of a crocodile.

I am convinced that you could eat a strawberry cake, and that you could play monopoly for 10 hours, but even though I have told you that you should not think of a crocodile, it is absolutely certain that this is precisely what you will do. The same thing happens when you give negative inputs to your children, or others close to you, instead of communicating to them what you want. That which we get, is highly dependent on how we say it. Always say what you want, not what you don't want.

From my own experience I know that this switchover can occur relatively quickly. Start today and monitor how you say something. Correct yourself when you notice it. Say the sentence again with a positive input. Do not get frustrated when you find yourself giving negative inputs at the beginning. I have two very lively sons and I often find myself giving them negative inputs, even if this only occurs on rare occasions.

Here are some statements that will show you how the watch-out method can determine your whole life. In these examples I have added another input – the non-verbal input, which strongly influences our behavior. Children particularly often think of what they should be like in order to be loved by their parents (grown-ups). Consequently children sometimes interpret words completely differently than they were originally spoken. Often however they also perceive the non-verbal input to be something other than what it really is. A message that we want to communicate to others, but which we do not trust ourselves to say out loud. However non-verbal inputs do not stop when we become adults.

Here are a few examples:

Watch-out language We say:	Positive input It would be better to say:	Non-verbal input Accompanying thoughts:
Doctors are good people.	I would really be happy if you studied medicine	I would be happy to tell many people that my son is a doctor.
Be glad that you have a job, given the present unemploymentsituation.	My experience has shown that it is better to accept a job, that is not quite to your liking than it is to be unemployed.	I would be even more of a failure if you get a job that you enjoy, as I never managed to do this.
Oh the things that I have done for you and given up for you.	Because your welfare was so important to me, I consciously put my needs on the back burner.	As soon as you are old enough, I want retribution from you.

In all these examples we can see that we are the product of these parental recommendations. Here the word parental should not to be taken literally, since these recommendations, which are anchored in us, could also have been spoken by other people. Please regard these parental recommendations for what they really are: as **recommendations**. Let's assume you have a twin brother and that he received the identical recommendations you received, this still doesn't mean that you both develop the same personality. Regardless of how many positive or negative inputs you have received in past years, all of these inputs have one thing in common: You can correct them!

But we don't just receive recommendations. We also give them out. This is why we must learn to be more careful with our language, because words create emotions, and emotions cause reactions. We can become victims or perpetrators through our words. If I say: "I think you're cool" it induces happiness in you. If I say: "I think you're strange", it induces irritation in you. If I say: "You make me sick", then most likely it would induce anger in you.

You see, if you are not aware of your strengths then you can easily be influenced by the people around you. However we can also consciously influence others, both in the positive sense and in the negative sense. We only want to deal with the positive sense here, and I would like to demonstrate how you can use words to influence yourself positively. It is significantly more pleasant for the person with whom you are conversing, if you say: "Mr. Miller saves a lot of work energy" instead of saying, "Mr. Miller is lazy", or instead of saying: "I am totally frustrated", simply think, "I find it a challenge that..." Try to replace the words in the left column with the words in the right column.

For example:

bad/terrible	interesting
hate	ignorance
deception	dishonesty
Nauseating	unusual
angry	not enchanted
fearful	somewhat uneasy / curious
disturbed	took a backwards a step
embarrassing	stimulating
tired	recharging
fear	wonder
frustrated	challenged/fascinated
injured	surprised
I hate	I prefer

insecure	questioning
have been insulted	have been misunderstood
jealous	love too much
lazy	energy saving
lonely	temporarily centered on myself
lost	searching
nervous	charged up
painful	uncomfortable
rejected	misunderstood
sad	ordering my thoughts

Basically look for new, positive, and intense words. Words that give a designation, that motivate you and other people, and which allow energy to flow to you. Consequently use words like: fascinated, enthused, excited, fantastic, extremely well, superb, unbelievably good, enchanted, phenomenal, loved, passionately, perfect, totally concentrated, explosive, gifted, unconquerable.

You can deepen the communication with focused questions and by analyzing the statements without value judgments. The conversation takes a completely different direction when you ask: "What can I learn from the fact that this thing has gone wrong", instead of: "Why did that have to go wrong again?" This aspect is very important if you have cancer, because it is the only way to achieve a state where you do not have to get upset about this or that, which blocks the flow of your energy, and this energy flow is very important for your healing.

Now that I have explained why it is so important to recognize your strengths, I would like to show you some techniques you can use to find out what you should change in your life in order to achieve your desired goals.

The balance-sheet technique

Just as it is usual for most companies to draw-up a balance-sheet at the start of a new year, I would also invite you to draw-up a balance-sheet of life. Prepare a profit/loss statement just as you would in a company. The difference is that for us there is no profit and no loss, since our entire life is profit, our calculation is a calculation of desire and profitability.

On the next page write down everything that was fun for you in life to this point, all that is currently fun for you, and all that you believe would be fun for you, even if you have never tried it. I request that you write down at least 10 situations that are fun for you. Do not stop until at least 10 lines have been filled in.

If it is difficult for you to fill these lines, then this is not because you are unaware of at least 10 situations that are fun for you, rather it is because you do not want to think of 10 desirable things. There may be several reasons for this. A lack of self-esteem, depressive moods, self-pity or a "the whole world is bad, mood" to cite just a few. **Stop these thoughts immediately** for at least 3 minutes and fill the next page with life.

Even if an inner voice tells you: "He's crazy" or "He should talk, I'm the one who is doing poorly", I would still like to tell you that there is nobody in the world who prohibit you from writing ten situations that have been fun for you, that you believe would be fun for you.

You can write, you can remember, and you can do it. OK, let's get going, do it now, immediately!

My daily work

1 _____

2 _____

3 _____

4 _____

5 _____

6 _____

7 _____

8 _____

9 _____

10 _____

Can't life be incredibly fun? Before you continue reading I would like to ask you to re-read your own words. Just read them again. Because it incredibly worthwhile on your path health, to know what is fun for you in life. I have placed the whole desire-page in one frame and have entitled it: *My daily work*, so that you are daily reminded of what you must really "work" at. I would like you to copy these pages and place them or hang them up where you can see them everyday. It would be even better if you could frame them and ensure that you "check-off" at least one point everyday. Please, never forget that we are not here on earth to be sad. And never forget that what is perhaps even more important for you: **your immune system will thank you for it!**

The next step in our desire and necessity calculation requires more effort, and in our business metaphor, this step is more comparable to collecting all the necessary documents for a corporate audit. The next page contains 3 columns. In the left column write down what you often do, which is no fun at all, however you do it anyway because you consider it to be necessary. In the middle column write down the advantage of this behavior. For instance in the left column you could have: "I go to work every day; it is a type of work that I do not particularly enjoy."

In the middle column: "My salary is actually OK. I have friends in the company that I would miss. Often I get to know interesting people through my job."

In the right column write down a number between 1 and 10. 1 means that you can live reasonably with this necessity, even if you should not be successful in pushing through important changes in the company, such as finally telling your boss what could be done to make your work more enjoyable.

The number 10 means that this necessity causes you a lot of stress and you only bear it because the advantages in the middle column are much, much, more important. You determine whether the item deserves 1, a 5, or a 10. Experience has shown that it usually takes longer to fill-out the middle column, because it is often not so easy to identify advantages associated with unpaid overtime, for example. However there are two reasons why it is worthwhile to take the time to do this.

First, with more precise consideration you will recognize many advantages that are very frequently and much too quickly forgotten, and second, learning to take something positive from those situations which on first glance only invoke negative thoughts, is an incredibly good exercise.

No desire in	The advantage	Evaluation

The balance sheet analysis that we do for ourselves is comparable to the balance sheet discussion with the tax consultant. The advantage is that you require neither a tax consultant nor an analyst. Quietly consider your numbers in the third column; take a marker and highlight all the numbers greater than 5. Now it is up to you to ensure that you either refrain from doing these things in the future or that you have somebody else do them for you.

Many people have told me that the balance-sheet technique has made their life a lot easier. If you use it often and develop a certain routine with this technique, then you will either keep both feet on the ground, or you will get both feet on the ground, and that which earlier piled up to be such a gigantic problem will suddenly collapse into its individual pieces. This makes the problem easier to understand and it is much, much, easier to deal with.

Cancer patients, in particular, do not have "just" the tumor problem to deal with, but many others as well. Consequently it is important here to be rational and to deal rationally. However this is not easy because the emotional involvement is very high. The balance sheet technique is ideal for cancer patients for precisely this reason, to prevent the forest from one day becoming obscured by the trees.

The tumor contract

Similar to the one-man Inc. now make a tumor contract with yourself. A contract between the person you are today, and the person you will be in 12 months. This may seem a ridiculous notion, to make a contract with yourself. But to be honest, haven't you done a lot of things in your life that are crazier than making a contract with yourself?

Before you sign this contract, talk to your tumor, after all it is part of you. Explain to it that its growth involves the risk that you will die, and this means that it also will die. Make this point clear to your tumor, and suggest to your tumor, that instead enter into an agreement that represents a benefit to both parties. The contract consists of just 3 paragraphs, and in the preamble of the contract you undertake to change the points that you list under paragraph 2, within the next three months.

Before signing the contract review your balance sheet, the Jefferson test and your desire list. Together they will help you identify what you really want to achieve in your life. Please take this contract very seriously and comply with it 100%. This is very important, otherwise your tumor will not keep its part of the contract either.

In recent years I have had extremely positive experiences with this contract, and the more I work with it, the better I understand the ingenious processes that occur in a person when he makes such a contract with the requisite **seriousness**. Consider: How is possible for a tumor to continue to grow? **You** yourself are the tumor! You are the person who determines what happens with your body, both in the negative as well the positive sense. Your tumor is only capable of continued growth, if you believe that some "bad" uncoupled cells inside you lead their own life.

My hope is I am able to some extent to explain to you in this book that tumors are not a second ego. They are a part of you, a part of you which for whatever reason, has been severely neglected. It's kind of like the situation in a large family, where one member "goes under", because he did not get enough attention. The tumor does the same thing. It creates its own attention through its "singular" growth.

Below you will find a sample contract which you should only fill out, when you have completely read this book and have slept on it for at least one night. The contract is very important and you require time for it!

3E Tumor Contract®

The following is agreed between

Tumor 1 and all distant metastases or cell changes
(hereinafter TUMOR)

and

_____

_____

(hereinafter CONTRACT PARTNER)

Preamble

Both parties obligate themselves to conclude a contract which stipulates in detail what each party will undertake so that they jointly can grow older in health and happiness.

§ 1

TUMOR warrants that it will become microscopically so small that CONTRACT PARTNER will no longer be consciously aware of it, or that other disorders are not caused by TUMOR.

§ 2

CONTRACT PARTNER obligates himself to execute the following changes in his life:

Starting today he will:

_____

_____

_____

In the next 14 days he will:

_____

_____

_____

In the next 3 months he will:

_____

_____

_____

§ 3 Severability Clause

Should compliance with for one or another of the provisions of this contract become impossible – for reasons beyond the control of either party – then the contract will still remain in force and both parties will look for a solution which most nearly approaches the original intent. This contract will be analyzed after 3 months at the latest, and it will be extended for an additional 3 months. These extensions will take place for at least 10 years and cannot be cancelled by either partner.

Date: _____

_____   _____
Signature TUMOR   Signature CONTRACT
                              PARTNER

The middle way technique

In the Benares sermon Buddha said: The enlightened one does not seek his salvation in self-mortification, nor does he look for it in a life of excess or self-indulgence. The enlightened one has found the middle way.

I cannot promise you enlightenment, but with application of the middle way, I can put a tool in your hand that will help you to make decisions of any kind more easily, and with more confidence. Moreover it is a tool that will allow you to bring your blood pressure down to a bearable level within seconds. In the future you will be able to make clear decisions without negative influences due to anger, or excitement. It is based on making decisions, within a few seconds and after mature, but nonetheless rapid consideration of extremes. The middle way technique developed by and Klaus Pertl and myself consists of three parts, or to be more precise, it consists of three successive thoughts.

1.   The question: "What will happen if everything goes wrong, and what will happen if everything runs optimally?"

2.   The Yin Yang symbol.

3.   The sentence: "God grant me the serenity to accept the things I cannot change, the courage to change the things I can, and the wisdom to know the difference."

This may seem to quite a lot at one time. Not by a long shot. Your brain is capable of performing thousands of actions in fractions of a second. What are three thoughts? Permit me to first explain the individual thoughts in more detail.

1. What will happen if everything goes wrong, and what will happen if everything goes optimally?
How often have you asked yourself this question? Not very often? That's too bad. Because it has an incredibly calming effect. Depending on the level of optimism or pessimism you take with you through life, you have often asked yourself a part of the question. "What will happen if everything goes wrong?", or you have only dreamed: "If everything goes positive then…". However there is nothing in the world that has one end only. This is why you must start taking both parts of the whole into consideration at the same time. Think about a line. Regardless of what you are thinking about, are agitated about, or what you must decide on. Think of an imaginary line, and think of your problem sitting precisely in the middle of the line.

Problem

―――――――――――――――――――――――――――――――――

Now imagine everything negative that you can think of on the left side of the line and everything positive on the right side line.

Negative   Problem   Positive

―――――――――――――――――――――――――――――――――

Be honest, how often have you done something unpleasant or put up with something unpleasant and have done it only out of the fear of penalties. If you have fear, or if you must bear something unpleasant, then first ask yourself what is the worst that can happen, if for instance you get a divorce, lose your job, make a fool of yourself, blush, stutter, are late, etc. You will quickly see that there is nothing that you cannot overcome. The question however does not just consist of: "What is the worse that could happen?", but rather the question has two parts, because the second part of the question is; "What will happen if everything goes 100% positive, simply goes optimally?".

Why? Because we undertake many things in life that are not nearly as positive as we imagine them to be. Haven't you ever said or thought, "And what did I get for doing that…!" Or haven't you fantasized something incredibly wonderful, and the reality turned out to be only half as nice. The possibility of leaving the real life behind is very high at both ends. Think of the rose colored glasses that lovers wear, or think of people who when they hear the words vacation and Dominican Republic, can only imagine plane crash and cockroaches.

Regardless of which fear is involved, regardless of which decision you must make, looking at both sides of the line brings you to the real middle, within seconds, and it is only from this point that you can make conscious decisions. By the way looking at both ends usually takes only a few seconds. You have certainly heard religious people say how important it is to find the center. Find your center as well, and start building the middle way technique into your life.

Let's take the example that you are afraid of losing your job. Perhaps spontaneous thoughts come to mind like: "How will I pay my rent next month – the next mortgage payment is due – what will my friends/parents/partner say – can I maintain my current standard of living – what a problem what will I do with myself all day long?"
However the following sentences also come to mind: "Finally, time for me and my family – Maybe I will finally dare to be retrained – Finally, I have a reason to visit my friend in Italy

– This is a real chance for a new career (or a private new beginning) – I never have to get upset about my colleague Mayer again, my goodness that's nice – Now I can take the time to figure out how much more money I can make than I before", and never forget: The wonderful *Harry Potter* books would never have been written if J. K. Rowling had not become unemployed.

We can only make real positive decisions when we consult both brain halves. But unfortunately in school we were only taught to think with the left brain (our rational) brain hemisphere and consequently we should not be surprised if the things that we associate with the subject of unemployment are almost exclusively negative. But it is up to us to learn how we can use our right (creative) brain hemisphere again, and this is where this exercise helps a lot.

2. Yin Yang

The second thought of the middle way technique is not a sentence, but rather visualizing the Yin Yang symbol.

It will be known to many readers. It describes the opposites in life and their interdependence. No health without illness, no wealth without poverty, no darkness without light. Yang describes the creative masculine and spiritual principle, while Yin stands for the feminine, nocturnal, and receiving principle. This symbol is important for our middle way technique because its presence it shows us that everything in life has advantages and disadvantages. There is never just the one. Always remember this, because it will bring you back to your center, regardless of where you are. If you are really sad then it will help you to feel joy again, because it tells you that there is a reason why you are so sad. A reason that you simply cannot understand at the present moment.

If you are doing really well, then it helps you remember that it has not always gone so well for you, or that other people are not as happy as you are. If we draw it with the arrow symbol, then the forces of Yin and Yang both tend towards our center.

Often people with cancer cannot discover any Yin in the Yang, because they believe that cancer is something that is fundamentally and exclusively negative. But then they hit on the idea that now they have "an excuse" to do this or that. Or they meet with other cancer patients and suddenly they hear things like; "My tumor was the best thing that ever happened to me in my life", and they begin to understand that the coin always has another side.

Yin   Yang

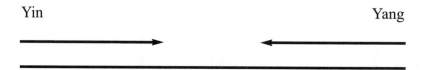

Does it often seem to you that traffic lights always turn red when you are about 30 feet away from them. Don't get upset. Be happy and think of Yin and Yang. You would probably been in an accident, or you would not have met your dream partner just because you arrived a minute too soon. Regardless of how upset you are, regardless of how sad you are. The knowledge that everything negative contains a positive aspect, and vise versa, always makes your life easier, and it will be a constant companion to you. Let **Yin** and **Yang** be your friends as well. They can not only move vexations out of your way, They can help you to not get depressed, or they can help you out of a depression. "Why me?", or "Why does this have to happen to me?" It is precisely at this point, when you no longer know what to do, your friends are at your side and give you the assurance that there is something positive behind these questions, which you just do not understand at this moment.

Don't forget your friends **Yin** and **Yang** the next time you are upset, or sad, or disappointed. They will help you see difficult moments in a new light.

3. God grant me the serenity to accept the things I cannot change, the courage to change the things I can, and the wisdom to know the difference.

This sentence originates from the work of Alcoholics Anonymous. Particularly the first part "God give me the serenity to accept what cannot be changed" will help you to see things more clearly, and to consider them from a different point of view. The word serenity alone has a very calming effect. The insight that it is easily possible to react with serenity to things that you cannot change, will give you an inner peace, which today may still seem impossible to imagine.

It is likely that you have also gotten upset about things that were 100% unchangeable, or that you have criticized yourself, although we certainly know that self-criticism always comes too late. This precisely where the word serenity can help you. If you get upset, then take a good look at the situation, and consider whether it can be changed or not. If not then is there any reason to get upset about it? The answer is clearly no! Unfortunately our genes play a bad trick on us at this point, because they still believe that they must increase our blood pressure, even due to little things, and put our whole body a state of alarm readiness, as in the cavemen days of the Neanderthals. Be aware that increased blood pressure prevents you from making decisions. And clear decisions are precisely what you need when you start to get upset.

An example. You are driving through town in your car. Someone rear ends you because he was driving too fast. What is your attitude when you get of the car? Just like Mr. Example: "We are lucky that nothing happened to us. Do you realize that we might have both been injured just because you were driving too fast?" The awareness that this accident cannot be undone helps you to react with serenity. A different example. Years ago a women hit my car door while she was backing up. I was with my wife at the outdoor market, and as we returned, the woman who caused the accident was very nervous. I asked her for her address, wrote down her license plate number, or insurance number and said good-by to her. A few seconds later she turned around and asked me if that was all. I said yes and wanted to drive away, but she spoke to me again and thanked me that I did not yell at her, and she said that it was hard for her to understand why I was still so calm.

However daily life is quite different. Who does not know a person who always curses other drivers when they are driving? Or have you yourself recently made an obscene gesture to another driver and got upset about a traffic jam on the freeway? Or how do you react to the gravy stain on your new dress? How do you react to the glass that your son lets fall on the ground or the F that your daughter gets in Geography?

All these examples have one thing in common. They obey the law of entropy and they can no longer be undone. Only if you do not get upset, can you calmly analyze and decide whether you can avoid these things in the future (the F grade) or not (getting rear-ended). Each idividual element of the middle road technique helps you to make clear decisions, to find out what you want, and particularly to simplify your life with the realization that you no longer have to get so upset. Combined however they are unbeatable. In their unity they can cover all areas of life completely. To start with, just note the following formula:

Irritation = Middle way + Yin Yang + tranquility

Practice it daily. Use any little thing. The toothpaste tube that your partner squeezes at the wrong place, your husband who reads the newspaper at breakfast, your wife's incapability to decide on a new dress, your children fidgeting at lunch, the traffic jam on the freeway, your overbearing boss, etc. Every day there are plenty of possibilities on your way to a healthy and fulfilled life.

Visualization

Visualization is perhaps the most important "single instrument" for moving your life in the direction that you would like it to go. It may be that today that this concept does not mean much to you, but I hope that by the end of this book you will understand that it is primarily visions that will make you better.

Everything around us was a vision at first. The glass that you are drinking out of, just like the house in which you live. Long before a house is built, there is the idea of building a house, and then the mental implementation, in the form of construction plans. Our entire life always runs on the rails of time and can never be turned back.

Past   Future

Please be aware of this. Everything around you was first a thought, an energy, a wave. It is very important to understand this, it is the only way to understand that energies generate matter. Just think of a hypnotist who can make you believe that the coin in your hand is hot, and then your skin gets red, in fact you can even get a blister. In this case existing matter is changed through thought alone. Would your skin have gotten red if you had imagined that you were holding a normal cold coin in your hand?

If your response is: Naturally not, then you have understood that the right thought can change the matter in your body within seconds. Why shouldn't this also be the case with a tumor? For many years visualization trainers like Carl

Simonton have been pursuing this question. I highly esteem his work (with a few limitations). In multiple studies Carl Simonton has demonstrated (just as has Lawrence LeShan, Bernie Siegel, or Andrew Weill), that some cancer patients live twice as long when they apply visualization techniques. Unfortunately Carl Simonton teaches that cancer patients should imagine how their white blood cells attack the tumor and destroy it. However my research has shown me that many cancer patients reject this type of visualization, and for many reasons I seriously doubt the correctness of this practice. First, it focuses the patient's attention on the tumor, and as we now know in terms of importance tumor is only secondary. Secondly the patient visualizes a war in his body and I am 100% certain that cancer patients require harmony and not fantasies of war.

In my discussions with many survivors I quickly noticed, that they were not (any longer) involved in confronting their tumor, but rather they were far involved dealing with their healthy future. Even if almost every person had his own "technique", the end result was always the same. Creation of their own future thanks to visualization. If there is one point in the 3E program that is more important than any other, it is this one, because if **we** do not create our future **ourselves – who else will?** Please consider our time line again and compare it with the thought-matter line.

Thoughts   Matter

$$\longrightarrow$$

Past   Future

$$\longrightarrow$$

Both lines can only proceed in one direction and there is no turning back. You can neither reverse the direction of one nor the other of these lines. Thus start today, start shaping your future yourself, by imagining it.

On the following pages I would like to show you a technique that I learned personally from my friend, and Europe's leading visualization trainer. Jack Black from Glasgow has taught his MindStore system to more than 50,000 people in recent years, and he is **the** consultant for leading personalities and firms. I can only recommend that every cancer patient participate in a seminar held by Jack Black (in English) or Klaus Pertl (in German), to learn visualization techniques that are unequaled in my opinion.

From many discussions I know that when a person has a tumor, he quickly believes that destroying the tumor is the most important thing, and that once the tumor is gone, then he will deal with a mental program. However this is a risky undertaking, and it is vital that you view the following visualization technique as part of your tumor destruction program.

The word **How?** also plays a significant role because, unfortunately it is this word which often holds you up from making important decisions. Usually people who have never meditated, or who are not particularly religious, have difficulties in understanding why visualization is so important. Thus do not make the mistake of starting to consider **how** such a thing as visualization can help you to destroy a tumor, rather please trust me and all the others, that it simply works.

Naturally there are many other teachers as well, (mostly NLP trainers), who teach good visualization techniques. Unfortunately there are also many others who are not really knowledgeable in dealing with cancer patients, and who are only out to dope you up mentally for a few days, and then you fall into an even larger hole 8 days later. Unfortunately there is no surefire method of recognizing a good therapist.

In summary I can say that my research has clearly shown that cancer patients with therapists should work on their future rather than on their past or present. Naturally, I know from my own experience that the future is easier to change when one is aware of one's past. But unfortunately cancer patients do not always have sufficient time to work analytically and consequently this portion of the mental work should be kept within an absolute and narrow timeframe.

I **am not** saying that you should not take a look at your past – please do not misunderstand. But in cancer therapy the emphasis is not on classic psychoanalysis and not on working with the here and now, rather in cancer therapy the focus is on creating the future. In the following pages I will explain how you can create your future.

The house on the right bank
In order to positively influence our body through our spirit, it is advantageous that you develop and "forward" your thoughts in a relaxed state. In order to do this you should be in a so-called alpha state. The word alpha is derived from the fact that we can record certain states of consciousness in the EEG, and alpha waves (7-14 hertz) indicate a relaxed state (the other waves are beta, theta, and delta waves). There are different relaxation techniques or meditation techniques. Courses in these techniques are offered in most communities or you can by a book/CD and learn them on your own. Alternatively you can also listen to classical music.

Once you are deeply relaxed then imagine the following situation: You are walking on the right bank of river and you turn to the right. There you see a green meadow, a blue sky, and a house with a red roof (please create your dream house). Enter your dream house and first go into a room with a shower. Under the shower rinse off everything that is negative. Afterwards bright sunlight dries you which streams through your entire body.

After you are dry go into your screen room. On the wall in front of you, you see three large screens.

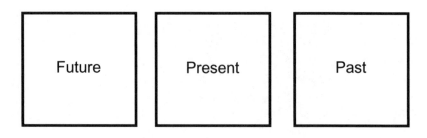

You sit down in front of the screens on a chair and you have a remote control in your hand. Regardless of the problem you have, you project it on the middle screen. Please consider it to be absolutely OK that you have this problem just as many people before you have had this problem. Then look at the right screen which shows your past, whether you have had this problem before and whether you found a solution for it at that time. In most cases you do not find a solution for your current challenges in your past, but often one encounters his problems two times in life and then it is very helpful to also look into the past for solutions. Now reduce the image on the screen to a mini image and "freeze" it. Now go back to the middle screen, use the remote control, and also reduce the image on the screen, and likewise freeze it.

Now look at the left screen and consider the solutions for the problem. View a situation in which your problem is already solved. An example: You have a tumor in the left thigh which prevents you from walking. View for example, how you are skiing with friends on the left screen. Feel the mountains, the snow, listen to your friends laughing and listen to your own breathing. Now enlarge the picture, make it brighter and imprint it in you. Every day when you return to your screen room, take a brief look at how you are skiing. In the future you do no longer need to look at the middle or right screens for this problem, just look directly at the left screen.

The next thing to do is to record the scene where you are skiing, on a video tape. Now take the video tape, insert it in your "universe" video recorder which is next to your screening chair, and send the recording out into the world. This is an important part, so that other people as well will learn of your goals. As through serendipity, other people who will help you to achieve your goals will then come into your life. Now leave your house and return to the bank of the river. Count to seven and end the session.

I realize that this may sound somewhat "incomprehensible" to some on first reading. However trust me, and you will quickly see the results. If you are still in doubt, then why not try this technique with something "small". Think of a parking place at the airport or railway station, or the exact result of a meeting with business partners. If this little exercise functions, then attempt a larger exercise, and do it until you have gained the confidence that you really can create your future yourself.

Please note that that end result must always be a situation that is useful for **all participants**. Everything that helps you **may not come at other's expense!**

Additional rooms in your house on the right bank

Naturally in your house on the right bank you still create other rooms, such as a room for total relaxation that can help you with pain, or a meeting room, where you meet with important people whose opinion you can ask. Thus it is conceivable that you could invite Jesus, the Pope, Einstein, Mother Theresa, Albert Schweitzer, to sit down at the same table together, in order to get their opinions on your problem.

If you have the support of a group (family, other self-help group) then invite this group into a room and role-play the following situation. The group is seated in a large room and looks at the rostrum where you are standing and telling an exciting story. This can be your ski vacation or it can also be an adventure vacation in Africa. In any case it is a story in which you are healthy and in which you have experienced something nice. The principle is that other people as well already see you as healthy and thus help you to create your future.

If you doubt the power of such a session then you can read the study conducted by UCLA in which prayers were offered on behalf of one group of heart attack patients, and prayers were not offered for a second group. Now guess which group not only had better results, but had results that were so much better that according to the opinion of the allopathic practitioners involved, that it bordered on a miracle.

Frequently I am asked: "How often should I go into my house on the right bank?", and my answer is always the same. "How often do you have to time for this?" Naturally there are no fixed rules here, but if you are suffering from acute illness, then you should visit your house several times a day.

Visualization generates an undertow in the health – in the right direction. It does not cost anything, and it is 100% effective. With this technique you have a powerful tool in your hand, regardless of whether you use it for your recovery or for your personal happiness, or financial success. Please ensure that in your desires you never injure, abuse, or otherwise treat anyone negatively. Always generate win-win situations. This is the only to way to ensure that it will bring you to where you would also soon like be.

Sexuality and Cancer

Besides football and cars, kitchen and shoes, sex is definitely one of everybody's favourite subjects – and this doesn't just go for Germans. But when the conversation turns to cancer and sex, then it appears that everyone is happy if no one raises the topic. Sex, not love, is however a very important subject for cancer, since almost everyone's sexual activity is limited when a breast is removed, when impotence and incontinence emerge after an operation, or when an artificial anus presents the challenge of a new relationship to your body.

Today we can certainly say that sex involves an exchange of energy. This exchange begins when you fall in love and ends with an orgasm. In-between, there are many different stages. When I use the word sex or sexuality, I mean an intensive 'flow' of energy in **our** bodies.

In this report you will often read that cancer is an energy problem. Orthodox medical practitioners are naturally aware of this, too, since they (must) repeatedly observe the collapse of their patients' energy. What is incomprehensible to me is that the subject of sex plays so small a role in classical oncology. At this point I do not want to discuss whether this is a product of most doctors not being trained to speak to their patients about this 'controversial' subject or whether this is fundamentally a result of our 'prude' Christian upbringing

It is only important for me to let you know that this subject is greatly undervalued in oncology and that you will generally have to obtain information about it on your own. This does not only apply to patients who have body parts cut out or changed, but for all cancer patients, since sex in itself is not as important as the build-up and deconstruction of energy involved in it. Having cancer means doing things that you didn't dare do in the past. If not now, then when? Be sure to take advantage of this, also with sex. Tell your partner **now** what you like and don't like. There will never be a better chance in your entire life, since almost every partner sympathises with your situation. If it turns out that your partner is one of the few who does not sympathise, then you should really consider whether you want to spend the rest of your life sexually unsatisfied with this person.

If sex has always played an important role in your life, then it should also do so in the future – irrespective of cancer. Definitely irrespective of cancer. I am only stressing this because I know how difficult it is for patients to enjoy sex with only one breast or an artificial penis. This goes for both partners, and you should be sure to discuss all your fears with your partner. There is no doubt that this takes courage; but it is worth while, since sex, happiness, activity and health often collectively guide the boat down the wild river, and if the boat should not capsize then it is necessary to keep everyone on board.

Knowing the importance of sex for your recovery should play a large role in your decision-making process for therapy. It is easily said: 'We'll operate the prostate once' and afterwards you will be impotent and incontinent. Patients usually only correctly understand the consequences of these 'side-effects' when it is too late. It is precisely in prostate operations that the most serious damage occurs in almost every case and, nevertheless, I repeatedly see that these 'side-effects' are barely touched upon in conversations with patients, as if being impotent were no truly awful development in the life of a man.

The decision to have a mastectomy (breast removal) is often made quickly, and many women develop a new, healthy self-image in time. However it is not just a few husbands who have more problems with this than their wives would have thought before the operation. So speak with your husband about it and listen to him with an open mind.

Masturbation

What do reading Yellow Press magazines and masturbating have in common? Many do it, but no one wants to talk about it. Why is it so difficult for us to talk about this? It definitely has something to do with our religious upbringing, while, from a psychological and social point of view, a variety of factors also speak against discussing this subject in public. If I do so nonetheless, there is an important reason.

Masturbation is still one of the cheapest, quickest and most enjoyable ways of letting energy flow freely. There is hardly a better one, since we should do everything to let the existing energy flow, and masturbation is ideally suited for doing just this. Try to see masturbation not as something 'indecent', as 'something that you don't talk about', as something 'dirty' and so on, but as a way of letting the energy in your body flow.

Spiritual energy

Whoever deals, or is forced to deal, with the issue of cancer, automatically has terms come to mind, such as: Death, pain, purpose of life, dying, why, God, etc.! The more people deal with this issue, the closer they usually come to their beliefs. Interestingly enough this applies for all religions. Basically I consider it to be necessary for the person affected on one hand, and for the entire human race on the other hand. Why for the entire human race?

I know a lot of people, who have put cancer or other "ordeals" like anorexia, or alcoholism behind them. 99% of these people have one thing in common: Expressed on religious terms, they have become "better people". They have started **first** to worry more about their own destiny, but **thereafter** they have also started to deal much more intensively with their fellow man. Parallel to this many of them have become "activists". They began to realize how important it is to leave something "behind" for the next generation. Whether it is a healthy environment or a better way to bring up children. In any event to this date I have not yet met a single person who continued his "not so positive life for mankind" after such an ordeal. Viewed from this perspective illnesses are **a way** to come nearer to God, or to a higher way of being, and to strike out on a new path.

But how does this help patients with cancer? Start now to reflect on your previous path in life. In intensive discussions I always note how little people realize, how rich they really are. Other than this "problem" with the tumor they have enough to eat, friends, parents, children, families, and often they even own houses, cars and many other valuable items. Why then are they not happy? Why are they lacking inner peace? Why are they looking for their center? Why? Questions on questions that I would like to bring to point: Being happy and balanced is the basic prerequisite for recovering your health. At first this sounds like a paradox; how can a person be happy if he has cancer, and with the thoughts associated with cancer is preparing for death?

I have worked intensively with a lot of patients and over time a totally different question is emerges: "Why shouldn't a be happy if he has a tumor in his body?" Even this question sounds confusing at first, but actually the answer to this question is on the tip of everyone's tongue. However this only applies if you considers cancer as it is portrayed in the media. The media portrays it as an incurable disease, a deadly fate, or "God's punishment". All three representations are incorrect and are more due to the fact that there is a large financial and political interest in the world that is concerned that we view cancer in this manner.

Regardless of what you have read about cancer to this point, it is an indisputable fact that cancer patients who have survived their illness, have pursued a course which made them into a happier person. The word forgiveness plays a major role in order for people to become happier. Every therapist knows what it means to deal with this subject. Forgiveness almost always involves two elements: first forgiving others, and second forgiving yourself. We will all be confronted with this issue at some point in our life. But at the latest when you are seriously ill and confront Christian issues like death, it is time to include the word **forgiveness,** because forgiving others is often the first step to a significantly happier life.

What words do you associate with the term forgiveness? Hate, heartache, years of contention, parents, children, brothers and sisters, injustice, spouse(s), or not to give an inch. I am sure that something will come to mind for you in conjunction with the word forgiveness. For this reason I would you to bring life into the next lines by first writing down **who** you could forgive for **what**. Please note that I have written could and not want. Forgiveness has a lot more to do with emotions than it does with reason. Consequently it is no use to move forwards rationally in this case and force yourself to forgive, but you should slowly feel your way toward this issue. Consequently write down now who you **could** forgive (since I assume that nobody would want to have anyone else read these lines, only write this in this book if you are sure that nobody else will have access to it. Otherwise copy the page, or simply write it on a blank sheet of paper).

Name	Why

Now I would like to ask you to write down what you would like to forgive yourself of. What have you done to others and to yourself that causes you and others pain today. Please write down which people have had to deal with negative things because of your actions (without value assessment).

Name	Why

And now please write down what you would like to forgive yourself of, what you are not yet capable of forgiving yourself of. Even if you believe that this is something that you could never forgive yourself of, I would still like to ask you to write it down.

_____

_____

_____

_____

_____

_____

As soon as all the things that you have written down on the last pages no longer effect you emotionally then I would like to ask you to destroy them in a solemn act. Naturally I know that such a process cannot take place in a few days. Therefore you should deliberately take time for this. Please do not believe that everything will suddenly resolve itself one day. Making this assumption could be a great mistake and it could impede your progress or even throw you further back on the path to health than you already are.

Work actively on this area until emotional changes set in. Obtain professional help from a spiritual leader, or from a person who for other reasons is not unfamiliar with the word forgiveness.

The healing field

or why system jumps are
so important for cancer patients

In recent years more and more is being discussed about morphogenetic fields, radionics, etc. and I believe with ever better data or theories. If you deal with cancer patients (not with cancer!) and particularly, as in my case, with patients who have recovered in spite of negative prognosis, then sooner or later you reach the conclusion that the immediate environment is very important for patients, but that the change of the patient's attitude relative to the world is much more important.

What do I mean by this? In my research I have noticed something which I earlier considered to be important but not **so** important. It is the fact that many cancer patients became better people in the religious sense of the word. Now I could naturally first assume that this is totally normal, because they now understand how beautiful life is how thankful they must be to God, etc. However I believe that this is only part of the story. I believe that there is something else totally different behind this. In this case I feel exactly the same about this as does on Rupert Sheldrake, who also cannot prove his theory of morphogenetic fields "scientifically". Nevertheless I would like to explain to you, what I understand when I refer to a healing field, in more detail.

We all live in systems. Our marriage, our job, our family, the house in which we live, but also our manner of thinking, loving, and even the manner in which we show this are individual systems. The whole functions like a clock mechanism with many small gears. However now we also know that a

547

clock can come to standstill just because one single gear no longer works the way that it is supposed to work. The same also applies to cancer. Most cells still act more or less normally, only this small part, into which a tumor grow, no longer participates correctly. And like a clock you only have to replace one gear in order for the clock to run again. But the questions come up, which gear is no longer functioning correctly and, and what brought the clock to a standstill.

Just as a clock smith pursues this question with filigree precision, we must also ask ourselves which gear of our life no longer runs true. This is why I have emphasized in this book that the mental part of a cancer therapy should not be short-changed, and why I place so much value on you learning how you can find out what you must change in your life. Even at the risk of repeating myself. **No final stage cancer patient can be healed, unless he is prepared to make system jumps.** By system jumps I understand that one leaves or changes certain systems. For one person this can mean that he must separate from his partner, or but the relationship on a new footing. For another it might mean that he does not go to the next family meeting, and for another person that he starts to accept that women can also be successful in professional life. Each change generates something new and this something new can now be positively evaluated.

However I have also become acquainted in recent years with many people, who certainly changed some things in their life and died nonetheless. In painstaking detail work I have worked on finding out, whether there was another difference and I have discovered that there was. It was the willingness to let their life flow, in deep trust, to a higher instance. Religious people call this a "deep faith", atheists would say that these people have absolutely "convinced themselves".

Interestingly enough I could not determine that there was any difference, whether people came to "their flow" through faith in something, or because they made a decision in their left brain – in this case a decision for life. The only important thing was that they gave themselves over to the flow.

Naturally I can understand that this sentence may be much too abstract for some readers and that they will not be able to do much with it. But believe me love, faith, and decision making are not simple to express in words, rather they must be experienced in order to better understand them.

I would like to tell you what is going on here from my perspective. The famous psychoanalyst C.G. Jung spoke of archetypes, and that we cannot disassociate ourselves from our history. This also means that not only are physical reactions, like increased blood pressure, anchored in our genes, but also that shared bodies of thought are passed on, or permanent fields/waves transmit this body of thought. An example: You go to an event and there you see many people who are congenial to you although you have never met them before in your life. A few days later you go to a different event and many of the people there are more uncongenial to you.

Now you could say that this is simply coincidence and totally normal. However there is also a different explanation for this. At the first event there were people who have a body of thought similar to you. These people generate a shared **field** in the room, and the radiation/wave length of the field generated there harmonizes with your own field. Just like in an orchestra where all the musicians are playing in the same key.

But what is happening in such a field and what does this all have to do with cancer? It's simple! Which event would you prefer to go to? On which of the two days did you feel better? Which was more fun? Of course it was the event with the congenial people around you? In simple terms because you simply liked it a lot better there. And this is precisely where you must be if you have cancer. To a field where it pleases you much better, and it pleases you much better for an extremely important reason. In such a field you consume significantly less energy and in addition you are capable of let-

549

ting the existing energy flow better. And now ask a cancer patient, whether he believes that he currently lives in such a field (environment)? But regardless in which energetic field you currently live, the hospital environment with energy robbing chemotherapy and irradiation is certainly worse for 99.9% of the population where a healing field is concerned.

I hope that I can show you in this book that cancer is always a problem of energy, and that the changed cells in your body cannot harm you as long as you are successful in getting more energy into you than the tumor robs from you. This is also the reason why people who understand that a tumor is not nearly as important as is usually believed, often live many years **with** a tumor before it goes away.

Previously I have explained the law of order or our various energy sources to you. Through the staying in a field that is "suitable" for you, you can indeed gain no additional energy, your "consumption" however will decrease drastically and possibilities of absorbing energy will increase massively. Two examples: In Ayurvedic medicine nutrition plays a major role, however great value is also placed on only eating when you are relaxed. We could also say happy, in a good mood, in nice company etc. Ayurvedic medicine recognizes good nutrition alone is not enough, but the field that surrounds a person while he is eating also plays a role.

We require a lot of energy "functioning socially". You know this too. One does this and does not do that, when he is with other people. But what is it like when you are in a ski cabin together with your best friends, or at your cousin's wedding? Where do you consume more energy just to exist, not for any activities? Naturally at the wedding. If you have cancer then you must pay attention to your energy budget. You cannot afford to withdraw too much from your energy account and an appropriate healing field can contribute a lot in this regard. I can recall an ham radio enthusiast whose dearest wish was to die at sea. But when she got on a ship again (she had spent many years on the sea earlier in life) she felt better and she was again capable of deciding for life. This decision for life had nothing to do with "wanting to live" but rather is a strenuous process, at the end of which there is a decision for life, **after** a person has more closely considered his life.

You have certainly been able to determine in this book that I am a very practical person, and consequently I would now like to tell you in simple words what you must do to generate a healing field around you.

First start immediately from this point on having only those people around you who you love and like. Haven't you wanted this for a long time? I am certainly aware that this is not always easy, but let's be honest. You certainly do not want to die, without having told your colleague at work what kind of a primitive he is? And believe me now is the time to do this. This does not mean that you should/must no longer talk with people who are not congenial with you. But it does mean that you become conscious of who robs energy from you. And you must strictly ban the major energy robbers from your life.

Then start speaking about your goals and desires with the people close to you, and not about your illness or what you do not want in life. I emphasize this so strongly because I know that too many people throughout the world always talk about that which they do not want. Don't make this mistake also, but speak exclusively about your goals and stop speaking about and thinking about everything in your life that is going wrong.

Experience has shown that only a very few people remain in the individual's environment with whom you can really talk about your goals, without having the feeling that you are really not being taken seriously. If you have such a partner or friend, then this is something to be happy about. Most people namely do not have such a friend or partner. But it certainly works in other ways. Go where you imagine that people with similar goals to yourself could be. I have been able to experience more than once how people come home after such a meeting (concert, seminar, conference, self-help group, continuing education, etc.) and simply said to themselves: "That is the right place for me". However it can also be that for this you must change your residence. Did you always want to live in the mountains or on the coast? Try it out now. Try it out, I do not say move. You can always move.

Now you are getting close to generating a healing field. But the most important thing is continuity. You require joy and healing fields around you on a daily basis and not just on weekends. In the meantime I know all the excuses standing in the way that this world has to offer: "I am a single mother", "I do not have any money for a seminar", "I still have got to do… and cannot be so egoistic", and so on, and so on. At the same time I have never experienced that a person who has really understood the importance of healing field, did not succeed in really finding it. As it says in the advertisement: *Just do it*.

For me it is often hard to see that people do not obtain for themselves the immense power that is in a healing field for themselves, because they continue to be prisoners of their thought systems and do not see that the door of their cell has been open for a long time. Often it is only a few steps to freedom, but these steps must first be taken. Earlier in this book I have written that cancer also has advantages, a person "may" pursue new paths, the proximate environment accepts, when a person with a tumor in his body changes his life – only do it, you must do it. Have the courage, visit (seek) your healing field and then finally become the happy person that you have seen in your dreams as a child. My best friend, Klaus Pertl, always asks in his seminars: "When did you stop living your dreams?" The answer to this question often contains the answer to the question: "Where do I find **my** healing field?" If there is one thing that I know it is that this field is already here. Get going looking for this field – it is worth it.

Daily 3E exercise

I have been involved in martial arts training since I was 14. I have been in Asia many times to train with well-known instructors, and with those that are not so well known. Moreover, I have trained with many different martial arts athletes around the world for more than 20 years. In this process I have been able to lean some things about breathing, body relaxation, and energy flow. Thus over the years I have learned, or forgotten, or relearned many techniques, but I have encountered a few exercises again and again, and these have proven to be effective for thousands of people. When I first learned of these exercises I did not understand scientifically why precisely these exercises were so good, nor do I understand scientifically today why they are so good. But that is no longer important to me, what is important to me today is the success of these exercises. And the success is something that you can quickly feel. However to motivate you to start the 3E daily exercise, I will also describe briefly why this exercise makes so much sense.

Here is the complete 3E exercise:

1. **Wake the meridians**
   First rub your hands together (1a) until the palms are warm, and then rub your ears (1b) with thumb and forefinger. This awakens your meridians to life, so to speak, and prepares them for the day.

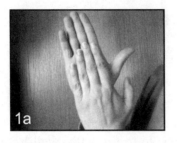

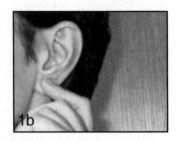

2. Open the chakras

The second part consists of a yoga exercise, Surya Namaskar, (description below) - better known as the sun prayer or sun salutation. Even within yoga this exercise has a special place because it is an ancient method of practicing several yoga positions in sequence in one procedure together with a controlled breathing rhythm. It would be too much to list all of the advantages offered by this exercise. However there are some effects of the sun prayer that I would like to point out: stimulation of stomach and bowels, promotion of blood circulation in the head, increase in breathing volume, lowering the blood pressure, and improvement of the nervous system.

3. Right spin

After the sun prayer turn yourself to the right several times on your own axis. Many of you will perhaps be familiar with this exercise from the five Tibetan exercises. Here however two additional exercises are added:

1) While you turn, massage your thymus gland. It is approximately in the center of the breastbone.

2) Then shake your fingers.

It is clear why you turn to the right. After we have opened our chakras (energy centers in the body) with the sun prayer we now support our cells with right turns, since we know that all healthy cells have a so-called right rotation in the body and that our excretory products such as urine or sweat are left spinning. Massaging the thymus gland supports our immune system and shaking the fingers prepares our brain for the coming activities of the day. Our fingers have direct lines to the brain, so to speak, and this simple exercise can significantly help our brain.

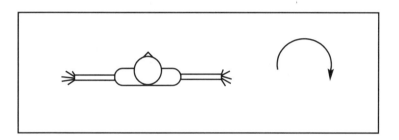

4. **Generate energy**

   Now that our meridians are awake, our chakras are open and our brain is ready for work, we want to generate some energy (which can now flow well). Position yourself and act like a karate fighter. Box alternately with the left and right fist in the air so that you increase your breathing and produce heat. The whole thing should last about 1 minute.

5. **Prepare your lungs**

   Now let your arms dangle briefly and do the following "tree breathing exercise". Imagine that you are standing in front of a tree and put your arms around it (5a). Exhale twice as long as you inhale. Thus you can prepare your lungs for the hard work that they will face in the coming hours. Do this for 1-2 minutes, depending how

well you feel when doing this exercise. At the end of the
tree breathing exercise push the energy that has formed
between your stomach and your hands, into your body,
by simply placing the hands slowly on the stomach (5b).

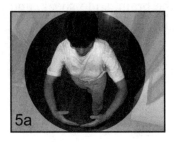 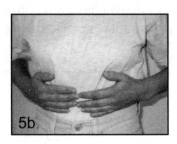

6. Bowel preparation

To conclude, prepare your bowels for the day.
Your hands encompass your stomach left and right from
below. Place the edges of your hands under the stomach
(6a). Now breathe deeply into the stomach and while you
exhale, lightly shake your stomach. This is done by
lightly moving your hands up and down without removing
them from your stomach (6b).

That's it. That was the entire exercise. You will quickly realize that you have a lot more energy when you do this exercise
daily. Taken as a whole, the entire exercise has many, many
more advantages. However for cancer patients, the primary
thing is that you get more energy through the 3E daily exercise, second, existing energy can flow better, and third, the
lungs and the bowels are prepared for the day. For a cancer
patient, an optimal way to start the day after waking up is to
rub ELDI oil "R" into your skin over the entire body, wait 15

minutes, and then do the 3E daily exercise, and then take a hot/cold shower.

Here are brief instructions for the sun prayer. Do not be concerned if you are not as supple as the young man in the photo. Neither am I, but the exercise still helps me better prepare for the day.

Some information on the sun prayer:

- The hands remain in the same position on the floor from the 4th position to the 9th position.

- A complete cycle of all 12 positions should not take longer than approximately 30 seconds. Try to do at least 3 cycles, in succession.

- Practice the positions individually at the beginning.

- As soon as you master the sequence, concentrate on your breathing.

Surya Namskar - sun prayer

1st position

Fold your hands in front of the body. Bring them from below starting slowly build tension in your entire body. Exhale and pull the stomach in while exhaling. Release the tension.

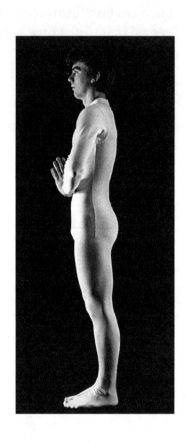

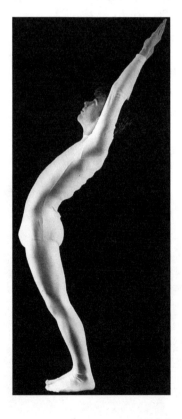

2nd position

Lift the arms over your head while inhaling. Bend backwards and push your pelvis forwards.

558

3rd position

Exhale slowly and bend the torso and both arms forward. Lay the hands flat on the floor with your knees unbent. If this is not possible for you, simply bend your knees slightly. Pull in your stomach while doing this. Now move your head close to your legs, stretch the neck and look towards your waist.

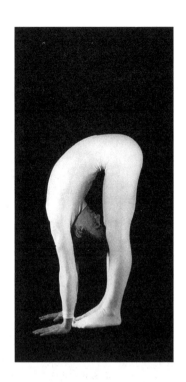

4th position

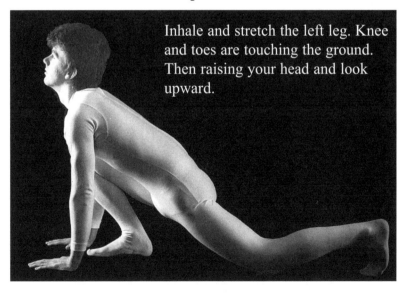

Inhale and stretch the left leg. Knee and toes are touching the ground. Then raising your head and look upward.

559

5th position

Hold your breath in, raise the pelvis, and place the right foot next to the left foot. The heels remain on the floor.

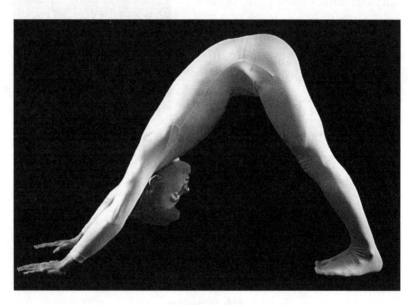

6th position

Exhale and lie on the floor. In this process, forehead, chest, knees, and toes have floor contact, however the hips do not. Pull in your stomach and press the chin to the collarbone.

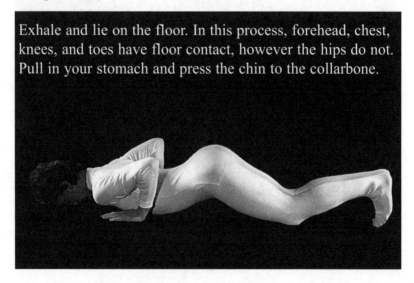

7th position

Inhale and stretch the arms until the upper body is straight. Keep your pelvis on the floor, bend the back backwards and look up, by bending your head back.

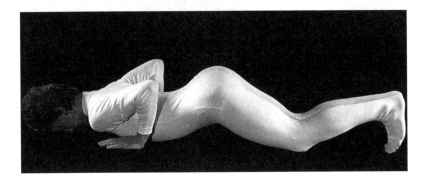

8th position

Hold your breath in. With this position you have returned to the 5th position and the first 4 exercises are then repeated in the reverse sequence.

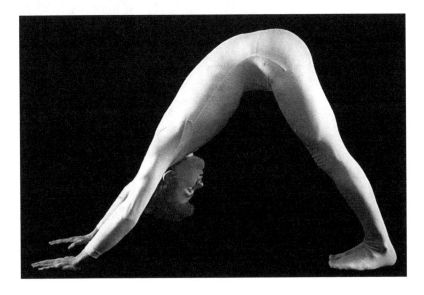

561

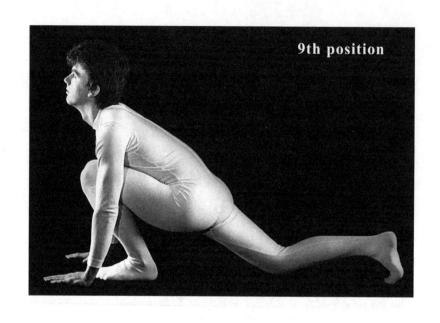

9th position

10th position   11th position   12th position

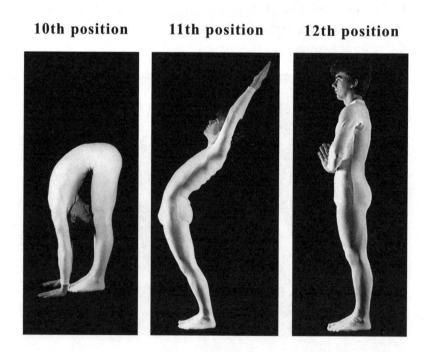

562

7

Non-
Conventional
Cancer Therapies

On the following pages I will introduce you to non-conventional cancer therapies. I have divided these therapies into two groups. A group consisting of "individual therapies" and a group of "supporting substances". I have further subdivided the individual therapies into three groups. Group one contains therapies which I believe to know will help you. The second group contains therapies which **could possibly** help you; and I advise against the therapies contained in the third group. However the reason why I mention the cancer therapies in the third group is that I am constantly being asked how successful they are.

I am confronted with the following sentence on an almost daily basis: "Mr. Hirneise are you also familiar with...? Naturally in this book it is not possible for me to describe **all** therapies that have been associated with curing cancer in recent years. But this is not so important, because there is no individual therapy that can cure cancer. I have made the following selection more on the basis of my personal experiences with therapies and due to the level of recognition individual therapies have attained. It may be that you are not familiar with many of these therapies, however most of the therapies mentioned have been available for many years, or decades, and hundreds of thousands of patients have been treated with them. If you are not familiar with these therapies even though they have been used to treat so many patients, then the question comes up again: Who actually controls what gets into the media?

Before I start with the individual therapies, I would like to say a few words about how they have been evaluated. My research is not the only research which shows that it is very risky to rely on individual therapies. Where this understanding of cancer is taking us, is evident every year in the increasing number of cancer deaths. I don't care which therapy is involved, whether chemotherapy or IAT (Immuno-Augmentative Therapy – see the corresponding chapter).

Cancer patients must understand that cancer is an illness of the whole person, and not a local degeneration in the form of a tumor. This is precisely why the following pages are not provided as a **self-help tool**! Please do not confuse this issue. I cannot repeat this enough. Cancer is an all-embracing illness and you need one (or several) therapists, who can treat you in an all-embracing manner. There is something else that is also very important. Mr. Smith's glioblastoma is not the same glioblastoma that you might have, and Ms. Jones' breast cancer is different than that of Ms. White. There is not *the* cancer treatment for a type of cancer, because physicians (should) treat people and not illnesses. Consequently neither is a treatment protocol that can be used for everyman. Do not make the mistake of believing that you can simply pull a few active substances out of this book and "brew-up your private cocktail". This book is designed to help you find a therapy, jointly with your therapist, and to enable you to sit across the table as an enlightened patient.

Naturally I am also aware that many patients will still "concoct" their own therapy. If you are one of these patients, then I would at least like to give you the following information to take with you on your path. **First** stick with the 3E's. Eliminate toxins from your body, stay on the oil protein diet, and execute the mental program that is introduced in this book. It is imperative that you visualize. You should only start studying various "additives" after these elements are in place. Absolutely avoid reliance on any kind of pills, whether vitamin C or some other kind of miracle cure, which may have helped others. My experience is that all too often people believe they can execute a colon cleanse with pills alone, or improve their immune system by taking some kind of tablets, which cannot even be absorbed by the colon or the cells. The likelihood that you will find out much too late that this little powder or that little powder does not make you healthy, unfortunately is quite high if this path is pursued. Again: There is no miracle cure, neither in the conventional world, nor in the non-conventional world. In collecting the following data I have made every effort to mainly use data from neutral sources and not the data from the manufacturers of these substances. You can imagine how difficult this is because basically there are no neutral sources. Most of the therapists mentioned have either been visited personally by myself, our team's personnel, or by my colleagues, and we have formed our own impression about who these people are, or what they do.

Many therapists or substances that are used I have investigated as executive board member of *Menschen gegen Krebs* e.V. jointly with *People against Cancer* in Iowa, or jointly with the *National Foundation for Alternative Medicine* in Washington DC. This usually involved going to the respective therapists with a medical team and investigating so-called best cases. Naturally I am aware that these cases simply cannot be applied to other people, on the other hand however, they do show us that people with a diagnosis of cancer that is 100% certain, and who are usually in a very advanced stage of their illness, have pursued a path that is different than that suggested by allopathy, and that these people were extremely successful. Allopathic practitioners always say that we should not draw conclusions about the effectiveness of a therapy from individual cases.

Basically I agree with this statement. However there is a huge difference here: These patients were all therapied-out, and allopathy had given up on them. Just go to a university and ask a professor there to tell you how many patients with metastasized cancer he has treated, who are healthy today. A long silence will be the answer, because chemotherapy and irradiation do not cure cancer in an advanced stage. Even allopathic practitioners admit this today.

The cases that I have investigated give me and others hope, again and again, and this is precisely what I would also like to achieve with this book. Never lose hope that you also will conquer your cancer, or that you will grow old along with it. I have personally become acquainted with many people, and I have visited many therapists who jointly know thousands of people who were in a hopeless situation, and who were healed thanks to the therapies or substances described on the following pages. Since I am aware that it is impossible for me to evaluate which therapy or which substance should be used first, I have included a summary at the end of this book, so that you do not lose time unnecessarily.

Non-conventional cancer therapies are often dismissed because they are "not recognized scientifically". What does this actually mean? Most doctors will then say that there were no double-blind studies. What they do not tell you is that there is no possibility whatsoever of performing such a study. First, you must know that it is very expensive to get approval for a new medication, and only large pharmaceutical companies can afford the approval process. Another problem is that many good therapies cannot be patented, consequently are of no interest to a large corporation. In addition, a medication can only be approved if it has been tested on people. Because cancer medications cannot be tested on healthy people (which is the usual procedure), due to the serious side effects, a so-called ethics commission decides on which human experiments (also referred to as studies) can be performed with cancer medications, and which ones cannot be performed. And now guess who sits on these panels? People like me, or doctors with holistic perspectives?

Certainly not, but rather professors, who are known to only represent one direction of medicine. In addition, members of the ethics commission must decide on applications submitted by colleagues, who may previously have decided on that member's own studies, or who will in the future decide on that member's own studies. Any thinking person knows what this means. How in the world can holistic therapies muster the "scientific" proof, when **to this day no study** has ever been approved in which non-conventional cancer therapies were compared with conventional cancer therapies. Such a study would certainly be simple to execute, I meet a sufficient number of people every month who would be happy to participate in such a study – in the non-conventional arm of the study.

However "to protect" cancer patients (and naturally pharmaceutical companies as well) such studies will not be approved in the future either, and thus the present situation will continue; in every study one toxin will do better than the other toxins. The next time your doctor says that this therapy, or that therapy, is "not-scientifically" recognized", then please ask him whether he might be aware of a possibility of how this could be "scientifically" determined. And if he has a serviceable idea of how an ethics commission, a university, and a health insurance company can be turned around, then I would be very pleased to get a call from you.

Again to avoid misunderstandings. I consider it unfortunate that non-conventional cancer therapies are not controlled with double-blind studies, and I abhor the whole-hearted promises made by representatives of many of these therapies, just as I abhor the lies about the successes of chemotherapies for epithelial tumors. It would be in the interest of all cancer patients if these studies would finally be executed, moreover many doctors would finally better understand, precisely which therapies really deliver on their promise. Unfortunately there is a gigantic financial and political interest in ensuring that these studies are never performed, and consequently there is zero chance that they will be performed. This is another reason why it so important that **you** form your own opinion.

Here are a few tips from the German Cancer Society (*Deutschen Krebsgesellschaft*), on how you can tell a "proper" cancer therapy from a quack therapy. It is interesting to note that publication of this list naturally resulted in non-conventional therapies being considered more "critically". But what would happen if the same criteria were applied to conventional therapies as well. Let's take a closer look at the points:

1. How long has this method been practiced? (If it has not been officially recognized after decades of practice then it is probably ineffective.)

My comment: As long as a group of people determine what is officially recognized, and what is not officially recognized, this naturally we cannot consider this to be a criterion. By the way, many chemotherapies have been recognized for many years, and to this day they still have not been proven to contribute to cancer patients living longer. What about these therapies?

2. Is the method unique, hard to understand, secret, linked to certain people or places? (The more secret, the higher the likelihood that it is not effective.)

My comment: What biochemist, to say nothing of what doctor, knows how chemotherapies really function? Do the pharmaceutical companies make all of their research available to the public, or can you think of any other field that offers more unique, non-understandable, and secret therapies than the field of oncology? The more secretive the more ineffective – in this case all chemotherapies must be designated as ineffective, because we are far away from understanding how these therapies function with people, or in most cases fail with people. And the personality cult within conventional establishments is much greater than it is in the non-conventional establishment.

3. Is the treatment predominantly successful or are failures also known? (If only successes are promised, then skepticism is advised.)

My comment: I can only agree. Therapies that only promise success disregard the complex nature of cancer. Thus be cautious if your doctor says that you only have a 50 or 60 % chance, or even an 80% chance of survival, if you undergo this or that chemotherapy or this or that irradiation. Isn't it precisely the allopathic practitioners who have been telling their patients how successful this or that medication is for years – until it suddenly is withdrawn from the market? And isn't it the allopathic practitioners who use therapies for decades without having real success?

4. Does the treatment also have side effects? (Without side effects, usually no effect can be expected.)

My comment: This statement must be absolutely refuted. High side effects have nothing, absolutely nothing, to do with high healing effects (a nice example in this case is high-dose chemotherapies). Pharmaceutical companies have planted this fairy tale in the heads of consumers for years, because they were fully aware that all their chemicals have fundamental effects on all cells, and consequently side effects must be calculated in. Free yourself from this false thinking!

5. Are strict dietary limitations required? (With due respect for a healthy diet, unfounded and invasive prohibitions must be rejected.)

My comment: Unfounded prohibitions must be rejected. I can only agree. Every therapist should be able to substantiate why he prescribes a specific nutrition therapy or he should find a new line of work. The sentence naturally is headed more in the direction of: Stay away from nutrition therapies. There are no cancer diets. This statement naturally reflects only the knowledge level of many allopathic practitioners, and from their perspective it is all too understandable. You can read that this statement is false, and why it is false, in detail in this book.

6. Do representatives of these methods fight against "allopathy"? (Attacks and defamations do not replace a lack of proofs!)

My comment: I cannot understand why a therapy should not be of value, just because a person uncovers errors in other therapies, regardless of whether allopathy or not. But there is a totally different intent behind this statement, which always comes to bear. "Dear patient, anyone who questions allopathy, is wrong." I am also against defamations and here my ideas conform with those of the writer of this sentence. However to be honest this statement should also be applied in the opposite direction. Just think of all the things that you may have read about Dr. Julius Hackethal. For years there were defamations and lawsuits. But do you know what the truth is? I was the first person in all those years, who went into the Eubios Klinik and said to Ms. Hackethal: "I would like to examine the files and find out what is really true." All of the other doctors, or all of the other organizations never bothered, they just attacked and defamed – without examining facts.

Personal opinion:

For many therapies at the end of the description I will provide my personal opinion. I have decided to make these comments because many patients repeatedly ask me: "If you were in my situation would you undergo this therapy or not?" Naturally I cannot answer this question in a way that is really satisfactory, because I know exactly what I would do, and this is actually irrelevant for you, because you must find **your** therapy. Nevertheless I have decided to provide my very personal response to this question.

If you have an older edition of a 3E book, and if my comments on some therapies change, this is because I have obtained new knowledge which impels me to make this change. A description's length is irrelevant. I have described some therapies in more detail because it is difficult to get more information about them, and because they are wholly unknown to many patients, and also to many doctors. It is better to use my personal comments as evaluation criteria, than it is to use the length of the description.

Successful Cancer Therapies

Group 1

The oil protein diet

For me, this therapy is still the most outstanding therapy and should serve as the basis every cancer patient's therapy. If I write this here, after all the experiences with so many cancer therapies throughout the entire world, then please understand that I do so after very careful consideration. You should study this therapy intensively regardless of which therapy you should decide on other than the oil protein diet.

Particularly for acute patients, if a person still has tumors in the body then, next to the Gerson diet, which is much more difficult to execute, I view the oil protein diet as a must. I know that even many non-conventional physicians will consider such a statement to be exaggerated, but the experiences that I have personally collected personally speak a very clear language.

The oil protein diet is explained in detail in the chapter *3E - Eat healthy*.

Frequency therapies

On the following pages I will introduce different frequency therapies. I am certain that these therapies will determine the future of medicine, because when we are able to measure the frequencies of our cellular communication, we will also be able to prescribe the correct frequencies to patients therapeutically. Until then we must all admit that we can only rely on the experiences of individual researchers. However these experiences are not bad at all, in my opinion. There are many promising approaches, and particularly there are therapists who have been able to gather positive experiences over years of research.

Scientists have understood for many years that they can influence the energy behavior of cells when they measure certain frequencies of the cells, and particularly they have understood that they can artificially produce these frequencies. Until a few years ago practical implementation was inconceivable, because fast computers were required that are capable of calculating millions of processes and tens of thousands of frequencies per second. For several years this has been possible and it will certainly be a significant influence on the future of medicine. This was only possible through the influence of modern quantum physics, because quantum physics could prove that invisible energy potentials, which were ignored for a long time by biologists, have a great influence on the form and the function of matter.

Conventional biochemistry is based on the belief that information is only transmitted through chemical substances, such as hormones. Now we know that force fields are not only capable of transporting information, they can also transport it faster and more efficiently. Image our body as a large planet on which billions of people (cells) live. Just like on Earth these people must communicate with each other in some way. Naturally the postal system (hormones, cytokines, etc.) is a very effective information system, unfortunately, frequently it is much too slow. It is precisely the same in our bodies. Our cells also do not just write letters, they also use a telephone (waves/light) in order to communicate with each other. Just like spies tap telephones, scientists attempt to tap our cellular communication. Unfortunately we are still in the beginning phase of our espionage activities, but I am certain that today we can already "tap" individual "conversations" and that the bugs will undergo dramatic further development in years to come, in the form of the most modern frequency devices.

There are hundreds of researchers, who have made wonderful contributions in this field and if I only mention three of them below, then it is only because I know more about these researchers relative to clinical application, or because I believe in their "theories". However this does not means that other researchers like Gorgun Suleyman in Istanbul, Dr. Fuda in Taiwan, David Spall in Australia, all die "successors" to Royal Rife throughout the world, Dr. Hans Kempe, Dr. Ludwig and Dr. Popp in Germany, and many many more, have not also discovered incredible things. However it is impossible for me to introduce all the work in this book, consequently in the following pages I describe only a few approaches in manner that is representative of many, of how a healing process can be promoted or stimulated with artificially generated waves.

Aquatilis Therapy

Dr. Essaidi is a nuclear physicist and former employee of Philips in Eindhoven Holland, where he worked in medical research. His therapy is based on binding free radicals.

Free radicals are atoms in which one or more electrons are not paired, and consequently they search for other electrons in the body. These radicals can be formed by the body, or they can also be formed by external sources. Unfortunately in their search for an electron, these radicals destroy our cells, and can thus trigger or favor illnesses, by attacking the receptors on the cell membrane, our mitochondria, or also our DNA (cell nucleus).

Usually our body has adequate defense possibilities against free radicals. However for various reasons often the cell can no longer offer sufficient defense and the damages take on dimensions that must be seriously considered.

Dr. Essaidi has developed a cabin that looks like a small pyramid with mirrors, and which is hot inside like a sauna. In this cabinet Dr. Essaidi generates a positively charged environment, which according to his theory, withdraws free radicals from the body or neutralizes them. At the same time the cabin represents a comprehensive detoxification therapy, because the skin pores are opened due to the heat.

First, toxins can thus more easily get out, and second, Dr. Essaidi adds special substances to the steam, which can thus be absorbed more easily by the body. Concurrently a precisely defined electromagnetic field is generated in the cabinet.

The treatment usually takes approximately 90 minutes with all preliminary and post-treatment procedures (the actual therapy takes between 30 – 40 minutes). An accompanying person can also be in the cabin. A session in the cabin costs between 70-100 Euro. Usually German patients stay in a motel or hotel near the center.

During the 4th German Alternative Cancer Day (4. Deutschen Alternativen Krebstag) in October 2004 in Stuttgart, the pathologist Dr. Frank Andä from San Remo / Italy presented his documentation on Dr. Essaidi's therapy for the first time. Over several years he took blood from his cancer patients prior to and after the Aqua Tilis therapy and determined the following:

* Elimination of circulating cancer cells
* Stimulation of T-cells
* Elimination of atypical microorganisms
* Elimination of blocking factors on the cell membrane functions
* Stimulation of the NKCs (natural killer cells)

The results clearly show that the Aqua Tilis therapy is a very intensive detoxification therapy, which has clear influences on the immune system.

Personal opinion: I consider Dr. Essaidi to be a very sincere scientist, who has perhaps invented something ingenious, and I wish that his therapy were accessible to every cancer patient. I view this an optimal beginning of a cancer therapy and find it tragic that here again financial interests hinder the spread of a successful therapy.

Synergetics

Synergetics is originally a term used in physics and means the "science of combined effect". Above all, this term has been coined by Professor Hermann Haken, mainly in connection with self-organisation. Professor Haken himself defines it thus: "There is a tendency today to subsume everything which has to do with self organisation under the heading of "chaos theory".

Chaos theory deals with a few levels of freedom or a few variables and stipulates that even when only a few variables combine together, a chaotic irregular behaviour results. One can therefore ask what indeed chaos theory has to do with self organisation, since self organisation arises from the cooperation of a great many individual parts. A liquid consists of many individual molecules, a society of many different individuals, an economy of many different players. Synergetics shows that even a complex system which consists of many individual parts can be described in terms of a few variables, which are then known as the ordering parameters. So once one has arrived at a few variables, they can be subjected to the laws of chaos theory. To this extent, chaos theory is a component part of synergetics."

What still sounds rather abstract coming from Professor Hagen has today, thanks to the physics engineer Bernd Joschko, become a guide to self-healing. As early as the end of the 1970's, Bernd Joschko, who originally worked as a profiler at the federal police department, collected numerous experiences relating to self-awareness therapies and holistic therapies. He was also positively influenced by the discoveries of a Dr. Hamers and, thanks to the rare combination of own experience on the one side and the logical thinking capability of an engineer on the other side, Bernd Joschko recognised that all remembered and symbolic images within our brain are in a state of constant interaction, and form patterns. If individual "inner pictures" are now altered, entire patterns are thus in a position to change. All of this knowledge is nothing really new, but Herr Joschko for the first time transferred the principles of synergetic pattern recognition over to the inner pictures which are "visible" under deep relaxation. In this manner, he found a way by which self-organisational processes can be triggered in people which simultaneously also lead to self-healing processes in the body.

In order to be able to trigger self-healing processes, one must first destroy the old structures, in the sense of: "We achieve order by creating chaos". In practice, this means that a person under the instruction of a synergetic therapist changes his inner pictures. For this purpose, one places oneself into a state of deep relaxation in order to be able to "address" larger areas of the brain, and is then led by the therapist through one's inner world.

In a similar way to the New Medicine, synergetics also believes that the three levels of brain, body and organs are in a state of constant interaction with each other and that permanent self-organisations take place. Another shared belief is that symptoms are nothing other than information structures anchored in the brain and should of course not be fought against, but used for better diagnosis and changed via the resolution of conflicts.

However, there are also clear differences from the New Medicine. The first is surely the active therapist who tries, using different regions of the brain from those in New Medicine, to find the anchored information structures and to change them. This addresses the strong desire many people who do not wish to just wait. Although the New Medicine does not of course consist only of waiting, many patients nevertheless perceive it as such.

A further difference is that, while Dr. Hamers only describes that a person has to be caught "on the wrong foot" for a conflict to arise at all, synergetics however asks why the situation should present any conflict for this person.

Personal opinion: I can only describe my personal experiences with synergetics as very good. Help towards self-help is exactly what cancer patients need. Of course I realise that many cancer patients do not understand what miracles changes of inner pictures can effect and that it will take a number of years before synergetics becomes accepted. But for all those patients who already understand this, and who are prepared to take an active part in the healing process, synergetics is certainly a true blessing.

More information can be found at: www.synergetik.net

PapImi Therapy

The Frenchman Charles Laville, (author of the book, „Le Cancer: dérangement électrique" – Cancer, an electrical disturbance), the Russian, Georges Lakhovski (1870–1943), the American, Royal Raymond Rife (1888–1971), the Italian, Antoine Priore (1912–1988) who lived in France, and the Greek, Panos Pappas (b. 1947) have developed devices for the frequency therapy of cancer in the last century. Panos Pappos, professor of physics and mathematics, who I visited personally in Athens in April 2001, and who introduced his therapy for the first time in Germany that same year at my invitation, experimented in the 1980s with strong electrical discharges. He was encouraged by the work of Prof. Graneau at MIT in the USA.

For many years Dr. Pappas continued his research and developed a high-frequency device with the name PapImi. With this device within microseconds, current values of more than 1000 amperes and frequencies ranging from a few Hertz up to 500,000 megahertz are generated, which can contribute to cancer cells normalizing themselves.

In recent years Prof. Pappas published quite a few "best cases" – these were cancer cases involving a wide variety of cancer types. PapImi was able to contribute to a shift in thinking relative to frequency therapy of cancer, because the approach of the therapy is: Give the body a huge variety of frequencies and it will take those which it needs. This contradicts the thinking of many researchers, which postulates that you must know which frequencies should be transmitted.

Otherwise Prof. Pappas assumes precisely (as do other frequency scientists) that cancer is not an autonomous illness, but rather like all other illnesses it is nothing other than an energy disturbance. If it would be possible to return these energy disturbances, (which could also be termed "electrical" disturbances), to their original line, then basically any illness could be therapized. By the way Prof. Pappas is of the opinion that cancer is a balance disturbance (see chapter: *What is cancer?* under balance theory) and can only occur when a cell is "hungry".

Personal opinion: Today I am not aware of any significant side effects of this therapy. However there are more and more patients who profit from the PapImi therapy. Doubtless studies are urgently needed here and I hope that these so necessary studies (particularly for breast cancer) are carried out soon.

Additional information: Since January 2004, a PapImi copy has been available on the market under the name *Rehatron*; it is produced by a former distributor of Prof. Pappas. However this is NOT a PapImi device and I can only warn against the *Rehatron*, because it produces different frequencies than those that are produced by the PapImi device. More information is available at: www.pappas.com.

Cluster Medicine

Prof. Ulrich-Jürgen Heinz, who studied philosophy, music and art history, had already made a name for himself in the field of spagyrics (in simple terms a type of homeopathy), before concentrating on his discovery, which he termed cluster medicine, in the early 80s. In this case as well, frequencies, cellular communication, and particularly the individuality of the person are involved. In cluster medicine, there are no classic diagnoses, rather each patient gets his cluster diagnosis, which however is matched to the individual past of the patient. Thus there is no breast cancer diagnosis, rather only the symptom of a tumor in the breast of a women, induced by certain events in the life of this woman.

Diagnosis is based on various processes such as our fingerprint, (hereditary disposition), a Polaroid picture of the face (life history) creating drawings (our conditioning), bodily substances like blood, urine, saliva, skin, ear wax, teeth, etc. (bodily status) and via the selection of geometric patterns (detecting physic events). Considering just the aspects of the diagnosis alone, it is evident that a very holistic perspective of illness is involved here. It is interesting to note that this diagnostic system can also be used for animals.

All evaluations of the diagnosis are translated via computer programs into a numeric sequence and are compared with over 300,000 sequences and approximately 6 million output combinations in a database. From this an "image" of the patient's currently valid situation is created; this image which sometimes runs several hundred pages. Cluster medicine goes to this effort because in its perspective a person is precisely the result of **all** content of his life, and that which allopathic practitioners refer to as an illness is nothing more than an expression of this life in the form of symptoms. Cluster medicine then networks this detailed evaluation with the symptoms or official illnesses, and by querying the psychological background, helps the patient to better understand his "illness".

In addition cluster substances in the form of an oral spray are produced individually for each patient. This spray contains information transferred to water, which is exactly tailored to the patient. In addition the patient is given special information about other things he can do to accelerate his healing process. This can be a certain piece of music, (individual CDs are made for each patient), relaxation exercises, colors, and much more. Also regulating the colon, i.e. revitalization of existing symbionts, plays a major role.

Personal opinion: It is not easy for me to evaluate cluster medicine, as I have too little data in the sense of traditional studies. Also the question arises in this case, as to whether such a comprehensive system could even be captured with the usual measuring methods. Nonetheless I am convinced that Ulrich-Jürgen Heinz is already on the path which must be pursued for a holistic cancer therapy – namely a narrow individual path for each individual patient.

NutriTherapy

This is a program which involves nutrition and detoxification of the body, and which is specifically matched to the individual bodily conditions of the person. NutriTherapy does not treat the cancer tumor directly, rather it attempts to optimize metabolic processes in such a manner that the body is able to help itself, or better able to accept help through other therapies.

The most modern computer technology is used to scientifically evaluate the nutrient requirement of people with cancer and other illnesses. The biochemical individuality of each person can be evaluated with this therapy in order to then provide focused assistance in the area of nutrition, body detoxification, and nutritional supplements. We have Dr. Kelley from Florida, and his work in the area of body chemistry, to thank for this development, which other therapies like the NutriTherapy are based on (Dr. Kelley was a dentist, who according to his own information, healed himself of pancreatic cancer in 1964).

Dr. Kelley recognized the importance of the fact that in the treatment of cancer patients therapies only work when certain processes in the body function more or less normally. Consequently his top priority was first to get these processes in line, or to optimize them, so that the body can defend itself against the illness. The optimal nutrition for each individual has priority here. In his opinion, the problem however is that no single "nutrition type" is equally suitable for every person. People have quite different nutritional needs. These vary and depend on: the illness, the severity of the illness, genetics, nutritional habits, how active a person is, the person's emotional condition, the daily behavioral pattern, and the general stress to which a person is subjected. The vegetative nervous system has primary control over our metabolism. It is divided into the parasympathetic and sympathetic nervous system. People who have a dominant sympathetic system tend for instance to have a lower metabolism and consequently need fast-burning nutrients, (this means primarily vegetarian diet). On the other hand people with a dominating parasympathetic system have a faster metabolism and possibly require nutritional products that burn more slowly (for example animal proteins). The primary therapeutic goal of NutriTherapy is to restore the metabolic balance.

Features of a typical program for cancer patients:

Phase 1: Body detoxification
Using homeopathic detoxification substances, vitamins, minerals, pancreatic enzymes and enemas, the liver and other organs are detoxified. This frees the immune system and normalizes the biological functional capability.

Phase 2: Substitution
If the body does not produce a certain chemical, then very specific nutrient substances are taken in the correct doses. For cancer patients there are often problems with metabolism of enzymes, hormones and various components of the immune system.

Phase 3: Stimulation
The organs and glands are stimulated using specific nutrients, vitamins, minerals, and phytotherapy (plant-based therapy).

Phase 4: Rebuilding
Nutritional supplement products are used to cover the additional nutrient demand due to the illnesses, and to strengthen the body's reserves.

Personal opinion: In recent years I have become acquainted with many patients who could be helped by NutriTherapy, (e.g. cancer patients with inoperable pancreatic cancer), for which almost all other therapies fail. Especially William Walcott´s programm (www.metabolictyping.com) is a serious one.

I am not surprised that this therapy comes from America. On one hand it is a very simple therapy, on the other hand it is not just Europeans who have difficulty in viewing capsules as a replacement for food and not as a nutritional supplement. At the beginning of the therapy 60-100 capsules must be taken per day. However the results speak for themselves and NutriTherapy is an option for anyone who can afford it (app. 200-500 Euros/ month in the first 3-6 months).

Moreover there is still a group of people for whom this therapy can be very effective: for all "energy savers" and for all those that do not want to change their life, or who cannot change their life. Again to avoid misunderstandings: I consider it imperative to follow the 3E program for cancer. But what do all the people do who for whatever reason, are just not interested, or do not understand how important it is. Naturally I could act as these patients did not exist – but the truth is that this group comprises the majority of cancer patients. It is easier for many people to take 100 capsules (later 20-30) a day, than it is to do without coffee with pretzels in the morning.

Naturally NutriTherapy functions a lot better in conjunction with the 3E program, however it is still significantly better than doing nothing, for this group.

Antineoplaston therapy

As a young scientist, Dr. Stanislaw Burzynski isolated various peptides (amino acid chains that are necessary for forming proteins) from human urine, and discovered that they are very effective in suppressing the growth of certain types of cancer. They belong to the arsenal of the body's biochemical defense system. They do not destroy the defective cells, rather they correct them or reprogram them, they carry good information to the abnormal cells, and tell them how they can develop normally. It has been determined that people with cancer only have 2-3% of the normal number of these peptides.

For more than 30 years Dr. Burzynski has been separating 5 different antineoplastons from human urine, these are substances that act against a neoplasm (an abnormal tissue change) – such as against a tumor. His explanation for this is that these molecules, viewed on a genetic level have a strong anti-cancer effect. Particularly they stimulate the activities of "tumor suppressing genes". Tumor suppressing genes are genes that switch off the activities of certain oncogenes (genes that support tumor growth). Thus they prevent cells from multiplying into a tumor in an uncontrolled manner. According to this theory cancer is the result of an antineoplaston deficit.

Supported by his scientific publications Dr. Burzynski was able to obtain funding from the National Cancer Institute (NCI) in the USA, in 1974. In 1977 he published the results of a study with 21 advanced stage tumor and leukemia patients, for whom there were no chances of survival according to conventional treatment methods. In a period of 9 months, four patients had a complete remission, and 4 others had partial remissions (tumor reduction of more than 50%). For 6 patients the illness stabilized – it neither progressed nor went into remission. 2 patients stopped the treatment after their tumors were reduced by less than 50%. Only 5 patients died as a result of their original illness. Dr. Burzynski was convinced after this study that his antineoplaston treatment could save the lives of people with cancer. Because the NCI funding ran out at this time, Dr. Burzynski decided to finance his research himself, and founded his independent cancer treatment center (Burzynski Research Institute) and started charging his patients for his, "experimental treatment", as he called it then. Thanks to these first patients he was able to survive the long years of research and development of the antineoplastons.

Since the early 1970s Dr. Burzynski faced bitter attacks from the allopathic establishment, until the US Supreme Court ruled that he could treat patients. His scientific studies and records were simply too clear to be refuted by the FDA (Food and Drug Administration).

In March 1990, at the 9th International Symposium on the "Future Trends in Chemotherapy" Dr. Dvorit Samid, declared that the antineoplaston AS2-1 sustainably suppresses the activity of oncogenes, as well as proliferation of malignant cells, however without being toxic for normal cells. According to scientific reports that were presented at the 86th annual convention of the "American Association for Cancer Research" in March 1995, it was recognizable that Dr. Burzynski's antineoplastons increased the activities of tumor-suppression genes. Today Dr. Burzynski produces his antineo-plastons in a production facility, that is approved by the FDA, in his clinic in Houston Texas. Currently Dr. Burzynski has more than 90 treatment protocols, and uses multiple antineo-plaston recipes.

The individual treatment protocols differ significantly in some cases and depend on the respective type and size of the tumor. Currently there is probably no other form of therapy that deals with this important mechanism in the occurrence of cancer. The irony is that Dr. Burzynski found virtually no recognition for his discovery, which is worthy of a Nobel

Prize. Instead for many years he was subjected to fierce attacks from the FDA and the Texas Medical Board. Today however his treatment is considered to be one of the most promising and most scientific non-conventional cancer therapies in the world.

The therapy consists of an intravenous infusion (at the beginning – later capsules). The patient carries a miniature infusion pump in a small fanny pack that introduces antineoplastons into the chest (24-hours a day). This procedure is painless and does not limit the patient's freedom of movement. As part of a study Dr. Burzynski used antineoplastons to treat 20 patients with an astrocytoma in an advanced stage. Approximately 80% had a positive reaction and some of them were still cancer-free after four years. Moreover animal studies in Japan showed that small doses of the synthetic antineoplaston A10 taken orally help prevent breast cancer, lung cancer, and liver cancer.

Personal opinion: Dr. Burzynski was in Germany at my invitation in 1999, and gave several presentations in which he supported his therapy with many cases. Other cancer organizations have investigated successful cases and they have come to the same results as I have. I can maintain without doubt that Dr. Burzynski's therapy should be viewed as the first option for brain tumors. Unfortunately the high initial costs of 2,000 to 3,000 Euro/month represent an excessively high hurdle and I hope that Dr. Burzynski's therapy will finally be recognized so that the costs can be reduced significantly.

Coley's Toxin

The New York physician, William B. Coley (1892-1936) discovered in the 1920s that certain infectious diseases – particularly those caused by bacteria – have a certain therapeutic effect against malignant ulcers, if they are introduced into the body in the form a sterile vaccine. Dr. Coley determined that the anti-cancer defense system of the body gets a lift in fighting cancer cells through this "toxin".

As a surgeon active at the Memorial Hospital (in New York City), Coley developed a bacterial vaccine. He refused to believe that cancer could not be cured; in his day cancer therapy mainly consisted of removing the affected body parts through operative intervention and amputations.

Dr. Coley used the bacteria streptococcus pyogenes and Serratia marcescens (which he cultivated in beef bouillon). He assumed that the body gets a lift through the bacteria and thus his anti-cancer defense could be guided in the right direction – namely against cancer cells. The theory behind this is that the immune system must first be mobilized against a less complex opponent, the bacteria.

Cancer patients were injected with the vaccine in the vicinity of the tumor, and Dr. Coley could thus achieve an effect. His patients not only had partial remissions but also complete remissions for a variety of cancer types. Patients who were given an injection (intravenous or intramuscular) in the morning first got a kind of ague which then was replaced by fever. Then in the afternoon a normal condition established itself with the patients.

After his death in 1936 his research disappeared from public interest for decades. What is interesting is that even during his lifetime, nearly 50 doctors in the USA (one of them in the Mayo clinic) and Europe treated patients with Coley's vaccine. The vaccine was prepared and distributed by the pharmaceutical company Parke Davis and Company. After Dr. Charles Starnes, an American immunologist, analyzed the vaccine for 9 months, he declared that he considered it to be the most promising cancer treatment. Dr. Starnes reported on Dr. Coley's successes with soft tissue sarcoma (more than 40 of 84 patients were still cancer-free after 5 years; 17 patients survived up to 20 years) and for malignant lymphonomas (19 of 33 patients were still cancer-free and 8 survived up to 20 years).

Unfortunately in 1962 there were changes in legislation which resulted in the fact that the vaccine could no longer be used in the USA. The FDA simply declared the vaccine was a "new medication". This meant that it would have been necessary to go through the usual astronomically expensive tests to obtain the approval. The funding wasn't there.

After Dr. Coley's death the vaccine was weakened by Parke Davis and Company to minimize the risk of a fatal reaction, and thus doctors' liability. However it became evident that the weakened version was not sufficient. Many cancer experts believe Coley's vaccine is not used in the area of conventional cancer treatment because it cannot be patented. Even though it is considered to be effective and cost effective.

We owe thanks to Dr. Coley's daughter, Helen Coley Nauts, that Coley's vaccine did not get lost. She collected approximately 1,000 patient reports and founded the Cancer Research Institute in New York and published several articles about the treatment of malignant tumors with Coley's vaccine, jointly with doctors. Tests conducted by the Memorial Sloan-Kettering Cancer Center in New York in 1976 showed that people with advanced Non-Hodgkin lymphomas who were given Coley's vaccine, had a 93% remission rate compared to 29% in the control group (who received a chemotherapy).

In Germany the preparation vaccineurin was the medication of choice for many years. Unfortunately production was stopped and the last vials are still being traded on the black-market. An alternative is the Japanese medication picibanil, which unfortunately is not very well known in Germany yet, although it induces a controlled fever curve similar to vaccineurin.

Since 2004, a new vaccine can again be purchased from a company in Hamburg, and I can only hope that this represents the beginning of new era of active fever therapy.

Personal opinion: My experience is that I know many patients who used an active fever therapy in a very advanced stage of their illness, with great success. I am often asked which would be better, hyperthermia, or an active fever therapy with bacteria. At this time, neither I nor anybody else can answer this question scientifically. Based on my experience however I must give preference to the active fever therapy with bacteria.

Hyperthermia

The word hyperthermia comes from the Greek and means over-warming (hyper: too much and thermos: warmth). The idea of hyperthermia naturally comes from the consideration that an artificial increase in body temperature is the same as healing fever. I cannot agree and my personal experiences show me clearly that there is really a significant difference between the body generating fever because bacteria is injected into it, as with the Coley therapy, or increased bodily temperature produced through artificially generated waves. There is another interesting aspect of hypothermia that is also very interesting; it is certainly a therapy, which has successfully found a place in allopathy through the detour of alternative medicine.

While allopathy for the most part only laughed at hypothermia until the end of the last century, today there is a close network of people who are studying this therapy intensively, at the University of Berlin, Charité, Campus Virchow-Klinikum, the University of Düsseldorf, the University of Essen, the University of Lübeck, the University of Munich, and at the University of Tübingen. Naturally the universities represent the opinion that hyperthermia only makes sense when it is combined with a chemotherapy. My opinion in this regard: Any other statement would have been surprising.

Here we cannot forget that the production of hypothermia devices and the therapy is an ever increasing business. For this reason alone active fever therapy hardly has a chance of survival. Please do not misunderstand me. I certainly believe that we can no longer imagine modern cancer therapy without hyperthermia, however I believe that this comes at the cost of active fever therapy with bacteria, whose effect is not doubted by anyone who has studied it in detail.

Basically there are the following forms of hyperthermia:

Local hyperthermia
The main application area are surface tumors like individual lymph node metastasis, breast cancer nodes etc.

Regional hyperthermia
The main application areas are larger areas of 20-40 cm. It can be used almost anywhere with the exception of the thorax.

Whole-body hyperthermia
Here the primary distinction is between moderate whole-body hyperthermia in which a body temperature of max. 40.5°C is achieved, and systemic whole-body hyperthermia in which a body temperature of over 42°C is achieved. Moderate whole-body hyperthermia involves more of an immune boosting effect or improved thermal regulation of the body, and the systemic whole-body hyperthermia involves supplemental direct destruction of cancer cells. Many physicians use both of these therapies together with chemotherapies, often in low dose. This form of therapy could be a possibility for reducing a hazardous tumor mass, if an operation is not possible.

Hyperthermal perfusion
With hyperthermal perfusion a pre-warmed liquid (e.g. the patient's own blood with chemotherapeutic substances) is channeled through the veins to warm the body part. This is used for tumors in the extremities (legs/arms).

Interstitial hyperthermia
This type of hyperthermia therapy is used for certain body cavities or within organs that are surrounded by bone (the brain for example) and it is executed via previously implanted catheters. In this regard microwave antenna are used almost exclusively.

Magnetic field hyperthermia

This process is still in the trial phase. Here magnetic materials are warmed by an alternating magnetic field.

Thermoablation

Here temperatures over $50°C$ are attempted, for example, for prostrate carcinomas via laser technology.

Warming for hyperthermia therapies can occur in different ways:

1. With two metal plates between which an electrical alternating field is generated (20 MHz to 70 MHz).

2. High-frequency with a frequency of over 60 MHz.

3. Infrared systems, microwaves or ultrasound.

Personal opinion: Doubtless hyperthermia has established itself in both camps, allopathy, and non-conventional. This was certainly only possible because of the many studies that show how successful this therapy can be. In addition to the fact that consequently active fever therapy has been displaced, hyperthermia has an additional disadvantage: Again the focus is placed on the tumor. Almost all doctors measure the success of hyperthermia by the size of the tumor. Do not fall for this error, never forget that with the exception of moderate hyperthermia this therapy is primarily concerned with destruction of the tumor and that the holistic perspective should not be forgotten.

Gerson Diet

Dr. Max Gerson (1881–1959) was one of the pioneers in the area of nutrition and disease. As early as 1929 the famous doctor Ferdinand Sauerbruch introduced the Gerson diet as a "breakthrough in the treatment of TBC patients". At that time Sauerbruch published a study in which 446 of 450 patients were able to be healed permanently.

Dr. Gerson, who cured Helene Schweitzer (the wife of Albert Schweitzer) of TB, emigrated to the USA in 1933. When Gerson died in 1959, Albert Schweitzer wrote: "For me he is one the greatest geniuses in the history of medicine. Those who he has healed, bear witness to the correctness of his ideas".

"There is no cancer in a normal metabolism", wrote Max Gerson, and this was also the basic principle of his therapy. It is only possible for cancer cells to grow abnormally if the liver, the spleen, and other parts of our immune system, are disturbed. Thus in order to treat cancer successfully the highest priority is placed on getting the disturbed metabolism back on the right track. This is accomplished through intensive detoxification and introducing important nutrients through a low-fat, salt-free diet. Although this sounds easy at first, in practice it requires considerable effort, since introducing the important enzymes, vitamins, and minerals mainly involves the patient drinking fresh-squeezed/pressed juice every hour (thirteen times a day) and having a coffee enema several times a day (see coffee enemas in the chapter on detoxification).

Gerson reached the conviction that many patients died because their liver was not able to eliminate all the waste substances which had accumulated in the body through the intensive enzyme therapy. In addition, patients are given thyroid preparations, potassium, liver extracts, beta-carotene, and other antioxidants. Meat is completely prohibited in the first weeks. Flaxseed oil and cottage cheese are also given. For Max Gerson the aim of his therapy was to restore the balance between sodium and potassium in the cell. Normally the liver, the brain, and the muscle cells must have higher potassium values. This is not the case with cancer patients. Consequently the Gerson diet is rich in potassium and it is virtually sodium-free.

Max Gerson was also concerned about increased oxygen metabolism in the cells. In his therapy this is done by introducing oxidizing enzymes through juices, fruits, and liver extracts. A remission of the tumor can be expected as soon as detoxification starts, the liver again produces enough enzymes, and a sodium-potassium balance is reached. As described above, the basis of the therapy is fresh-pressed juices and coffee enemas. Please be aware that you will require help, as this is quite strenuous.

If you have carefully read the cancer theories, then you will readily understand why Gerson's views were so revolutionary and successful. With his views on potassium and sodium he was many years ahead of his time.

The Gerson Therapy is not possible if you have just gone through a chemotherapy. Thus do not start this therapy on your own, without instruction.

As the research director of the National Foundation for Alternative Medicine in 1999, I had the opportunity to personally witness the effectiveness of the Gerson therapy. Our team investigated more than 30 cases and documented them for a Best Case Series, in accordance with the guidelines prescribed by the National Cancer Institute in the USA. Moreover, I know many patients in Germany and in England who survived thanks to the Gerson therapy. I do not want to hide the fact that the Gerson therapy demands a lot of effort; it is a full-time job to make 13 fresh-squeezed/pressed juices per day, and to perform 6 coffee enemas. On the other hand it is also a full-time job to undergo chemotherapy.

Personal opinion: The Gerson therapy has certainly helped many people. I know a few of these people personally and I have no doubt whatsoever concerning the effectiveness of the therapy. Because it is becoming increasingly difficult to get biological fruit, unfortunately the effectiveness of the therapy is somewhat reduced, and this point is one of the crucial factors for its success.

Dr. Paul Gerhard Seeger's
10 point program

Dr. Paul Gerhard Seeger was a researcher and cancer specialist, and he did not accept Otto Warburg's theory that a cancer cell is irreversible and thus incurable. Seeger produced the evidence that cancer cells could be cured.

In order to understand Seeger we should take a very close look at a body cell. The cell wall is called a membrane. The cell membrane lets certain substances through, otherwise the cell cannot take nutrients from the blood. Imagine the cell as a nylon stocking. If a protein particle approaches then the nylon stocking opens. The cell membranes have a negative electric charge, the cell nucleus on the other hand has a positive charge. The cell has an electrical potential of -90 millivolt. Within the cell there are cell salts like magnesium and potassium. Outside of the cell of membrane there is sodium. Thus the cell is a miniature battery. Also the mitochondria are inside the cell. They are the breathing organs and contain the respiratory ferment, the cytochrome oxidase.

Seeger discovered that this respiratory ferment is lacking in the cancer cell (see also the work of Dr. Johanna Budwig in this regard) and consequently no oxygen combustion takes place. This lack is due to the fact that the blood has become alkaline through many kinds of toxins and through other causes. The blood acid level is no longer neutral. This causes the red blood corpuscles to become diseased and the tissue cell is damaged as a result of insufficient supply of oxygen. Cell membranes are permeable. Because mitochondria can now move out of the cell, the number of mitochondria in the cell is reduced. Through the diminution of the respiratory organ the cytochrome oxidase quantity is also reduced and these are precisely the elements that ensure oxygen combustion.

Through the disturbance in permeability sodium gets into the cell from the blood serum, while magnesium and potassium leave the cell. Consequently the electric potential is reduced.

Seeger's therapy consisted of introducing substances into the body which activate cellular respiration. These substances are:

1. Vitamin A in high doses
2. d-lactic acid (L+)
3. Ozone peroxide
4. Polyunsaturated fatty acids
5. Free radicals
6. Betacyanin, the red coloring of red beets
7. Anthozym, an enzyme drink

Seeger is also of the opinion that cancer is an illness of the soul. Healing the psychological disorder, in his view is just as important as the physical therapy. He cites the following psychological causes for cancer:

1. Fear or suppression of feelings
2. Protracted stress
3. Depression
4. Hopelessness
5. Conflicts
6. Anger, worry
7. Sexual problems
8. Social need
9. The loss of a loved one

In 1965, Seeger proposed a 10-phase therapy based on his experimental biochemical and electro-chemical findings, and based on his experience with cancer patients.

1. Phase	Resolution of interference fields.
2. Phase	Detoxification of the body and nosodes treatment.
3. Phase	Reversing the dysbiosis and normalization of the intestinal flora
4. Phase:	Activating cellular respiration through hydrogen acceptors.
5. Phase:	Activating the body's own immune system.
6. Phase:	Activating the immune system and desensitization.
7. Phase:	Cytoplasmatic therapy and activation of the antibodies
8. Phase:	Inhibiting glycolysis
9. Phase:	Changing the diet.
10. Phase:	Support of heart and circulatory system.

The Seeger therapy is organized logically. Resolution of interfering fields and detoxification of the body are the top priority. The "garbage can" must be cleaned out first! (I can only agree with this view; it proves how important detoxification measures were to Dr. Seeger as well.)

The second step in the Seeger therapy is normalization of the intestinal flora. The intestinal bacteria must be built-up with the assistance of physiologic intestinal cultures such as the acidophilus, bifidus, and the thermophilus bacteria (d-lactic acid bacteria). Then Seeger activates cellular respiration with cellular respiration activators. These are preparations that bring oxygen into the cell and in this way influence the glycolysis process. Vitamin A and betacyanin, the coloring of the red beet, are two important substances for this. In 1916, professor W.F. Koch wrote about the significance of Vitamin A relative to cancer. For cancer patients it is difficult to convert the provitamin Carotene into vitamin A. Thus they must take liquid vitamin A as a nutritional supplement. In addition Seeger prescribed one liter of red beet juice a day for his patients.

Personal opinion: There is no doubt that Dr. Seeger was the man who did more research with cancer cells than perhaps all those before and after him. He was probably the greatest cancer researcher of the 20th century and every doctor or homeopathic practitioner should have read Seeger's book: *Krebs, Problem ohne Ausweg (Cancer, Problem Without a Solution)*. In this book he not only describes his own experiments, he also describes those of many other cancer researchers. In my opinion, every oncologist who has read this book has just two courses of action:

1.   He must stop treating patients
      conventionally, or

2.   Refute Dr. Seeger's work.

Unfortunately the fact is that there is a schizophrenic attitude among many therapists. On one hand they do not have the knowledge to refute Seeger's work, on the other hand, they prescribe chemotherapies on a daily basis. To this day I do not understand how a person could read Seeger's work and then simply continue on as before. But this is precisely what goes on in German oncology on a daily basis.

Homeopathy

The founder of homeopathy was Dr. Samual Hahnemann, who lived from 1755-1843. Homeopathy means, "similar suffering" (homoion = similar and pathos = suffering). Hahnemann believed that an illness should be treated with a medication that would induce "similar suffering" in a healthy person. His statement in Latin: „Similia similibus curentur", in English: "Let likes be cured by likes" has gone down in medical history.

Hahnemann assumed that the disease symptoms are not the illness itself, rather they are reactions to the causes of the disorder. These causes are nothing more than the body's attempt to regulate. Thus homeopathy does not try to suppress the symptoms, and thus the regulation attempt, rather it attempts to stimulate the self-healing powers of the body.

The medications used are traditionally designated in Latin. The name is followed by one of the letters D, C, or LM, plus a number. Occasionally the character Ø is used or alternatively the term, mother tincture is used. Example: Avena sativa D 12 or Cardius marianus Ø. This somewhat complicated nomenclature indicates the "potency" of the substance used.

The extract of a medicinal plant is produced in accordance with a formulated guideline in the so-called homeopathic book of methods and gets the name mother tincture with the abbreviation Ø. Then an alcohol/water mixture is added to the mother tincture and the mother tincture is shaken. This produces the first homeopathic potency scale, which depending on the mixing ratio is designated mother tincture/alcohol water mixture. A mixing ratio mother tincture/alcohol-water mixture of 1 :10 corresponds to the first potency scale D 1, 1:100 corresponds to the first potency level C1, 1 : 50,000 corresponds to the first potency scale LM 1. The next potency scale is attained if the produced first potency is again mixed in the same ratio with an alcohol-water mixture. Depending on the mixing ratio this produces D 2, C 2, or LM 2.

There is no "pure homeopathic oncology", because homeopaths treat each cancer patient differently, since they view cancer for what it is, a symptom. Also I personally do not know a single homeopath who treats cancer patients with homeopathy only, **and** states this publicly. Naturally this would be very difficult, for legal reasons alone. Interestingly enough there were studies in the first half of the last century that were quite positive. For instance in 1931, a study was published (Homeopathic Recorder, vol. 46, 674–649) in which of 225 cancer patients, who were exclusively treated homeopathically, 66% were still alive after 6 years.

In Switzerland and in Southern Germany there are two cancer clinics that view homeopathy as the basis of a cancer therapy, and that also treat many cancer patients exclusively on a homeopathic basis.

Personal opinion: Without doubt homeopathy has a legitimate place in oncology, and whoever maintains the contrary has certainly not studied Hahnemann's work. Hahnemann deserves recognition just for his approach that a tumor is a self-regulating mechanism of the body. What is difficult however is to find a homeopath who is knowledgeable about cancer, and who can use homeopathy not only to relieve side-effects of the "proper cancer therapies", but as partial treatment or the main treatment of a holistic cancer therapy. I cannot imagine that Hahnemann would have prescribed chemotherapy and Gelsemium sempervirens D 12 for the concurrent fever therapy. Usually a homeopath is a good choice, however for a different reason: He/she usually will spend more time with you than is the case with most allopathic practitioners.

IAT
(Immuno-Augmentative Therapy)

IAT was developed in the 1960s by Dr. Lawrence Burton at the St. Vincent Hospital in New York City. On the basis of animal experiments Dr. Burton was able to identify and isolate tumor suppressing factors that also were effective with humans. Dr. Burton identified and isolated blood protein components, which he assumed were associated with the occurrence of cancer.

These were: Tumor complement (a substance that is developed from the blood clots of cancer patients. This factor, which is also referred to as the C3 complement, then activates 2 tumor antibodies (TA1 and TA2). A fourth protein, the blocking protein factor (DPF), comes from the blood serum of healthy donors.

When these 4 blood protein components are in balance, then the body, according to Dr. Burton, should be capable of conquering the cancer on its own. If they are not balanced then the body cannot adequately defend itself. If, for example, too much of the blocking protein is present, the tumor antibodies will be suppressed, and then they are no longer capable of neutralizing cancer cells. Dr. Burton explained that all cells release a blocking protein when they die, which prevents additional activities of the tumor antibodies.

Dr. Burton determined that a remission for different types of cancer could be induced when he injected his patients with a certain number of these components. Even for types of cancer which apparently were thought to quickly end in death. However he also declared immediately that his treatment was no cure for cancer. Rather he compared it with insulin for diabetics. It controls the cancer and the patient can live for many more years. Dr. Burton astounded the oncological world in 1966. At a seminar in Phoenix Arizona, he injected his serum into mice with very large tumors. The tumors disappeared within two hours. In the same year he repeated this experiment in front of the skeptical New York Academy of Medicine, whose members doubted the Phoenix experiment and brought their own mice. Here as well the tumors of 16 mice disappeared within two hours.

Although a book published by the American government agency, Office of Technology, **Unconventional Cancer Therapies,** explained that IAT was not able to clearly demonstrate tumor reductions, it did accept the results of a different study (coordinated by Dr. Barrie Cassileth from the University of North Carolina – a critic of alternative cancer therapies and a representative of the American Cancer Society). In this study 79 patients with advanced (metastatizing) cancer were give IAT. 60 patients (63%) survived an average of 65 months (more than 5 years after the diagnosis). The 20 patients who died survived on average 59 months (i.e. almost 5 years).

These results were astounding because the normal chances of survival for the majority of these patients was 36 months. Consequently it could be determined that Dr. Burton's IAT approximately doubled the survival chances as compared with the survival chances of patients treated with conventional cancer therapies. Another study published in 1977 with 277 patients, most of whom had a hopeless prognosis, showed that 18% were still alive after 5 years. This number is also astounding because the one-year survival rate of these patients was less than 1%.

As with almost all non-conventional therapies, patients are usually subjected to other conventional treatment methods, and it is only after these have been unsuccessful that patients decide for IAT. Dr. Burton knew this and yet was still able to send 4 – 6 patients out of 10 home with improvement. According to Dr. Burton's information IAT achieved a tumor reduction or total remission in 40-60% of the patients that he treated. His results were particularly good for people with advanced colon cancer and for mesotheliomas. According to the standard statistics, chances for 5-year survival are zero for these cancer types.

Dr. Burton reported on the successful treatment of 11 patients with pleural mesothelioma, a form of cancer (usually triggered by asbestos), which we know is fatal and incurable. The American Medical Association was certainly alarmed about this statement and immediately proclaimed that IAT must be a quack remedy.

Patients come into the IAT clinic every morning; they stay in apartments or hotels. In the clinic blood is taken and analyzed every day. After the evaluation a new serum is determined and created daily (a protein from the serum of healthy donors is used, which improves/strengthens the blood of the patient). The patient then leaves the clinic and administers the injections himself in the course of the day. Daily injections are administered for 6-12 weeks. Afterwards the patient can return home where he continues with the injections.

Personal opinion: *People against Cancer, the National Foundation for Alternative Medicine, personnel from the Office for Alternative Health* in Washington, and I myself, have been to Freeport/Bahamas several times to examine the patient data. There is no doubt that hard facts confirm that Dr. Lawrence Burton has found something phenomenal. Unfortunately to this point a holistic approach is lacking in the clinic, and I would be more than pleased if someday a holistic approach was added. If you decide on this therapy, then you must ensure that you plan a holistic therapy on your own. It should certainly be legally punishable not to recommend this therapy for pleural mesothelioma.

Galvano Therapy
Bio-Electro-Therapy

Although cancer treatment with galvanic currents is far more widespread in China today than it is in Germany, it is a European to whom we owe gratitude for this therapy, Dr. Rudolf Pekar from Bad Ischl in Austria. Pekar was already known as the patent holder for "Obtaining vaccines for an immune therapy" when he discovered that he could render tumor cells harmless with direct current.

First he started to reverse the polarity of tumors in the bodies of mice with direct current and then he started treating the first patients. Today this therapy is even used in the form of an electro-chemotherapy, i.e. in conjunction with chemotherapy.

According to Dr. Pekar, who I personally met first time on his 88th birthday, he had major success with malignant melanomas (skin cancer), mamma carcinoma (breast cancer), prostrate carcinomas, spinaliomas, lymphomas, and tumors in the genital area. Also, bio-electro-therapy should be considered instead of an operation where tumors sit directly on the skin.

In the therapy two platinum wire electrodes are introduced directly into the tumor, or into surrounding tissue, or in the case of melanomas, platinum platelets as electrodes are placed on the skin. Then a weak direct current flows between both electrodes, which reverses the polarity of the cancer cells in the tumor tissue and allows the cancer cells to die.

The idea behind this therapy is that tumor cells are negatively charged, and consequently in the treatment they are attracted with direct current by the positive electrode. The current then works on each individual cell of the tumor tissue directly on the cell membrane and induces the repolarization of each cell. Afterwards macrophages can again recognize the cancer cells, which previously hid themselves, so to speak, behind an excess negative charge. In addition, the surrounding tissue becomes highly acidic (pH value 4-5) which likewise reduces the survival chances of cancer cells.

However, Dr. Pekar is aware that cancer is a systemic event and that destruction of the tumor is only a small part of the treatment. Consequently he recommends the following therapy to his patients, in addition:

* No meat, no foods containing carbohydrates,

 no sugar (also no real sweet fruit). Instead

 daily in any sequence:

* Quark, mixed with vegetable oil (flaxseed oil is even better)

* Sauerkraut (raw or cooked), sauerkraut juice

* Brewer's yeast mixed with yoghurt

* The juice of two lemons, taken proportionally in herbal tee

* Onions, garlic, mustard

* Red beet juice

* 2 almonds daily

* A+E Mulsin, 10–15 drops daily

* Vitamin C as an effervescent tablet

* Selenium, magnesium, beta carotene as tablets

* Jodonorm tablets, 1 tablet, three times a week.

Personal opinion: Galvano-therapies are certainly an interesting approach for tumor destruction. This is why an increasing number of physicians and homeopathic practitioners are using this therapy in Germany. For me it was very interesting to note that 20 years ago Dr. Pekar still advised his patients to have operations, and in summarizing his more than 50 years of work as an oncologist he said, that today in most cases he would no longer advise an operation, because he frequently could see that particularly women with breast cancer lived much longer if they did not have an operation. (Now other therapists also represent this opinion).

I do not want to hide the fact that in the meantime I have become acquainted with patients who experienced rapid tumor growth after several galvano-therapies. It is hard for me to evaluate whether this growth was exclusively stimulated by the galvano-therapy. At the outset I would not exclude the possibility that tumors "defend themselves" against this treatment, particularly after several galvano-therapy sessions.

Govallo's VG 1000

The Russian immunologist Dr. Valentine I. Govallo found that cancer has a unique characteristic, which enables it to avoid or prevent attacks from the human immune system. He discovered that this particular factor is present in the placenta, which surrounds the fetus, and he developed a vaccine from the blood of the placenta (which he removed immediately after birth). He uses this vaccine to strengthen the body's immune system so that it can better master the cancer and the cancer's defense mechanisms.

Cancer immunologists have always assumed that if the immune system can be stimulated in a specific manner, this stimulation could stop the cancer or possibly even reverse it.

In Dr. Govallo's view this is because cancer has a unique immunological characteristic. This is why cancer is usually successful in withstanding the attacks of the human immune system. Dr. Govallo, who has published more than 250! scientific articles, and written more than 20 books, was the director of the Laboratory for Clinical Immunology of the Moscow Medical Institute. Over the years he discovered that after miscarriage, many women had a problem in the general dismantling of the fetal placental immune system – caused by environmental toxins. Dr. Govallo's therapy is based on his understanding of how the fetus communicates with its mother (on the immunological level).

Even if babies are totally dependent on their mothers, the fetus still has a primitive immune system with features that deviate very slightly from the mother's immune system. The immune system of the fetus and that of the mother are practically in a competition with each other. It sounds almost unbelievable but the immune system of the mother could consider the fetus as a foreign protein and eliminate it. Under normal conditions the fetus however is not rejected, because its placental immune system is capable of blocking or bypassing the local immune system of the mother.

A miscarriage occurs because the immune system of the mother recognizes the antigens of the father in the fetus. Because her immune system assumes that a foreign invader is involved the fetus is rejected. Environmental toxins that are especially prevalent in Russia, exacerbate this problem, because the immune system of the mother is increasingly stressed with external proteins and materials and thus the fetus is subjected to even greater hazards. For Dr. Govallo this knowledge was an important part of the solution to the cancer problem. It became clear to him that just as the placenta produces "factors" to ensure that the baby is not rejected by the mother, in the same manner a tumor could also be capable of outfoxing the immune system, by using a type of immunological protection mechanism. To prevent a rejection through the immune system of the carrier, the tumor uses the same technique employed by the fetus.

Today scientists know that tumors produces "defense factors", and proteins are involved in some of these factors, which, so to speak, are stored by the tumor after it comes into contact with the immune system of the "host". For example a form of the tumor protein can switch off the activities of the natural killer cells (NKC). The secretion of these defense factors involves a mechanism with which the tumor cell gains an advantage relative to the anti-tumor reactions of the "host". Consequently tumor cells are capable of fending off the counter-attacks of the immune system.

Thus the cancer has found a way to switch-off the host's immune system, like a burglar can switch-off the alarm system of a house. This could be the reason for the biological survival capability of the tumor. If the cancer's protective shield can be successfully penetrated, then the body should be able to neutralize the growth of the tumor, or even destroy it.

The healthy human placenta contains factors that are capable of suppressing the defense system of malignant cells. The vaccine produced by Dr. Govallo from the placenta makes it possible to "uncover" the tumor. Govallo's vaccine is produced from the placenta tissue immediately after the birth of a baby. The most active parts of the placenta extract are used in order to neutralize the protective defense factor (which is produced by the primary tumor). This is why the treatment is referred to as IPT (Immuno-Placental Therapy). The vaccine really became known however as VG 1000.

Dr. Govallo warns every patient and treating physician that if the tumor is destroyed too quickly, then large quantities of toxins are released in the body, which in turn are capable of killing the patient. This is referred to as a *tumor lysis syndrome*. The killed-off tumor cells are absorbed in the blood and in the lymph channels and must be eliminated from the body. However this can overload the detoxification capacity of the body. This is why the body must be supplied with sufficient nutrients in order to improve its detoxification capacities. In a study with advanced cancer VG 100 demonstrated a survival rate of 77% after 5 years, compared with a 6 % survival rate on the basis of other immunotherapeutic procedures. Quality of life improved for all patients who took VG 1000.

Doctors at Duke University in the USA observed a 50% survival rate over a period ranging from 7-32 months after 25 leukemia patients (mainly children) were given a placenta blood infusion. Even if all 25 patients required bone marrow to replace stem cells, through the use of the placental blood there was a better survival rate compared to that offered by a standard bone marrow transplant. Through VG 1000 recipient and donor were better suited to each other (New England Journal of Medicine – July 1966).

Personal opinion: *People against Cancer* personnel were in Moscow several times with American patients to obtain VG 1000 from Dr. Govallo. I personally know the wonderful case of a man who already had a scheduled operation for bladder cancer, and who received a VG 1000 injection 8 days prior to the operation. On the day of the operation no tumor could be found.

Without doubt there are hard facts that speak for Govallo's therapy and VG 1000 is an option, particularly after an operation. Dr. Govallo's original therapy consisted of only 2-3 injections. The present manufacturer recommends injecting VG 1000 over a longer period; moreover the manufacturing process has changed. I cannot evaluate the extent to which this impacts the effectiveness.

Laetril

Laetril, also referred to as amygdaline or vitamin B17 is a nitriloside and caused quite a furor in America in the 1970s. An active ingredient, which particularly occurs in the seeds of apricots or apples became so well-known as an anti-cancer agent, that first the Sloan Kettering Center in New York, and then even the Mayo Clinic in Rochester performed their own studies. "Naturally" with the result that the predominantly positive studies produced by biochemist, Dr. Kanematsu Sugiura, in which he was could prove that Laetril was able to particularly stop the growth of smaller tumors, could not be correct. Rubin also proved that patients with breast cancer or bone cancer lived longer.

Only much later was it disclosed that virtually inactive isoamygdaline was used in the Mayo Clinic study. Most of the patients had already undergone chemotherapy and irradiation without success and after stabilization occurred for app. 70% of all patients within 3 weeks, in spite of advanced disease, the treatment was changed to oral doses of Laetril instead of intravenous Laetril.

This is another prime example of how a positive study result, or a negative study result can be generated with any medication in the world. In Germany since the death of the famous cancer physician Dr. Nieper, who treated well-known people like Caroline of Monaco or John Wayne, Laetril unfortunately has again sunk into oblivion. The current Laetril center is the Contreras Clinic in Tijuana where Laetril has been used for more than 25 years.

We have Dr. Ernest Krebs to thank for the discovery of Laetril. His theory was that trophoblasts (cells that develop at the beginning of fertilization) which normally are destroyed through the enzyme chemotrypsin, survive and years later these cells can develop tumors, if the pancreas no longer functions correctly. Laetril consists of 2 glucose molecules, a benzaldehyde molecule and a cyanide radical molecule. The glucose molecules are replaced in the body by glucoronic acid. This process has negative effects on cancer cells, however it does not have negative effects on healthy cells, because the enzyme glucoronidase which occurs in high concentrations in cancer cells, splits the glucoronic acid and thus loses the benzaldehyde then cyanide, which kills cancer cells.

As opposed to cancer cells, healthy cells also have the enzyme rhodanase which adds a sulfur atom to each free cyanide, in order to form harmless thiocyanate. Although there are other studies by Tatsumura (1987) or Kochi (1985) which confirm the positive effect of benzaldehyde on cancer cells, today Laetril is an almost forgotten cancer medication.

The book by Phillip Day: **Cancer: Why we're still dying to know the truth**, has brought Laetril back into the headlines in Germany. What is less well known is the fact that in 2003, a physician in Hannover, "was advised" to stop treating his patients with laetril, and currently I only know of one other doctor in Germany who administers this medication intravenously. Taken orally it is uncertain whether Laetril can work at all, and unfortunately taken in larger amounts you overtask your gastrointestinal tract very quickly.

Personal opinion: During my stay at the Contreras Clinic in Mexico, I had the opportunity to speak with many patients and doctors who have had good experiences with laetril. It certainly belongs in the hands of an experienced physician. Unfortunately there are very few of these and it appears as if laetril will disappear from oncology in a few years.

Gonzales Therapy

Dr. Nicholas Gonzales learned his therapy program from Dr. William Kelley, who claimed that he had had pancreatic cancer, and healed himself with his therapy. Dr. Kelley became famous through his cases and Dr. Gonzales was the first to examine his cases in detail. After 5 years he had examined more than 1300 cases and had interviewed 450 patients, all with pancreatic cancer. He published this work in a 300-page volume titled: One Man Only.

The results that he documented were so convincing to him that he soon started treating his own patients with Dr. Kelley's therapy. Precisely like other doctors, such as Dr. Krebs, Dr. Kelley was convinced that our immune system was not the first immune mechanism of cancer cells. For this reason he prescribed large quantities of enzymes that are normally produced by the pancreas.

For years Dr. Gonzales was attacked from various sides, sued, laughed at, and called a criminal. Then came the day in 1999 when the American NIH (National Institute for Health) made more than 1.4 million dollars available to Dr. Gonzales to compare his therapy with other pancreatic cancer therapies. From this day on he was again considered to be established, because everyone knew that he only got this money because he could demonstrate better successes than could be demonstrated by allopathy. But perhaps it was also due to the study that had been published previously, that of 126 patients with pancreatic cancer who had been treated with chemotherapy, after 19 months all 126 patients were dead - as opposed to the Dr. Gonzales patients.

The Gonzales therapy consists of up to 150 capsules, vitamins, enzymes, and minerals per day, and at least two coffee enemas and a drink made of black walnut. The usual "diet" consists of vegetarian meals, and in many cases meat as well, because he was a firm believer that many people need meat.

Personal opinion: With his therapy, Dr Gonzales proved that pancreatic cancer could certainly be treated differently and more successfully than it can be treated with chemotherapy. Unfortunately there is an enormous interest in keeping his therapy as limited as possible and consequently there is a precise prescription as to which patients he may treat in America and which he may not treat. It is very difficult for German patients to avail themselves of his therapy. However NutriTherapy, which is also based on Dr. Kelley's work and which is available in Germany, represents one alternative.

Patients with pancreatic cancer must study this therapy or NutriTherapy, because unfortunately there are not many physicians who can demonstrate success with pancreatic cancer.

Transfer Factors

Dr. Giancarlo Pizza from Bologna has been treating cancer patients for more than 25 years with an immuno-therapy developed by his institute that contains various cytokines. His successes are very good with metastasizing kidney cancer, large-cell lung cancer, recurrences of bladder cancer, and for metastasizing prostate cancer. However his therapy is basically promising for all other types of cancer. Since April 2001, a study has been underway conducted jointly with American Universities to collect the successful data of Dr. Pizza.

In June 2000, Dr. Pizza introduced the results of his examinations in a presentation to the US Congress in Washington DC, where I was personally in attendance. I have also examined documents in Bologna and can confirm Dr. Pizza's published data.

Origin and features:
In research conducted by the urology department for immune diagnosis and immunbiology at the Orsola-Malpighi Hospital in Bologna, Italy a possibility was discovered for producing so-called special transfer factors, that are produced from human blood. Currently these transfer factors are only produced in Bologna, and may only be used under the supervision of the Italian Ministry of Health. In parallel Dr. Pizza uses interleuken-2 , interferon and human antibodies produced in vitro, to stabilize and-or improve the immune system.

Treatment procedure:
Unfortunately Dr. Pizza may only use his therapy (which is virtually free of side-effects) in Bologna; he cannot send it to other countries. Consequently you must travel to Italy for the first injection. Usually you get the two syringes for the next two months in Italy (1x month). The costs are adjusted indi-

vidually, however the costs for a 3-4 day stay including blood test, LAK (Lymphokine-Activated Killer cells) production, IHL, 2-inhalation and intralymphatic punction of IL2 and LAK PLUS transfer factors for two months' therapy, are between 1,000 and 2,000 Euro.

Personal opinion:
I have known Dr. Pizza personally for many years and I am not the only person who has examined his work many times. He can show very good data, particularly for kidney cancer. I would be very happy to see his therapy integrated within a holistic therapy, unfortunately this is not possible for political reasons.

Reduced L-glutathione

Glutathione is a protein which is formed from the amino acids cystein, glutamic acid and glycin which all of us produce in our livers. It occurs in two forms, firstly as reduced glutathione and secondly as oxidised glutathione. The reduced form in particular is very important as a medication. In organic chemistry, by the way, oxidation is the uptake of oxygen or the emission of hydrogen - reduction is the exact opposite.

It has been known for decades that there are so-called mitochondrial gates, a complex transfer system for the flow of protons and electrons and for many and diverse metabolic products. What has only been known for a few years is that these mitochondrial gates are controlled by a mixture of gases consisting of nitrogen monoxide (NO) and superoxide ions, i.e. the "waste products" of the oxidative respiration chain in the mitochondria. Interestingly, the energy preparation in certain phases (late cell-division phase, early wound-healing phase and the initial embryonal phase) switches over to fermentation. This takes place in order to protect the genes, which are sensitive to oxygen compounds during these cell division phases.

Reduced L-glutathione plays a major role here, for the flows of protons or electrons to take place at all. Unfortunately, this tripeptide can be destroyed by many medications or everyday toxins which we ingest more and more frequently. In addition, there is often a lack of cystein and glutathione due to excessive cystein and glutathione consumption or insufficient absorption of cystein. This can lead to the formation of cancer cells, since not enough oxygen can be utilised for the preparation of energy and the cells must therefore switch over to fermentation in order to survive.

In the meantime, there have been some quite positive investigations to find out what happens when reduced L-glutathione is administered to animals or humans in large quantities. Many different studies can be found on the Internet in which the positive effects in animal trials are described, either when administered alone or in combination with chemotherapy. The dosage recommendations in this context vary between 500mg - 5,000mg per day. Most authors however recommend a daily dose of between 1,000 - 2,000mg. However, this also means a monthly cost of between 200 - 400 Euros per month, depending on the preparation.

Personal opinion: The importance of reduced L-glutathione for cancer patients is in my opinion beyond doubt and the fact that many people, above all advanced cancer patients, have a lack of this has been established by many doctors for themselves. But as regards whether the solution is simply to introduce reduced L-glutathione, I am not quite sure. In the first place, reduced L-glutathione is very unstable and easily destroyed. Of course I know of the discussions concerning which is better: S-acetyl glutathione or just reduced glutathione. Naturally I also know of the question of whether it would be better only to administer the whole thing intravenously, or just the individual amino acids instead of the entire tripeptide. For me, however, these questions are of secondary importance, since it is much more important WHY a person has too little glutathione their body and what one can do to make the body use less or produce more L-glutathione. The administering of reduced L-glutathione alone cannot possibly be the solution.

However, this does not mean for me that a temporary substitution of reduced L-glutathione would not make sense, quite the opposite. Instead of paying out a great deal of money for vitamin pills or miracle teas from Brazil, I am rather in favour of "investing" this money in reduced L-glutathione. In the long term though, a better glutathione balance can only be achieved by nutrition and detoxification.

The biofield test

The biofield test belongs to the category of radiesthetics, which according to Brockhaus is the science of purported radiation effects which radiate from animate and inanimate objects and which can be detected by particularly sensitive people (radiesthetes) using divining rods or sideric pendulums (sideric = iron). While many people in western countries dismiss radiesthetics as "ridiculous fiddling about with rods" or "pendulum quackery", the spiritual world and its significance form part of everyday life in other countries. One only has to think of the term Feng Shui in China. Many of us have also forgotten that radiesthetics has always been a component part of our culture. We all know the story of Moses, who caused water to flow from a rock by means of a staff, that even in our latitudes pendulums have been found in old burials as grave goods, or that the divining rod is mentioned in the Nibelungenlied and in Parzival in German literature.

More and more during the last century, physicists have also concerned themselves with radiesthetics. However, it was not until 1982 that the physicist Alain Aspect brought a somewhat more "scientific approach" to radiesthetics, when he was able to prove that "non-locality" actually exists. That which Einstein still regarded as impossible suddenly became common knowledge within universities in 1982. Non-locality means that two or more photons from the same source do not forget each other, i.e. that each knows of the other what it is doing and that they react to an alteration in the other immediately - completely independently of how far from each other they are.

The biofield test was developed at the end of the 80's by the physicist Dr. Paul Schweitzer as a test of the stresses caused by biophysical and physical fields. In cooperation with doctors, the test procedure has been further developed into a valuable medical testing and diagnosis procedure in which doctors and healing practitioners have been trained since 1991. In Germany alone, over 500 specialists work in this field. The test device concerned is an tuneable horizontal pendulum (H-dipole). Since in the past this test apparatus has always been prone to subjective results, Dr. Schweitzer has developed a special substance, the so-called suppressor. This stabilises the own field of the tester, so that no methodological errors occur and the test results become reliable and above all reproducible. As test preparation, readily-available potentiated organ preparations and nosodes are used (nosodes are preparations made from altered organs or organ parts in accordance with homeopathic process technology).

From the viewpoint of biofield testing, toxins and microbes produce three different forms of stress:

· genetic stresses

· genetically induced stresses

· acute stresses

The genetic and genetically-induced stresses are sub-clinical and can only be measured using the biofield test, or by procedures in which the person is included in the measurement process. Using the normal diagnostic procedures of conventional medicine, these stresses cannot be detected, which again also explains the poor record of conventional medicine in the case of chronic illnesses. Therapeutically, the appropriate media for compensation of the stress factors are established with the tolerance test of the biofield test. The compensation media thus ascertained are, incidentally, preparations of 16 salts and their mixtures. The salts are the phosphates, carbonates, chlorates and sulphates of the elements sodium, potassium, calcium and magnesium.

Personal opinion: Although there are certainly an impressive number of therapists in Germany alone, there are still relatively few patients to whom the term biofield test means anything. This is principally because of the fact that many therapists do not tell their patients that they are using the biofield test. The reasons for this are difficult to ascertain, but more than understandable to insiders. I wish here too that "official" studies were available, so that myself and others could better evaluate the biofield test.

Breuß diet

Rudolf Breuß was a homeopathic practitioner from Bludenz in Austria, who dared to take a stand against the prevailing opinion that cancer patients should not fast. While his "teachers" like Dr. Otto Buchinger were vehement proponents of the 21-day fast, he was of the opinion that the usual 21-days were much too short and that patients should fast for 42-days. The idea behind this therapy is that during longer fasts the body will get rid of everything that does not belong in it - including tumors. Breuß repeatedly stated that had healed over 1000 cancer patients and thousands of other persons with serious diseases.

I cannot confirm Breuß statements, because I know too few of his patients. On the other hand in my daily work, I frequently meet people who have fasted in accordance with the Breuß therapy and who have truly wonderful things to report. I take this seriously; I do not maintain that the many people who highly praise this therapy are liars. Personally I do not believe in the theory of starving out cancer, but still I must say that again and again I find patient reports that are extremely positive, and they including the curing of cancer.

Total cancer cure according to Rudolf Breuß

Ingredients for a fresh-pressed juice mixture of 500 ml daily:

3/5 red beets (300g)

1/5 carrots (100g)

1/5 celery roots (100g)

Add a little radish and a potato the size of an egg. All vegetables should be pressed through a juice extractor and the juice should be poured through a fine tea sieve or linen cloth.

After waking drink fi cup of kidney tea slowly. 30-60 minutes later drink 1-2 cups of sage tea with St. John's wort, peppermint, and melissa. 30-60 minutes later take some vegetable juice and do not swallow it immediately but move it around in your mouth! 15-30 minutes later take a small swallow again and repeat the process up to 15 times.

At noon drink fi cup of kidney tea, and then depending how you feel, take a small swallow of vegetable juice at any time.

Before sleeping drink kidney tea again but only for the first three weeks. Complete instructions are available in the book: The Breuss Cancer Cure: Advice on the Prevention and Natural Treatment of Cancer, Leukemia, and other Seemingly Incurable Diseases.

Personal opinion: With his therapy Breuß adheres to the highest principle of traditional medicine, which is not to harm the patient. From the energy perspective it certainly helps the patient at the beginning of his 42-days. I am not sure of its effects over the entire period; at least this could be a significant problem for many patients. Even if I do not back it personally, the starving out theory is an interesting approach that can even be found in Indian medicine.
Successful Cancer Therapies

Successful Cancer Therapies

Group 2

Alloplant

The ALP Project was most likely one of the greatest projects in Russian medical history. Behind this name is Russia's former fear of a third world war and the associated consequences for Russia. It was clear sure that such an inferno would leave many seriously injured people in its wake. Consequently many years ago a team composed of the best researchers in Russia, under the direction of Prof. Muldashev, were "freighted" to Siberia to develop medications to treat the most serious burns and injuries. Because research with human cells had a long tradition in Russia this research was immediately intensified, and after a few years the team was able to manufacture a "second skin" for burn victims, from human cells. However, they quickly found out that these cells could also be used very successfully for cancer.

The western world only learned about this discovery a few years ago when Russia tried to sell this material (which today is primarily used in eye surgery) to western countries.

Because (and not in spite of) the fact that tens of thousands of patients had been treated successfully treated, the sale of these cells is still being fought successfully to this day. Considering that thousands of people in Germany alone go blind through macular degeneration (and Alloplant represents a safe therapy), and application areas like melanoma, or liver cancer also come to mind immediately. Once again I am shocked to see all the measures that are taken to ensure that sick people do not learn anything about successful therapies, or to ensure that these therapies are denied to them. For example, in a published study 892 patients with skin cancer were given Alloplant, of this number, 798 patients were controlled and 89% were treated successfully (observation period 1-15 years).

Personal opinion: Because it takes a lot of effort to get this material, and because there are too few studies, currently I would not recommend this for everyone. In the case of macular degeneration I would recommend it to my best friend. Also its use for therapy-resistant melanomas is totally conceivable.

Di Bella Protocol

Prof. Luigi Di Bella was born in 1912 and was a surgeon. Since the mid 1960s he has been working on his new cancer therapy. He held numerous conferences in various Italian cities in which he presented the ideas of his therapy methods for blood and tumor diseases, which he has used on more than 10,000 patients since 1966. This therapy became well-known through his televised debate with the Italian Minister of Health, Bindi.

The components of Di Bella's therapy:

High-dose multivitamin preparation
This preparation is a special composition of vitamins A (in pure form, as well as retinoic acid) vitamin E, vitamin C, as well as beta carotene.

Somatostatin
Somatostatin is so-called releasing hormone which inhibits the synthesis of the somatotrope hormone (STH) in the hypophyse. STH, also known as Somotropin, is a growth hormone. With cancer diseases STH is co-responsible for the growth impulse of cancer cells. Di Bella sees a connection between STH and cancer, for instance in the fact that children who were treated with the growth hormone later got cancer.

Melatonin
To increase the level of resorbtion, as well as the biological availability of melatonin, it is mixed with adenosine and glycine. This not only makes it water-soluble and it can be more easily resorbed, but it also promotes transport via the circulatory system.

Matrix
A Mucopolysaccharide (glycosaminoglycan) a high polymer combination of amino sugars, which particularly occurs in connective tissue. In the Di Bella cocktail, matrix has the job of increasing the synthesis of the body's own cortisone.

A.T. 10
This preparation also has the job of stimulating the adrenal glands to an increased production of the body's own cortisone. A.T. 10 is taken orally in drops.

Calcium
According to the Di Bella protocol the patient is given calcium (2000 mg) daily.

Vitamin C
In addition to the above-listed multivitamin preparation the Di Bella protocol also prescribes taking 5 grams of pure vitamin C per day.

Parlodel 2.5mg
The main active ingredient of this preparation is bromocriptine, which in the Di Bella cocktail handles the suppression of the prolactine synthesis. Bromocriptine is also used for Parkinson's disease as dopamine antagonist with effect on the central nervous system. With the Di Bella therapy bromocriptine is thought to contribute to suppression of undesired cell growth in close association with the somatostatin.

Glucosamine
Glucosamine is a carbohydrate and special basic nutrient which is used in the human organism as an important structural substance.

Endoxan
The main active ingredient of this preparation is cyclophos-phamide, which is a strong cytostatic agent. In the Di Bella therapy, endoxan is given in tablet form.

Synacthen
Synacthen is a polypeptide with which corticotropic effect, similar to ACTH. As it inhibits protein synthesis, it promotes protein catabolic degradation and thus should block uncon-trolled cell growth.

Personal opinion: Much of what Di Bella says makes sense, and without his personality the topic of non-conventional can-cer in Italy would never have made it to television. However I cannot accept the basic use of endoxan (cyclophosphamide). This chemotherapy can disrupt the entire process of the ther-apy he describes. In addition allopaths say correctly that all of Di Bella successes, naturally were due to the use of Endoxan. In 1999 a *People against Cancer* team, visited Di Bella in Italy and it was interesting to hear, that he did not believe that cancer was a problem of the immune system. According to Frank Wiewel, President of *People against Cancer* in the USA, Di Bella was a highly motivated doctor who always gave his patients hope. For me naturally the question comes up as to whether his successes were due to the endoxan or because of the endoxan.

Dries Diet

In 1997 I met Jan Dries for the first time at a cancer conference in London, where he gave a presentation on his nutrition therapy. It mainly consists of dividing certain food groups into 7 different categories and mixing them according to certain plan.

Here raw foods, particularly fruits from warmer climates, play a significant role, because according to Jan Dries, the important thing about food is how many biophotons we ingest. In other words, he says calories are not important, what is important is whether or not we absorb enough light. According to his theory, matter in our body is built-up through light, and also perfect cellular communication can only take place if sufficient light is in the body, absorbed through daylight and through food.

I absolutely agree with this opinion, as other researchers (Dr. Budwig, for example) have reported in detail about this aspect of nutrition or light. According to Dries you can categorize food into the following groups ordered according to biophotons:

Group I:
Pineapples, avocados, raspberries, honeydew melon, pollen, comb honey.

Group II
Blueberries, kiwi, cherries, persimmons, apricots, melons, hog plums, papaya, almonds, mushrooms, honey.

Group III
Red and black currents, strawberries, lychees, passion fruit, red and green grapes, peaches, sunflower seeds, pumpkin seeds, wheat, sprouts, liquid brewer's yeast.

Group IV
Bananas, gooseberries, green melons, Brazil nuts, coconut, vegetables, dairy products.

Group V
Oranges, mandarins, apples, pears, plums, and grapefruit, (these fruits are viewed as supplements).

Group VI
This group mainly consists of different vegetables.

Group VII
Avocados, nuts, and seeds of any kind are the best suppliers of fat because they contain fat in an organic structure.

For whoever would like to know about this I recommend the book: *Lebensmittel richtig kombinieren* (Combining Food correctly). ISBN 3-926453-89-3. In addition the more interesting book for cancer patients is available in English: *The Dries Cancer Diet* – ISBN: 1862040923.

Personal opinion: I have personally become acquainted with two of Mr. Dries' patients who said that they were alive because of Mr. Dries. Unfortunately I have no meaningful data, thus I cannot say much about the Dries diet. However I value his approaches dealing with the importance of light.

Hulda Clark

Cancer patients ask our *Menschen gegen Krebs* office about Hulda Clark on a regular basis, because she states in her books that she can cure any type of cancer. This is said to occur when a parasite (Fasciolopsis buski) which is in the colon of cancer patients and does its mischief there, is destroyed through a diet, detoxification measures, (avoidance of propylalcohol) and through so-called zappers. A zapper is a small device that transmits different frequencies and is said to be capable of destroying the parasite, or viruses and bacteria.

The approach of effecting a positive influence via frequencies is certainly correct, and it was due to Hulda Clark that this approach again attracted wide-spread attention. Unfortunately investigations around the world have demonstrated that the incidence of this parasite is extremely rare. To my knowledge, most users who want to destroy this parasite with a zapper, do not test to know whether this parasite is even present in the patient. In 1987 for example the NCID in America tested 216,185 people for this parasite and found Fasciolopsis buski in only one person. Similar investigations were made in China, Taiwan, and Indonesia, and they always came up with the same devastating result.

Personal opinion: If I overlook the zapper, and Ms. Clark's theory, which often comes across as somewhat self-righteous in her writings, then the Clark therapy is a good therapy, just based on the comprehensive detoxification measures (removing amalgam fillings, avoidance of many toxins, getting toxins out of the body), and the diet recommendations, and as a consequence must it must produce good results. However I am absolutely against telling cancer patients they should just: "Zap for 3 x 7 minutes and they will be healed", which I regularly hear from patients, unfortunately. The parasite theory is not close to being proved, however this does not necessarily mean that the theory is false. But I do date to doubt that Fasciolopsis buski is always the culprit. I certainly consider it possible that parasites can play a role in cancer, and this theory should not be simply be dismissed as crazy. Naturally the logical question can be raised as to whether the parasite is the trigger or the result of the cancer event. For me this question has certainly not been answered.

Unfortunately to this day I have no data which prove Clark's theory, although Ms. Clark promised the *National Foundation for Alternative Medicine* early in 2000 that she would make this data available. I also called on the adherents of Ms. Clark in Germany in 2000 to make data available to me, unfortunately without a response that could be evaluated in terms of best cases. But whoever is capable of reading books and theories critically, can find good approaches with Ms. Clark.

Clark's new book: *The prevention of all cancers* confused many practitioners, because she is recommending in the book many things totally different than before, f.e. she is now against flax seed oil or other healthy things like olive oil, red cherries, bananas...

Hoxsey Therapy

The Hoxsey therapy consists of a herbal tincture developed in the 19th century with which Harry Hoxsey treated cancer patients, since ca. 1920. It all started in 1840 on a horse farm in Illinois. Apparently John Hoxsey the great grandfather of Harry Hoxsey, who was in charge of horse breeding had a horse that was sick with cancer. The horse was lead out to a paddock to die. After 3 weeks John Hoxsey determined that the tumor in the horse had stabilized. He observed that that the horse ate unusual plants. Within a year the horse had recovered completely.

John Hoxsey started to experiment with the herbs on animals and was very successful. The formula was handed down within the family and the father of Harry Hoxsey was the first to use the formula on humans. Harry Hoxsey opened his first clinic in 1924 in Illinois and immediately became a target for allopathy. A bitter fight broke out between the two camps and Hoxsey was finally forced to go to Dallas Texas. Hoxsey was called the greatest quack of the century. However his adherents called him an effective healer who was persecuted by the establishment.

In spite of the harassment in the 50s his clinic in Dallas Texas was the largest privately-held cancer center in the world. He had a total of 14 clinics in various states. His treatment was supported by senators, judges, and by some doctors. The therapeutic value of his treatment was confirmed by two court rulings.

Harry Hoxsey invited the American Medical Association (AMA) and the Food and Drug Administration (FDA) to examine and evaluate his therapy. Both the AMA and the FDA refused these invitations even after Hoxsey declared his willingness to bear the costs for such a study himself. All the herbs in the Hoxsey tincture are listed as plants that are used in fighting cancer in the book (***Plants used against Cancer***) written by the chemist, Jonathan L. Hartwell. By the way Jonathan Hartwell worked earlier for the American National Cancer Institute (NCI).

In August 1954, a book published by the New York *Man's Magazine* reported on the effectiveness of the Hoxsey therapy (at this time Hoxsey had more than 12,000 patients) with 100-pages of extensive documentation. At this time a group of 10 physicians also visited the Hoxsey clinic in Dallas to personally investigate the Hoxsey therapy. They reached the following conclusion: "We were able to determine that the examinations have shown to our satisfaction that the Hoxsey clinic successfully treated pathologically proven cases without the aid of operative interventions, radium, or irradiation".

The AMA laboratory analyzed the Hoxsey tincture in 1943 and came up with the following analysis. The primary active ingredient is potassium iodine (which makes up 3/5 of the entire tincture). In addition it contains red clover (Trifolium pratense), buckthorn bark (Rhamnus purshianus), burdock roots (Arctium lappa, which we know has antimutagenic characteristics), queensroot (Stillingia sylvatica), barberry bark (Berberis vulgaris), chaparral (larrea tridentata), licorice root (Glycyrrhiza glabra), Cascara amarga (Picramnia antidesma) and ash bark (Zanthoxylum americanum).

A number of investigations were able to prove the biological activity of different substances from the Hoxsey mixture; i.e. that these substances had anti-tumor characteristics. Harry Hoxsey died in 1974 at the age of 73 (he was the most arrested person in American Medical History – even though he won every case). Hoxsey gave his formula to his long-time colleague and one-time nurse, Mildred Nelson (who became acquainted with Hoxsey in 1946). She began treating cancer patients with the Hoxsey therapy in the Bio Medical Clinic in Tijuana/Mexico in 1963. Unfortunately Mildred Nelson died in 1999. The Hoxsey therapy as it is practiced today in the clinic in Tijuana consists of the Hoxsey herbal mixture for internal treatment and special pastes for external treatment, that are combined with a special diet. Yeast tablets, vitamins, garlic, thyroid gland extracts, liver, SOD, D.M.S.O., Schultes medicinals, BCG (tuberculosis vaccine), shark cartilage and hormones. I also noticed during my stay at the Bio Medical Clinic in Mexico that there are almost no doors in the clinic, so that the "energy can flow".

Personal opinion: The available data are not adequate for me to be able to recommend this therapy as a first therapy. However this may be due to the lack of data rather than to Hoxsey's success. Once again great knowledge is being lost and after the death of Mildred Nelson I believe that Hoxsey's therapy, unfortunately, will no longer be practiced one day.

Issels Therapy

Without exaggeration we can say that Dr. Joseph Issels is the best-known cancer physician in Germany. In 1951, he was the first German doctor to open a clinic for cancer patients using immunotherapy, and he contributed to the fact that established medical practitioners started thinking more about the holistic aspect of cancer diseases. Over several decades he primarily treated cancer patients for whom conventional therapies failed. He spent the last years of his life in Florida or in San Diego where his wife still lives. She has been president of the Issels Foundation since his death in 1999.

Dr. Issels was born in 1907 in Mönchengladbach Germany. After studying medicine and after residencies in various hospitals he opened his own practice and in 1951, later the famous Ringberg Clinic in Tegernsee, and there he treated thousands of patients. Most of these patients came in a final stage of cancer, after conventional cancer therapies could no longer help them. Although Dr. Issels was attacked again and again by the cancer establishment and was even put in prison, he fought until he died on February 2nd 1998, for the view that tumors are not cancer diseases, but that cancer diseases generate tumors.

Dr. Issels whole-body therapy mainly consists of two points. He differentiated two complexes of causes:

*   Factors that transform a normal cell into a cancer
        cell

*   Factors which are responsible for the occurrence of the
        immune weakness and thus also for the formation
        of the tumor

It follows that every cancer, whether initial tumor, recurrence, or metastasis, is a collapse of this defense. In treating cancer it is very important that the therapist attempt to treat both factors, i.e. resolve all causes of the illness, in order to thus provide the basis for a healthy immune system, **and** fight the symptoms, in other words, the tumor.

Both factors must always be approached together. In fighting the causes Dr. Issels was primarily concerned with:

* Eliminating all causes such as malnutrition and undernourishment

* Residual infections in the teeth, jaw and tonsils

* Restoration of the intestinal flora

* Dyslocation of vertebrae

* Spiritual and mental well-being

Desensitization takes place through injections of vaccines from infected teeth, tonsils, pathogenic colibacteria, and from the blood of the patient. In addition the immune system is strengthened by overwarming and fever therapies, oxygen ozone therapy and through enzyme therapy, neural therapy, and organ therapy. Symptoms (tumor) are treated through operation, irradiation, or in rare cases also through chemotherapy.

This basic therapy has the task of restoring or bringing the body's four defense zones into balance without side effects.

Dr. Issels identified 4 defense zones:

* Location-specific microflora outside of the body
* The totality of epithelial surfaces

* The lymphatic system including spleen, thyroid, liver, lymph nodes etc.

* The mesenchyme (soft connective tissue).

Each of these 4 defense zones has specific tasks, and they are subordinate to direction through the neruohormonal control organs. Dr. Issels started to work in a consultative role in the CHIPSA Clinic in Tijuana 2-3 years before his death. He particularly considered his work in combination with Max Gerson's nutrition treatment to be very promising.

Personal opinion: Dr. Issels certainly is one of the greats in the field of cancer therapy, and he was the first to establish a consistent holistic approach in a clinic. Primarily his consistent removal of infections e.g. from teeth treated with root canals (!) or tonsils, and the associated successes were able to demonstrate the importance of comprehensive detoxification.

His successes in general speak for themselves. Issels' vaccines are only used singly and are probably doomed to disappear from the market completely one day.

TUMORSPECIFIC IMMUNO-THERAPY
developed by Dr. Klehr

Cytokines are natural information carriers that bear certain markings on their surface. These messenger substances of the blood imitate white blood corpuscles and remain unknown to the immune system, similar to tumor cells. Dr. Klehr's therapy, so-called human own-blood cytokine injections with interferons and interleukins, has the objective of changing a portion of the cells of the patient's own blood in the laboratory, in such a manner that when the removed blood is returned to the body, a defense reaction occurs in order to wholly or partially destroy the tumor.

In detail this involves tumor necrose factor a, interferon, and the interleukin-2 receptor (s/L2-R). Today researches believe that they can prove how interferon activates the macrophages, killer cells, or suppressor cells. In accordance with the classical model of our immune system this would naturally be a good thing, if a cytokine injection causes these cells to be present in the body in increased number. Also the present research with dendrite cells or tumor vaccination proceeds from this concept and it plays an increasingly significant role in oncology.

As there are few meaningful studies about this direction of oncology today, it is very difficult to evaluate how important all these therapies are Furthermore a lot of money is earned here (app. 2,300 Euro for approximately 3 months with Dr. Klehr) and this does not make things easier.

Personal opinion: Dr. Klehr is considered to be a charlatan and con man in many circles in Germany. I have been in his Munich lab several times and I have also examined his documented cases. Dr. Klehr showed me multiple cases in which a protracted stabilization phase could be seen after his cytokine injections.

I consider it to be unfair to praise all the cytokine research at the universities and at the same time position Dr. Klehr as charlatan. Anyone who does this should consider is own motivations carefully. I am certainly the last person who would want to position myself in front of or behind Dr. Klehr. But the manner in which non-conventional practitioners and allopathy go against Dr. Klehr is certainly a boomerang which could hit anybody one of these days.

Today's immune research is still in its infancy, and regardless of how of Dr. Klehr's successes or failures are evaluated, for years he has been one of the few researchers in this field who was also able to gather practical experiences. We are certainly still a long way away from developing specific attack weapons against cancer cells. But certainly mutual attacks, instead of an exchange of information, will not bring us forward.

Since 2004, Dr. Klehr has also combined his therapy with the therapy of Dr. Fryda, detoxification therapies, orthomolecular medicine, and homeopathic medicine.

Tumosterone

The biochemist Dr. Erich Klemke has been working for more than 30 years in the field of cancer research, and has discovered a natural substance, or more to be more precise, a cholesterol derivative from the thyroid gland, which he called tumosterone. In addition he tests the actual cancer event with an hydroxylamine test developed by Prof. Neuenhoffer. Hydroxylamine is a waste product of active cancer cells and can thus be verified in urine, often long before a tumor can be verified through the usual processes. Unfortunately the problem here is the test, because if cancer cells are not very active then little hydroxylamine is produced. Consequently for patients a negative test certainly does not mean that a tumor is not present, on the other hand, a higher hydroxylamine value does indicate an active event.

Below is Dr. Klemke's statement on what cancer is and how it should be treated. Please understand this is all "somewhat scientific", unfortunately there is no other way to explain it.

Dr. Klemke determined that cancer cells generate considerable quantities of H_2O_2 (hydrogen peroxide). It was impossible for him to accept that the DNA mutation hypothesis could be correct, as the chromosomal DNA is out of the question for H_2O_2 production. In addition he is of the opinion that returning the cancer cell to normalcy is no longer possible because chromosome aberrations are triggered through the endogenic hydrogen peroxide production. The deluge of H_2O_2 from cancer cell mitochondria is the actual reason for the oxidation of proteins already present in cytoplasma – particularly those of the strongly alkaline histones with their sulfhydryl (HS) groups to disulphide S-S bonds. These cancer cell proteins are then oxidized on the peptide connections from -CO-NH- to -CO-N-OH.

Both types of oxidative mutilation are responsible for chromosome breaks and chromosome aberrations during the next cell cycle, as these are known for example from the so-called Philadelphia chromosome, where the long arm of chromosome 22 has been transferred to chromosome 9. This mechanism becomes even more clear in the HeLa cells with 70 to 80 small chromosomes. This phenomenon has attracted little attention to this day. No obvious conclusions are drawn in this regard.

Prof. Neunhoeffer noted that approximately every 50th peptide bond of a protein is hydroxylized on the nitrogen, where the peptide bond, which previously had a neutral reaction, takes on acid characteristics. In the case of the oxidative disulphide formation of the histones, branching form, also to other chromosomes. If such proteins which are now acidic instead of alkaline, and chemically-branched, get into the cell nucleus, whose job it should be to neutralize the growing-up acidic DNA double helix as presented beads on a string, these cause a catastrophe at the next cell division, due to their branched node points and their now acidic characteristics, because the DNA is not neutralized at certain points. This means that genetic information, which does not belong to the cell type, is open for transcription, while other genetic information of the affected cell type is suppressed. The chaos is then even greater, in Dr. Klemke's view, because chromosome breaks and aberrations occur on the created node points because the disulphide bridge represents a stop signal. Then the repair mechanisms used by the cell, the endonucleases and exonucleases cut the strand. In this manner there is a transfer of genetic information from the affected chromosome onto a different chromosome, while the genetic information itself remains completely unchanged.

From this perspective the malfunctions of the cancer cell are not triggered through point mutations on the DNA, but rather are problems of the respiratory chain in the mitochondria. This is because their cytochromes must act together in pairs in order to generate a pair of electrons. If one of these is blocked by a toxin, then instead of forming H_2O_2 this results in formation of H_2O_2, or of hyperoxide radical $*O_2$. Consequently the misconduct of the cancer cell cannot be a problem whose cause is sought in the primarily in cell nucleus. In the cell nucleus defective presented hydroxylized proteins, which the growing-up DNA double helix finds present, must necessarily result in a cellular catastrophe of the type described.

Dr. Klemke also notes during the tumosterone therapy that breakdown of the tumor should not belie the fact that the defective immune response continues to exist. In order to make the immune defense functional again, and at the same time eliminate the vagabonding blocking factors in the serum of cancer patients, (these are soluble tumor antigens, antibodies, and antigen antibody complexes), which hinder the formation of specific antibodies against the affected tumor cells, a biochemical complement therapy is required. This complement therapy gives higher doses of reduced L-glutathione, L-cystein, trace elements, vitamins, particularly vitamin B1, B6, B12, C, and E, zinc orotate, selenomethionine, choline hydrogentartrate to prevent the metastasizing, omega-3 fatty acids such as the 20:5 omega-3, eicosapentaenoate acid and the 22:6 omega docosahexaenoic obtained from fish oils. Sugar in any form is contraindicated.

Personal opinion: Tumosterone could be helpful in conjunction with the complement therapy, particularly at the beginning of a cancer illness. I would also like to see tumosterone in a study as intravenously injected medication, since some approaches speak for this form of administration. Unfortunately there are very few physicians who test tumosterone and who also inject it intravenously. The fact that tumosterone has also found significant interest in allopathy is indicated by the research performed by physicians of the Freiburg tumor clinic, who examined this substance in a 1999 study. Why their positive results were only published in a Greek journal (Anti-cancer Research 19/1999) is only understood by insiders and is not important for this book. Moreover there are additional studies by Dr. Steinkellner in Austria and Prof. Masato Koreeda in the USA, which would substantiate the use in oncology. Unfortunately once again patent rights and financial interests are more important than the good of mankind.

The Reglin publishing house in Cologne has published a special booklet: "Theoretische Betrachtungen zum Krebsproblem" (Theoretical considerations on the cancer problem, issue 12/200). This 32-page booklet lists Dr. Klemke's view on how cancer occurs in the most minute detail for all biochemists. Unfortunately I cannot evaluate whether what is written in this brochure is correct or not. Although I have requested several "experts" to provide their opinion on it, none of them could tell me whether Dr. Klemke's observations were correct or false.

Urtherapy

Most people in Germany know Franz Konz because of his bestseller: *Steuern sparen* (Save Taxes). What many people do not know is that Konz is a first-class observer of the medical scene and has distanced himself from the diplomatic approach for some time. Anyone can read what this means in his book, which is almost 1,500 pages long: *Der Grosse Gesundheits-Konz* (The Konz Health Conpendium). In this outstanding book he presents his views on medicine in a manner that is totally unique.

At first glance his urtherapy (ur = original) may seem a bit crazy, as it says that the patient "finds" his food for himself everyday. But if his book is considered from a holistic viewpoint, the reader quickly understands why this therapy simply has to be effective.

Whoever looks at his therapy in detail will find elements in common with other nutrition therapies. Konz however pursues an extremely consistent path, which not even Dr. Johanna Budwig requires in this manner. However after many years in oncology I must say in favor of Dr. Budwig or Mr. Konz, that I can readily understand their attitude. However I cannot recommend their manner of conducting a dialog, particularly with very ill patients, from a psychological perspective.

Nevertheless Konz also describes how important it is to detoxify, live happily, and pay attention to diet. In other words: He is another specialist who describes a 3E path, even if such a path will never experience a breakthrough because it is too far removed from "normal" life for 99.99% of the population. Unfortunately Franz Konz has also totally distanced himself from the "diplomatic world" and mixes private matters and medical matters in his therapy description in such a manner that I am not the only person who has difficulty separating the important things from the unimportant things.

Personal opinion: I find the personal extremism of Franz Konz quite unfortunate, as he certainly has a lot of good approaches and his therapy could help many more people. On the other hand, as previously mentioned, I can readily understand people like him, Dr. Hamer, or Dr. Budwig, as I have often considered leaving the diplomatic paths, in order just to be there for a few people. In any case his book is interesting, it clears up many myths, and every cancer patient should have it on his bookshelf.

Livingston Therapy

Dr. Virginia C. Livingston, who died in 1990, was one of the few female doctors of her time. In 1936 she was the first female assisting physician at New York Hospital in the USA. She developed a cancer germ theory and vaccines which she used successfully for patients with cancer. Her theory developed out of her experiences with tuberculosis and leprosy. She recognized a certain relationship between these diseases and cancer.

As researcher she discovered certain organisms that were similar to tuberculosis. In this process she discovered after she had examined a wide variety of cancer tissue, that a similar microorganism was present in all these tissues. She was able to prove with scientific methods that a bacteria with the name of Progenitor cryptocides promotes the development of cancer. According to Dr. Livingston's information, from birth on we all carry this P. cryptocides in us (it is also present in animals). Normally it is held in check by our immune system. If our immunity is suppressed due to poor diet, chemical toxins, stress and other impacting factors, this idle microbe can multiply and promote the growth of tumors. Dr. Livingston's research revealed that P. cryptocides were present in high concentrations in cancer patients.

Dr. Livingston described this microbe as an organism which is capable of changing its form and which can develop in different forms. After the microorganism was identified as a cause for cancer, it was clear that a vaccine was required for treatment.

However Dr. Livingston's theories and clinical results were challenged by allopathy. She was subjected to enormous pressure and finally she was forced to close her laboratory in New York. Then she founded the Livingston-Wheeler Medical Clinic in San Diego in 1968, one of the few non-conventional therapy clinics in the USA that is still active today. She continued her research and developed a cancer vaccine after she successfully treated a patient with a malignant tumor in the thyroid gland. Her treatment is based on using the bacteria in the patient's body to fight the same bacteria. This is why each vaccine is prepared individually for each patient.

Each vaccine also contains vitamins and minerals to strengthen the immune system. In addition to vaccines patients are put on a vegetarian raw food diet, they take gamma globulin, vitamin and mineral supplement preparations, and have their teeth examined. Thermal therapy and detoxification measures are also part of the Livingstone therapy.

Dr. Livingston reported that she successfully treated many types of cancer in an advanced stage, and she presented numerous case studies of remissions for metastasizing illnesses. However she never performed controlled studies, or other confirmed statistical research on people. If a localized tumor is involved like prostate cancer or breast cancer the remission rate varies between 70% and 95% according to her own information. If the cancer has moved into the bones or local lymph nodes, then the remission rate sinks to 40-50%. For patients who have no chances of survival with conventional therapies (and perhaps have 3 more months to live) a 20% remission rate was obtained (source: Livingston Foundation).

Other researchers also report successes with the Livingston vaccine. One of these researchers is Dr. Speckhard from Norfolk Virginia. In a study with 40 patients he observed that 3 patients had a complete remission. For 4 patients the vaccine contributed to a drastic partial remission.

Personal opinion: The data available to me are not meaningful enough to recommend this therapy as first therapy. In the listing of "supplemental therapies" like raw food diet, dental examination etc. naturally the question arises as to whether these might be the "main therapies".

In this case the problems associated with good non-conventional statistics are manifest, and we see how difficult it is to evaluate such statistics. Livingston certainly has something to prove, but the theory of the therapy can be dismissed by anybody as crazy, because it cannot be substantiated scientifically.

Macrobiotic diet
(Michio Kushi)

This is a special diet and nutritional philosophy which is based in traditional Chinese medicine, and which is primarily practiced in Japan and the USA. The diet has the objective of maintaining the energy values of fresh, whole foods in balance, to ensure that the Qi force important for life is maximized. Macrobiotics means "magnificent life"

Macrobiotic theories were introduced in the US by George Ohsawa (1893-1966) a Japanese teacher who studied the writings of the physician Sagen Ishizuka (1850-1910). Ohsawa is said to have cured himself from a serious illness, by changing his usual diet to a simple traditional Japanese diet (brown rice, miso soup, sea vegetables and other traditional dishes). He developed the macrobiotic philosophy by combining western and eastern elements.

In the 70s and 80s there were changes in the focus and content of the macrobiotic movement, which to a great extent were introduced by Michio Kushi who emigrated to the USA from Japan in 1949. Kushi and other leaders of the macrobiotic movement adhered to some of Ohsawa's elements, but at the same time they introduced a variety of more complex components into the macrobiotic philosophy. The macrobiotic standard diet was developed, which Kushi described in 1983 in his book: **The Cancer Prevention diet**. According to the macrobiotic teachings of Kushi, cancer is caused by nutritional factors, environmental/social factors, and personal factors. He writes that cancer is not the result of extraterrestrial influences over which we have no control, rather it is the result of our daily behavior, including our thinking, our lifestyle, and what we eat daily.

Diet components:

50-60% of the daily diet includes boiled organically grown grain (e.g. brown rice, barley, millet, rye, wheat, buckwheat, etc.).

5-10% soups (app. 1-2 large cups daily with vegetables, grains or beans, seasoned with miso or Tamari soy sauce)

25-30% should be local, biologically produced vegetables (e.g. cabbage, broccoli, cauliflower, watercress, carrots, etc.)

5-10% in the form of different types of beans.

Occasionally fresh fish (flounder, snapper, trout) as well as **local** biologically grown fruits and nuts can be eaten. Foods to avoid are: Meat and poultry, animal fat, eggs, dairy products, refined sugar, chocolate, molasses, honey, soft drinks, artificial drinks, aromatic or stimulating types of tea, coffee, all artificial colorings, preservatives, injected or chemically treated food products, all processed or polished grains and flours, canned food, frozen food products, hot spices and alcohol.

The therapy first determines whether Yin or Yang dominates the illness. This is determined by the locality of the primary tumor in the body and the locality of the tumor in a specific organ. Then a diet is selected to return this state of imbalance to equilibrium. Different cooking instructions are prescribed depending on the type of illness.

Success statistics
In one study Carter and colleagues compared the survival time of 23 patients with pancreatic cancer who were given a macrobiotic diet, and comparable patients who were given conventional therapies. The authors reached the conclusion that

average survival time significantly longer in the macrobiotic group. (Source: Carter, Saxe & Newbold, 1990, Tulane University, New Orleans/USA)

Personal opinion: Certainly the macrobiotic diet is a comtemporary theory of modern nutrition. Unfortunately there is insufficient data relative to cancer patients, so that cancer patients are better advised to rely on the oil protein diet or the Gerson diet. This is not a negative comment assessement of the macrobiotic diet, it is just an assessment based on the available data.

Moermann Diet

Dr. Cornelius Moermann was a Dutch physician who was treated as a charlatan in the Netherlands and who was attacked in the meanest manner. His "crime" was describing in detail that cancer was a side-tracked metabolism and that it could be treated through diets and by administering substances that are lacking, like vitamins.

Dr. Moermann experimented a lot with homing pigeons and through these experiments he came to the conclusion that 8 substances played a significant role in their health: Vitamins A, B, E, D, as well as citric acid, iodine, sulfur and iron. The same holds true for humans however with one exception: Vitamin C is not on the list for pigeons because they can produce it themselves.

Moermann has an interesting view of what cancer really is. You will readily identify elements that are common to the theories of many other scientists:

1. You must completely separate yourself from the old view which says that the cancerous tumor is of a local nature, and that the tumor is the point of departure for the subsequent course of the illness.

2. You must become familiar with the new view which states that the entire organism is sick with cancer, before the actual tumor is formed.

3. You must bear in mind that all the cells of our body – like trees or other plants – can only flourish in a very life-specific medium.

4. Even in an optimally healthy body, cancer cells occur here and there, which however are eradicated by suppressors, so that tumor formation does not occur.

5. Because we can get a cancer tumor, the logical conclusion is that this only possible if the person's health is no longer optimal. Thus first the entire organism gets sick. This inhibits the suppressor in its activities. And at this point only can a cancer tumor occur.

6. Under no circumstances should a therapist make the body which is already sick, even more sick by administering toxic substances e.g. cytostatic agents. Rather the body's healthy state must be restored by reactivating the suppressors.

7. Operative intervention is possible; however it should be not associated with the idea that removal of the tumor, to a certain extent equals removal of the illness. A real improvement in the patient's condition is achieved exclusively through administration of the 8 substances (iodine, citric acid, yeast = vitamin B complex, iron, sulfur as well as vitamins A, E, C, and D).

8. Irradiation handicaps the immune system, which is so urgently necessary for the patient's healing. The immune system must be activated instead of handicapped.

Based on these 8 facts Moermann's treatment was as follows:

First: The patient is given dietary guidelines, because it is understood that he cannot continue with the cancer-promoting incorrect diet. It is an error to believe that cancer can be healed with the Moermann diet alone. His diet takes replaces a diet with non-whole foods?? (i.e. foods that have been robbed of vital components through chemical or mechanical processes) that provide a boost to the occurrence of cancer.

Second: The healthy state of the entire organism must be restored and indeed the aforementioned 8 substances are the prerequisite for optimal health.

Third: If the cancer patient is in the reversible stage (i.e. capable of improvement), then the therapeutic introduction of the 8 substances mentioned effects a recovery of the organism which results in reactivation of the suppressor, and thus of the total defense system, including melting of the tumor, this means that the cancer cells are then destroyed and the patient is healed.

Unfortunately Dr. Moermann was constantly persecuted in Holland, although he published many successful cases. Even the protection of other doctors did not help, so he certainly goes down in history as one of the "misunderstood oncologists". For more information: see Dr. C. Moermann's book: *Cancer.* ISBN: 3-591-08310-0

Personal opinion: I consider Dr. Moermann to be the forerunner of orthomolecular medicine. I believe however that Dr. Moermann, if he were still alive would certainly "adapt" his therapy.

Naessens 714X

Dr. Naessens discovered that tumor cells produce a substance (cocancerogenic factor K, CFK), that handicaps the immune system. 714X neutralizes CFK and thus makes it possible for the immune system to better identify and destroy cancer cells. 714 X does not destroy cancer cells, rather it blocks them so that they can no longer feed themselves.

Gaston Naessens, who is French, developed an optical microscope which is called the Somatoscope. With this somatoscope scientists can observe living organisms at a high resolution. Thus Naessens could reveal small particles in the blood that nobody had ever seen before. He called these particles somatids (little bodies). These small units of life are the precursors of DNA and according to Naessens they are capable of transforming matter into energy.

He discovered that somatids go through a 3-phase micro cycle. Normally the somatids are harmless, but when the immune system is under stress, damaged by toxins, or impacted by illnesses, then the somatids develop malignantly as part of the micro cycle. The results are cancer, multiple sclerosis, lupus or other illnesses. According to Naessens, 714X can reduce tumors, help with gaining weight or losing weight, or, contribute to reduction or elimination of pain, and it can extend life. Usually the therapy consists of 3 consecutive treatments with 714X injections that are injected directly into the lymph nodes in the abdominal area, once a day for at least 21 consecutive days. Then there is a 2-day pause. For advanced cancer the treatment can also be more intense.

Dr. Naessens collected hundreds of case studies, in which 714X was used successfully against melanomas, carcinomas, malignant lymphomas, osteosarcomas, and other types of cancer. Many cases are published in the book by Christopher Bird: ***The persecution and trial of Gaston Naessens.***

Dr. Naessens by the way was not the first person who discovered little blue particles under the microscope, many years before him it was Dr. Wilhelm Reich, who called these particles bions

Personal opinion: I personally know patients who were treated by Dr. Naessens, who swear that they would not be alive without 714X. However evaluation of 714X is not easy, as long as there are no larger studies. For this reason I cannot make a statement either in favor or against 714X.

Systemic Cancer Multistep Therapy (sCMT)

The Systemic Cancer Multistep Therapy developed by Prof. Manfred von Ardenne (1907-1997) is a combination of the following therapies:

* Extreme whole body hyperthermia – with anesthesia app. 42.0 to 42.5 °C over 60-90 minutes

* Induced hyperglycemia (high blood sugar level)

* Relative hyperoxemia (high oxygen content in the blood)

More than a few doctors combine this therapy with chemotherapy or biological cytostatic agents in order to directly damage cancer cells. This occurs because cancer tissue accumulates lactic acid when the blood sugar level is extremely high (hyperglycemia), as cancer cells transform glucose (grape sugar) to lactic acid to a greater extent in the presence of oxygen. This over-acidification probably makes the cancer cells more susceptible to overheating (hyperthermia) while the other body cells cannot be so easily attacked by glucose in the presence of oxygen. Temperatures around 42.0°C directly damage cancer cells and an increased oxygen partial pressure (relative hyperoxemia) stabilizes the functions of all vital organs.

What appears important to me here is the warning that large quantities of toxins can be released through rapid destruction of the tumor. If your therapist does not instruct you to pursue an intensive detoxification therapy, then do this yourself, otherwise a toxic crisis could occur.

Results:
By the end of 1998 over 900 patients with different cancer diagnoses had been treated in the Ardenne clinic in Dresden. According to the clinic a positive therapeutic influence could be achieved in more than 50% of the treated cases. Similar results are cited for the Japan Whole Body Hyperthermia Center in Tokyo. Unfortunately the Ardenne Clinic ceased to exist in July 2000. More information is available in the book: *Systemic Cancer Multistep Therapy* (ISBN 3-773-1297-5).

Personal opinion: sCMT could be a therapy for young "healthy" patients, and it is a possibility for fast tumor destruction. Unfortunately it is very expensive, because it can only be performed under narcosis (see also: hyperthermia).

Oxygen and Ozone Therapy

Ever since Dr. Warburg recognized in the 1920s, that cancer cells have an acute oxygen problem, there have been a wide variety different approaches aimed at healing or relieving cancer by administering oxygen and ozone. Doubtless the theoretical background is interesting. However I am against simply accepting this therapy as a given and administering oxygen and ozone to every cancer patient. We should not forget that both substances can be fatal, and that these therapies only make sense if oxygen really gets into the cells. From the chemical perspective this involves O_2 or O_3 and both substances produce free radicals in the body, which we know can play a negative role with cancer. In addition, oxygen influences the oxidation of glucose and this process also can be important in a cancer therapy.

This is why I consider that oxygen and ozone therapies are only appropriate if they are integrated within a holistic concept, and particularly if a nutritional therapy is followed at the same time. Increased oxygen in the blood can cause more harm than good without nutrition therapy.

The following therapies are used today.

1. **Oxygen Multistep Therapy developed by Manfred von Ardenne**
   Here virtually pure oxygen is administered with light physical activity and (usually) prior administration of vitamins.

2. **Ionized oxygen**
   Here oxygen is administered either with positive or negative oxygen ions.

3. Hematogenic oxidation therapy (HOT)

Dr. Wehrli from Switzerland first introduced this therapy, in which blood is foamed with medical oxygen and then irradiated with UV-C. In this process a small portion of ozone is produced, a singular oxygen and O_2 gas.

4. Self-treatment with ozone

In what is usually referred to as the "big own-blood ozone treatment" usually 50-150 ml blood is channeled out of the vein into a bottle where it is combined with an ozone-oxygen mixture. Then the enriched blood is reintroduced into the vein. So that it continues to flow, it is previously treated to be non-coagulating with a suitable amount of heparin or citrate.

In what is usually referred to as the "minor own blood therapy" only 3-5 ml blood is taken from the vein and and combined with an oxygen ozone mixture.

This mixture is then injected into the muscle and it is supposed to stimulate the immune system. Less often ozone is injected in the artery or gasses are injected into the muscle. However frequently ozone is still being used locally e.g. for ulcers   or for disinfection.

Personal opinion: Animal experiments show that tumors grow when oxygen is administered. Giving oxygen and simply hoping that this oxygen will also get into the cells through the blood is not enough. Oxygen and ozone therapies belong within the framework of a holistic therapy and if a nutrition therapy is not included, then I would stay away from approach. So please speak first with your therapist.

Revici therapy

This involves a biological non-toxic "chemotherapy" which is matched to the metabolism of the respective patient, with the goal of strengthening the body's cancer fighting ability. Dr. Revici (born in 1896) practiced medicine in a private practice in Rumania from 1920 to 1936. From 1937-1938 he was acting director of the Pasteur Institute in Paris. Due to the Second World War he emigrated to Mexico in 1942 where he founded the Institute for Applied Biology (for treating cancer patients) in Mexico City. His work came to the attention of physicians in the USA, and 4 years later he was invited by the medical faculty of the University of Chicago to publish the results of his research. Then he moved to New York where he founded the *American Institute for Applied Biology*. Its primary goal was to transfer breakthroughs generated in the laboratory as quickly as possible to patients. He published more than 30 scientific articles on his cancer theory.

Dr. Revici's therapy explains that metabolism consists of two fundamental phases. Anabolism is the build-up phase (this phase is associated with growth, energy, production of organic substances like enzymes, hormones etc.) and catabolism is the destructive phase (in which things are decomposed and energy is used).

According to Revici, health is present if a balance exists between these two competing metabolic phases. Usually the body alternates back and forth between these two phases. However if the body remains too long in one phase, this can result in illnesses (see Dr. Hamer as well). Another concept plays a very significant role in Dr. Revici's therapy. He describes the body's immune system in 4 consecutive phases:

1. Enzyme phase: Decomposition of foreign bodies (antigens) by enzymes.

2. Lipidic phase: In which neither fatty acids or sterols are produced.
3. Coagulant antibody phase: In which antibodies collect around the foreign body.
4. Globulinic phase: In which foreign bodies are completely neutralized.

According to his theory, cancer occurs when the immune system is interrupted in the lipidic phase. When this happens, then either too many fatty acids or sterols are produced, which in turn promote the development of cancer. The therapy is divided into 2 programs: A program for patients with anabolic dominance and a program for patients with catabolic dominance:

Success statistics:
In 1984 Dr. Eduaordo Pacellin (Naples/Italy) presented his results with 372 cancer patients (with 6 different types of cancer), based on using the Revici therapy. None of the patients were considered curable. 186 of the patients had lung cancer; their expected survival time was 80 days. Through the Revici therapy survival time was extended to 172 days (45% lived longer than 172 days).

53 had stage 4 breast cancer and doubled their survival time to 180 days with the Revici therapy. 57 had cancer in the intestinal area. Their survival time increased from 60 days to 245 days. 278 had fallopian tube cancer. With this group the survival time with the Revici therapy increased from 90 days to 270 days. Almost all patients reported less pain and improved quality of life.

Personal opinion: Here as well it is difficult for me to evaluate the Revici therapy and will remain difficult until studies that are more precise are available. For this reason I cannot make a statement in favor or against Revici.

Rife Therapies

Royal R. Rife (1888-1971) is certainly one of the top frequency researchers in the field of oncology. He started his work under the microscope in 1920 and opened a clinic in 1934. Over the years he treated several thousand cancer patients, and many other patients some of whom were seriously ill. His misfortune was that his ideas did not fit in well with the prevailing concept of the 1930s and thus he was prohibited from treating patients in the future, although he had demonstrated great successes.

It was only after quantum physics was recognized in scientific circles in the 1950s, that some researchers remembered the work of Rife, Antoine Bechamp, Günter Enderlein or Wilhelm Reich, and recalled that they had seen "other things" under their special microscopes. Today even dogmatists can no longer avoid admitting that connections from cell to cell can be overcome by the transmission and reception of electromagnetic signals via receptors.

Rife's primary concern was to prove that cancer occurs through viruses and bacteria. Today, for example SV 40, hepatitis B, papilloma, Eppstein Barr, or herpes viruses, are recognized as carcinogenic, but in Rife's day this idea was a revolution and he was only laughed at. Rife's next thought was to determine how these viruses could be killed. His idea was to eliminate viruses and bacteria by using specially selected frequencies, and he started research in this area. Thus he discovered that tuberculosis bacilli dissolve when the appropriate frequency was applied, and viruses were produced. He was then able to culture these and find the appropriate frequency to dissolve the virus.

Through many years of research, Rife found special frequencies to influence viruses and bacteria. These frequencies or the frequency generator developed by Rife, are used today by many therapists around the world. But this is not all. Without people like Rife, perhaps there would not be any new approaches like that of Hulda Clark, for instance.

Personal opinion: I am firmly convinced that Rife was on the right path. Not so much in terms of bacteria and viruses, but his approach of influencing cells through artificially generated waves is right on target. Naturally this does not apply to cancer alone, it applies to any illness. The fact that little research funding flows in this direction today, certainly has nothing to do with the field of study, rather it is because if Rife's work should be confirmed, then manufacturers of pharmaceuticals would sooner or later go bankrupt – and who is interested in that?

Stockholm Therapy

Research by Dr. Karl Folkers at the University of Texas and Dr. Knut Lockwok in Denmark show that Co-enzyme Q10 (CoQ10) combined with other nutrients and with a diet that is principally vegetarian, could reduce many types of tumors, or even eliminate them.

Both researchers studied breast cancer and discovered that the cancer could be eliminated if high doses of CoQ10 were used in conjunction with selective antioxidants, fatty acids, nutrition and diet. And it could be eliminated even if the cancer had already formed liver metastases. Coenzyme Q10 (CoQ10) is also known as ubichinone and belongs to a family of substances that are called chinones and which occur widely in nature. All life forms that use oxygen require chinones to produce energy from ATP (adenosintriphosphate). The body produces its own CoQ10, however some foods, like fish (particularly sardines), soy beans, sesame, pistachios, walnuts, spinach etc. are also important sources for this coenzyme.

In one study 32 cancer patients were given 90 mg of CoQ10 daily over a two-year period. All patients survived and 6 had a partial remission. One person with a partial remission was then given 390 mg daily for 3 months, whereupon the tumor disappeared completely. There are proofs that patients with tumors in advanced cancer breast cancer had a total remission through CoQ10 (including patients with a variety of metastases of the liver). CoQ10 plays an important role in the antioxidant system of the body. In conjunction with Vitamin E, selenium, and beta carotene, CoQ10 can significantly reduce the damage free radicals cause to the tissue of the liver, kidneys and the heart. The entire therapy consists of the following supplements:

1. Coenzyme Q10 nutrient mixture of:

   300 mg   Coenzyme Q-10
   300 I.U.   natural vitamin E
   6,500 mg Flaxseed oil (that contains app. 3,500 mg
                Omega 3 fatty acids)
   5.0 g   Borage oil (that contains approximately 1,200
                mg gamma linoleic acid (GLA))

2. 3,000 mg Vitamin C (powder capsules) plus calcium,
   Magnesium, potassium, ascorbate with
   Bioflavonoid rutin, hesperdin, quercetin and
   lemons)

3. 2.500 I.U. Vitamin E (gel capsules – D-alpha tocopherol
   with mixed tocopherols)

4. 25,000 I.U. Beta carotene
   (gel capsules – from a mixed carotinoid
   complex)

5. 200 mcg selenium capsules of selenium methionines
   (100% yeast free)

6.   Liver supporting – nutrient mixture,
   consisting of:
   600 mg lipoic acid
   600 mg curcumin
   300 mcg selenium of selenium methionine
   600 mg silymarin (milk thistle extract)

By the way Dr. Folkers warns that the dried form of CoQ10 which can usually be obtained in health-food shops is almost useless, as it is practically impossible for the body to absorb it in this form.

Personal opinion: Lockwok and Folker's results are certainly demonstrable however the studies are too small for this to be considered a sensation. Amidst all the euphoria don't forget that the Stockholm protocol is no miracle cure. Nevertheless internal examinations conducted by *People Against Cancer* have shown that the Stockholm protocol could represent a sensible combination for the 3E program. For many patients it had positive influences on tumor markers, tumor size and the energy findings.

Ukrain

Ukrain is a mixture of chelidonium majus L. Better known as greater celandine and the cytostatic agent, thiotepa. It contains different types of alkaloids whose concentration is seasonal, similar to mistletoe, and it is approved as a medication in the Ukraine and in White Russia. It *was discovered by the* chemist J.W. Nowicky from Vienna, *who is also the chairman of the Ukrain Institute for Cancer* in Vienna, which I visited together with Frank Wiewel for the first time in 1999.

Mixing a cytostatic agent with herbs at first sounds somewhat unusual. But according to the Nowicky's information the mixture has been substantiated by chemical tests which have now been published. The following processes occur in the mixture: From the chemical perspective thiotepa works through its alkalizing properties. In English this means that its three aziridine rings split off and enter into a chemical combination with the cells, which inhibits cell division. Now if these rings are split off in the test tube and are combined with the alkaloids, thiotepa loses its toxic characteristics. Thus no thiotepa can be found in Ukrain.

In Germany it is primarily Dr. Burkhard Aschoff, owner of the Villa Medica Clinic in Edenkoben, in the Palatinate who has been using Ukrain for many years. He also attracted a lot of attention through two cases, when he successfully treated a 10-year old girl with an Ewing sarcoma, and in 1998 when he successfully treated a 2-year old child with a neuroblastoma using hyperthermia and Ukrain. The available data show successes with breast cancer, colon cancer and particularly with bladder cancer, and individual cases show successes for several other types of cancer. Thus 90 patients with pancreatic cancer were treated at the University of Ulm. The survival rate after 6 months with Ukrain was 65% compared to 26% for patients who were given Gemcitabine

Also Prof. Zemsko at the University of Kiev was able to achieve a clear extension of life for 42 patients with pancreatic cancer using a combination of Ukrain and vitamin C.

While Ukrain is not approved in Germany, it can nevertheless be obtained with a doctor's specific prescription. Unfortunately there are few doctors who have studied Ukrain intensively, there are however many doctors who think that they know Ukrain does not work, and that only quacks use this preparation. The fact is that worldwide there are more than 100 studies using Ukrain and there are indications that it is entirely capable of fighting tumor cells. More information and all studies are available at: www.ukrin.com.

Personal opinion: Dr. Aschoff has had good experience with Ukrain, and also the many studies made by Dr. Nowicky allow us to surmise that ukrain could be an effective medication for certain types of cancer like prostate cancer, breast cancer, or colon cancer.

Galavit

In 2000 the term galavit appeared often in the press and in oncology discussions in Germany, most of those who wrote about it however did not even know what Galavit was. Chemically it is: 2-amino-1,2,3,4-tetrahydrophthalazine 1,4-dione sodium salt, which naturally means nothing to a lay person. In Russia it is approved as an infection inhibiting medication (non-specific immunotherapy), however it has been used by many therapists for many years even in oncology, as was confirmed to me by different physicians during my stay in Moscow in March 200.

In Germany it was first considered to be a miracle cure, and later it was considered to be quack remedy. Moreover out of profit motivation Galavit was first sold at a very high price, although in Russia it only costs 10 Euros per ampule. Galavit is no miracle cure for cancer, (which is what many greedy physicians told their patients), however it is important not to dismiss it as various cancer organizations have done. Galavit is a preparation that many Russian physicians have been using for years, and like all chemicals, it belongs either in the garbage can, or in the hands of a responsible therapist. By the way long before Galavit appeared in the press, there were therapists in Germany who had integrated Galavit into a holistic therapy program and who continue to do so today.

Galavit is also a good example for how the press deals with cancer and how organizations cannibalize something that they know little about for their own purposes.

Personal opinion: Galavit belongs in the hands of an experienced therapist and should only be used as part of a holistic therapy.

Urea & Creatine Therapy

Urea and creatine can contribute to the collapse of tumors, and to our immune system's ability to destroy cancer cells. In the 1960's Dr. Evangelos D. Danopoulos (professor on the medical faculty of the University of Athens/Greece), did pioneering work using urea in the treatment of cancer. Urea is a natural by-product of protein digestion and has a major antioxidizing effect. Products derived from urine have been used since the 1940s in cancer treatments, even if they continue to be controversial. Dr. Danopoulos and his daughter Iphigenia have been able to determine substantial clinical advantages in the treatment of liver cancer with urea.

In 1954 Dr. Danopoulos declared that urine had an anticancer effect. The active component in urine is urea – a by-product of protein metabolism. The theory behind this therapy is that it can change the chemical characteristics of cellular surfaces of malignant cells and thus interrupt the process, which is necessary for uncontrolled cell growth. Dr. Danopoulos reported that this combination therapy was effective for 100% of the patients, after 46 cancer patients with a large tumor in the eye area received urea injections and the tumor was removed surgically. In the 1970s he discovered that oral administration of urea was effective for liver cancer. When 18 patients were given 2-2.5 g urea 4-6 times daily, orally, the patients survived on average 26.5 months – five times longer than expected.

According to Prof. Danopoulos this is/was the most effective treatment of liver cancer and inoperable types of cancer that have metastasized in the liver, and which in most cases cannot be cured with conventional methods. When urea is taken orally concentrations in the liver can be achieved that are large enough to suppress cancer growth in the liver. Particularly urea appears to work because it destabilizes the stroma (supporting tissue) of the tumor. In addition it is effective against formation of new blood vessels in tumors. The latest research shows that the effect of urea is improved through absorbing creatine monohydrate. This likewise natural substance is associated with muscle activities.

For treatment of liver cancer, usually 15 g of urea are used at the beginning, which is dissolved in 1 liter of water or juice, this is then divided into eight 125 ml doses, which are taken every two hours throughout the day. The objective is to reach a blood/urea nitrogen value of 35-40 mg – which is 3-4 times the normal value. At the same time 25 g of creatine monohydrate is taken (in 1 liter of liquid). The creatine solution must be strongly shaken as creatine does not dissolve completely in the liquid.

Because the liver is the only organ that shows high concentrations of urea after oral administration, it could certainly be possible that this therapy is mainly suitable for livery cancer and liver metastasis. However the low cost of production has certainly contributed to the fact that this therapy is almost unknown throughout the world today.

Personal opinion: My experience is that most physicians have never heard of Prof. Danopoulos. The few doctors who I have met who were familiar with his work met were to some extent even enthusiastic. It would certainly be necessary to give this cost-effective therapy a new chance in the form of a study. Unfortunately this therapy cannot be marketed because all substances are freely available and consequently the chances are not very good.

Bach Blossoms

The English bacteriologist Edward Bach apparently cured himself of his spleen cancer and devoted himself in the 1930s to intensive research of various blossoms. For him illness was nothing more than a tool used by our soul to get us back on the right path of truth and light, so that we do not have to suffer even greater harm. This is an interesting observation which is 100% in harmony with the thinking of other holistic oncologists.

As an adherent of pyschoanalysis he divided his blossoms into seven (architypical) areas:

* Uncertainty
* Fear
* Excessive care
* Lack of interest in daily life
* Oversensitivity to influences and ideas
* Lack of courage
* Lonliness

Bach's blossoms are supposed to intervene energetically in our regulation system similar to Hahnemann's therapy (see homeopathy). For Bach in a cancer therapy it is crucial that the Bach blossom therapy motivate the patient to confront himself and the psychological backgrounds of his cancer illness. In addition to aiding psychological crises, individual Bach blossoms also help as supporting treatment after operative interventions and in situations of particular stress.

Personal opinion: Bach blossoms belong in the hands of specialists (homeopaths).

Mistletoe

In recent years, there is not a single non-conventional therapy that has been successful in finding official acceptance in conventional medicine. Not one – no, that's not right. The famous exception is mistletoe. Oncology would not be the same today without the substance Rudolf Steiner experimented with in 1917. Unfortunately most doctors who prescribe a mistletoe preparation apparantly have not understood the teachings of Rudold Steiner, or they are at least of another opinion, because in Steiner's anthroposophy the tumor is exclusively understood to be a symptom. Mistletoe today is the substance which is prescribed most frequently **in addition** to conventional therapies. This manner of thinking continues in hundreds of studies on mistletoe. In most studies the focus is on improving the side effects of conventional therapies and this even though there is no other substance whose content has been more precisely investigated than mistletoe.

Starting with viscin, the sticky and eudermic adhesive and extending to oleanols, cerotine, linoloc acid linoleic acid, arginine, glycogalactopentosan, these are the substances that some people maintain are the strongest cancer inhibitors in misteltoe.

However here we must take a good look at who is responsible for these statements. Is it a company like Weleda which sells Iscador and which naturally maintains that all ingredients only work in combination, or for example is it the company Madaus, which maintains for the competing product Lektinol that it is mainly lectins (plant proteins) that have a tumor-inhibiting effect. For me and particularly for a patient without a specialized background it is absolutely impossible to form an objective opinion about mistletoe in the light of all the differing statements. There is no doubt that mistletoe can show some things in oncology. In 1938, F.E. Koch was able to induce a cure in 47% of his mice that were injected with the Ehrlich carcinoma. Over many years famous cancer researchers, like the phycian P.G. Seeger, confirmed the tumor-inhibiting effects of mistletoe and countless therapists used it in treating their patients.

What you propably will not hear is that there are also opponents of mistletoe, even in non-conventional oncology. I have personally heard from therapists more than once that mistletoe promotes tumor growth particularly with advanced tumors, this is especially the case for liver tumors and brain tumors which can experience explosive growth. The argumentation is similar. Usually people argue that mistletoe is a toxin for our body biologically speaking, and the increase in the immune sysstem (leucocytes, lymphocytes, T4/T8, etc.), which is always positive evaluated is nothing more than a totally natural reaction of the body to the introduction of a toxin, which can be seen by a reddening of the skin with the injection. As a consequence the detoxification function of the liver (which is already overloaded) is burdened even more through the toxin of the mistletoe.

The information provided by the manufacturers, who naturally for financial reasons "as well", recommend injecting mistletoe over many years, must also be viewed critically. First the countless injections certainly do not promote your immune system, and second there is the resistance issue. Some doctors are of the opinion that if there is no reaction (reddening) of the skin, then it is likely that no immune stimulating effect can be achieved either, and thus that mistletoe only represents a stress for the liver.

However one aspect which must always be very positively evaluated in a cancer treatment is the temperature increasing effect of the mistletoe. Ita Wegmann first described this effect. P. Wolf, N. Freudenberg und M. Konitzer also described this effect in their book on the effect of high dosed Viscum Album infusion therapy, published in 1994. Every holistic thinking oncologist is pleased with fever reactions of his patients and clearly delimited studies are necessary, particularly in this area. Unfortunately however, manufacturers of mistletoe preparations are not at all interested in such studies, because naturally they can sell their products much better as a complementary therapy. The mistletoe preparations used most frequently are: Iscador, Helixor, Eurixor, AbnobaViscum and Lektinol.

Personal opinion: Oncology would not be the same without mistletoe and this is good, considering all the studies. With the exception of leukemia, there is no differentiation relative to whom, when, and particularly, how long mistletoe preparations should be given, and nobody wants to use the word "resistance" in conjunction with mistletoe. A lot of work is still necessary here, and until this work is done, I do not dare make a statement about when mistletoe should be administered, in which doses, and particularly for how long it should be administered.

Essiac & Indian*Essence

In 1922 a Canadian nurse by the name of Rene Caisse obtained the recipe for a herbal medicine from a patient with breast cancer, who had been cured by a medicine man. She called this recipe Essiac, which is simply her name spelled backwards. After she successfully treated cancer patients with this herbal mixture, in 1940 she was given official permission by the Canadian Minister of Health to use this therapy on cancer patients.

This mixture has only become known since 1977, just prior to the death of Ms. Caisse. Specifically it involves:

* Greater burdock — recognized in alternative medicine as an immune stimulating substance

* Garden sorrel — recognized in alternative medicine as a diuretic and blood cleaner

* Medicinal rhubarb — recognized in alternative medicine as a laxative and for cleaning the colon

* Redelm — recognized in alternative medicine as a substance against infections

Greater burdock in particular is not unknown in oncology. In 1966 the Hungarian researchers C. Dombradi and S. Földeák discovered the cancer-inhibiting characteristics of this plant, and in 1984 researchers K. Morita and M. Namiki from

Nagoya University in Japan confirmed these effects. Medicinal rhubarb has also demonstrated that it can suppress the activities of the sarcoma 37 line in animal experiments. Many patients also reported a softening of the tumor and a clear reduction of pain. In 1983 Dr. Bruce Hendrick, a neuro-surgeon at the University of Toronto, requested permission from the Canadian government to finally perform a study on Essiac, after 8 of 10 of his patients required neither chemotherapy nor irradiation after a treatment with Essiac. Naturally the Canadian government rejected his request, as it was clear that Essiac would soon sink into oblivion anyway after the death of Rene Caisse.

After the death of Ms. Caisse there were doctors who repeatedly reported on fantastic results with Essiac. One of the best known was certainly Dr. Charles Brusch, personal physician of John F. Kennedy, who repeatedly emphasized that he healed his own colon cancer with Essiac.

Indian*Essence is an alternative to Essiac. This "Tea" which is marketed by the *Indian Wisdom Foundation*, which obtained the recipe from the Ojibwa and Cree Indians, contains all the ingredients in Essiac, plus:

* Genuine blessed thistle   - recognized in alternative medicine as harmonizing and a support for the digestive system

* Mistletoe   - recognized in alternative medicine as supporting cancer medication

* Brown algae   - recognized in alternative medicine as as a detoxification agent

*   Genuine water cress   - recognized in alternative
                                             medicine as a blood cleaner

*   Red clover blossoms   - recognized in alternative
                                             medicine as a strengthener of
                                             the immune system

Another product that contains almost the same ingredients and is also marketed in Germany is Flor-essence, which is marketed through the publishing house Ernährung & Bewusstsein (Nutrition & Consciousness).

Personal opinion: If the cost of Essiac is not considered then in my opinion there are some things that speak for the substance. Interestingly enough many people also use Essiac as a detoxification agent (see the book *Radiant Health* by Prof. Peskin). It is not possible for me to evaluate whose recipe is now the "genuine" recipe, should such a thing exist. There are hard facts about Essiac which have been collected by Rene Caisse and many doctors. Indian*Essence claims to have 9 ingredients instead of 4. Since both products are marketed commercially, it is very difficult for me to provide an evaluation.

Hackethal's Buserelin

Dr. Julius Hackethal was a revolutionary and it is a tragedy that his entire concept of a "healing clinic" no longer exists. Dr. Julius Hackethal has been pursuing an independent path of hormone blockade since 1985, by daily injecting buserelin (suprefact) a so-called hormone blocker (GnRh), in high doses (20-40x higher than recommended). Usually buserelin was given for 6-24 weeks and thereafter for 3-6 months with pauses. I was the first person to examine over 30 successful cases and I have documented 13 cases which clearly demonstrate how successfully Prof. Hackethal was able to treat cancer.

To what extent these results came about because Prof. Hackethal injected Buserelin or were due to his holistic therapy in general, neither I nor anybody else can evaluate. According to Hackethal it was primarily due to the total hormone blockade, others doubt this, as Buserelin contains N-acetyl neuramine acid, in addition to carbohydrates. Thus the biochemist Dr. Klemke says that this acid is split off through enzymes and that naturally the hormonal effect is also lost. His long-time companion Dr. Axel Weber has had his own clinic in Bavaria since 2001, where it possible to have the Buserelin therapy prescribed.

Personal opinion: Whether the Buserelin theapy alone results in similar successes as those experienced in the ParkKlinik I cannot answer, the future must show. However there is no question that Professor Hackethal was an absolute anomaly, whose life to the very end represented all that he recommended to his patients. His holistic approach was outstanding and his books helped many people avoid hasty decisions particularly for prostate cancer and breast cancer.

Hydrazine Sulfate

Hydrazine sulphate is a gluconeogenetic (new sugar forming) blocker which is used for cancer, and particularly the cancer cachexia (loss of strength and loss of weight). Expressed in scientific terms: It influences the phosphoenolpyruvate carboxykinase reaction. Research indicates that this non-toxic and valuable medication is an important substance in treating cancer.

It involves a simple freely available chemical product which can contribute to a dramatic reversal of the chachetic process (when cancer patients become weaker and weaker and which causes the death of most cancer patients). It can help prevent growth of malignant tumors, and help them regress, and in some cases, particularly for early phase cancer), it can contribute to their complete disappearance. It can be used for all types of cancer and in all phases of cancer. Dr. Joseph Gold from the Syracuse Cancer Research Institute in New York (which he founded in 1966) discovered in 1968 that hydrazine sulphate can suppress the weakening process and tumor growth in cancer patients. After many years and many confrontations with allopathic organizations, hydrazine sulphate was finally crossed off the "black list of unproven methods". Hydrazinsulphate finds an increasing number of adherents (whose results after 10 years of analysis support the effectiveness of the medication) particularly in Russia, and to some extent in America

In principle cancer has two major effects on the body. On one hand there is tumor penetration into vital organs and the associated destruction of the the organ's function. Most people believe that this is the main reason why people die of cancer. In reality this destruction is only responsible for 23% of cancer fatalities. The second effect is the cachexia (loss of strength and loss of weight). The cachexia in most cases precede the penetration of the tumor and people die for this reason.

Dr. Gold's strategy is to stop the cachexia, and not to attack the cancer cells directly. Cachexia occurs because cancer cells need about 18 times the amount of sugar that normal cells require. This sugar is mainly produced by the liver, by changing lactic acid into glucose. When cancer cells use sugar (glucose) as fuel, then they only partially process it. Lactic acid remains behind as a waste substance of this incomplete combustion. The lactic is introduced into the blood and absorbed by the liver. The liver then processes this lactic acid into glucose and the sugar is consumed in greater and greater quantities by the cancer cells. This causes a vicious circle. The healthy cells starve and the cancer cells grow like crazy. To stop this process Dr. Gold looked for a non-toxic substance to suppress the gluconeogenesis (recycling lactic acid back into glucose) and he found the suitable substance in hydrazinsulphate.

In a clinical study with 225 cancer patients in a final stage (with a variety of cancer types) who previously had shown no more reaction to all the other cancer therapies, Hydrazinsulfat was administered for at least 6 weeks. In this group 65.2% had a subjective positive reaction (weight stabilization, increased appetite, reduced pain) and 44% showed anti-tumor results (stabilization of tumor growth and reversal of growth). In an experiment at the Petrov Institute in St. Petersburg/Russia 46 patients with a malignant brain tumor were treated with hydrazinsulphate. A therapeutic effect of 61% was reported in the hydrazine sulfate group, and hydrazine sulfate was described as an absolutely safe mediaction for treatment of brain tumors. It was demonstrated that it improved the quality of life and extended the chances of survival. Even conventional practitioners in America like Dr. Chelbowski from the Harbor-UCLA Medical Center in California who combined hydrazine sulfate with chemotherapy for patients with small cell lung cancer, published in the Journal of Clinical Oncology in 1990 that on average his patients lived almost 60% longer.

Although hydrazine sulfate has proven in many studies how successfully it can be used, in Europe it is all but unknown. Pharmaceutical companies for logical reasons have no interest in hydrazine sulfate because it is much too cheap and cannot be patented. At the same time it cannot be used very well for self-medication because the patient must follow the administration protocol precisely, since it belongs to the group of MAO blockers and cannot by taken together with alcohol, tranquilizers, barbiturates or old cheese (that has a high proportion of tyrosines). Also when taking this substance it is recommended not to take more than 25 mg vitamin B6 and 2000 mg of vitamin C.

Allopathic practitioners maintain that hydrazine sulfate is not effective because the Sloan-Kettering Center in New York brought out a study that showed no advantage for 29 patients. What those doctors who cite this study most likely will not tell you is that Dr. Gold found out in an unannounced visit that the doctors were not following his guidelines and varied the dose as they wished. This is another good example of how the result of a study is pre-determined, even at the outset.

Personal opinion: Personally I only know a few patients who have taken hydrazine sulfate, and who did not participate in a holistic therapy at the same time. For this reason I can neither speak in favor of the medication or against the medication. If it is true that the phosphoenolpyruvate-carboxykinase reaction is suppressed, then this could however help cancer patients and should be more closely investigated.

Bio Pro

Bio Pro is a supplementary preparation whose task it is to replace missing thymus proteins and to strengthen the immune system. It consists mainly of a natural thymus protein which is produced with the help of living cells in the laboratory (by the immunologist Dr. Terry Beardsley who discovered the protein 23 years abo in his cancer research).

The isloated and cleaned protein originates form cattle thymus cells. The thymus is the the small gland directly behind the breast bone which produces proteins that are essential for normal T-cell immunity functions. The "T" by the way stands for thymus. Dr. Beardsley has a taken out a patent for his discovery and isolation of the protein.

Our immune system is a complex network of very specific organs, glands and cells, when they function properly they can protect our body from foreign cells such as cancer cells. There are two basic subsystems, the humoral (through bodily fluid) and the cell transmitted system. Each of these systems has its own specific methods of protecting our body from diseases.

The humoral system uses antibodies in a type of "chemical warfare". B-lymphocytes (which are produced and mature in the bone marrow) are used to produce antibodies that protect us from pathogens. The cell transmitted immune system uses T-lymphocytes (T-cells) as "shock troops". They are produced in the bone marrow but they mature with the assitance of proteins, which are produced in the thryoid gland. Both components of the immune system must function correctly in order for our body to have an optimal reaction relative to penetrating pathogens. The activities of the T4 lymphocytes (helper cells) are crucial for effective immune reaction and these activties are triggered when the T4 cells detect an antigen (which originates with a penetrating pathogen). When activated, the T4 cell produces interleukin proteins and interferone proteins, which are also referred to as cytokines, these in turn activate or program T8 lymphocytes (killer cells) to find the specific antigens of the invading pathogen and to kill them. In addition due to the activated T4 cells, the antibodies of the B cells are produced more effectively.

Before a T4 cell can detect an antigen and trigger this chain reaction of activities, it must be programmed by a specific thymus protein, whose special task it is to switch on or activate newly formed T4 cells. The thyroid gland produces proteins that program the T-lymphocytes. The importance of this gland has only become known to doctors within the last 20 years. The function of the gland declines with age. In addition, other factors like chemicals, irradiation or chronic illness accelerate the decomposition of the thyroid function.

Personal opinion: BioPro should not be viewed as treatment for a specific illness. However it could strengthen the immune system and for this reason it might play a role in preventing future illnesses.

Yeast Cells

The fact that cellular respiration in our mitochondria plays an extremely important role in cancer therapy, is known to every interested oncologist. Consequently, protection, or regeneration of mitochondria consequently is daily practice in oncology. Yeast cells are an active ingredeint that can contribute to this. It is not just that they have a cell membrane and a nucleus, but they also have a composition that predestines them for a supplemental therapy.

Professor Jurasunas from Lisbon discovered how successfully yeast cells can be used in cancer therapies. In many presentations and many books he described the successful use of yeast cells in cancer therapy, in detail. However the first work dealing with the positive aspects of yeast did not come from Lisbon, but from Dr. Paul Seeger and Dr. Stephan Wolz from Germany.

Yeast cells contain vitamins, different trace elements, calcium magnesium, potassium, amino acids, including cystein and methionine which have high sulphur content and are important in conjunction with essential fatty acids, enzymes and other biological substances like glucans, mannane, glutathione, etc. Jointly these substances stimulate cellular respiration and improve utilization of available oxygen. But the support of the natural intestinal flora also depends on these substances.

Personal opinion: The experiences of Dr. Seeger, and particularly those of Prof. Jurasunas, speak very positively for yeast. However is hard for me to evaluate whether it has to be preparations like Zell Oxygen Plus, or whether less expensive products are just as good. In any case yeast can have a very positive effect.

Bacillus Calmette-Guérin (BCG)

BCG is a vaccine that was introduced in the fight against tuberculoses in 1921. It involves highly weakened tubercolosies microbes that are supposed to have a strong immune reaction against cancer.

In an aggressive form of bladder cancer (transitional cell carcinoma in situ) the BCG vaccine causes a strong immune reaction in the form of a healing fever.

Dr. Burton Waisbren (leader of the Waisbren Clinic in Milwaukee) explained that the main advantage of BCG and other immune therapies like Coley's toxin or transfer factors (TF) is the capability of preventing the recurrence of secondary cancer. Also many German doctors such as Professor Hackethal have had positive experiences BCG.

Transfer factors (that are produced from the immune system of healthy donors) have been able to demonstrably improve the clinical reaction of breast cancer patients (Book of the National Academy of Science, 1974 – see also transfer factors). A study by Dr. Waisbren with 22 lung cancer patients showed that a combination of the aforementioned mentioned vaccines was helpful in delaying the recurrence of lung cancer. In his study, cancer patients who received the vaccine lived 9 months longer than patients in a control group who were not given the vaccine. In Oncology Magazine in 1995 a study of bladder cancer (transitional cell carcinoma in situ) was published in which 20% of the patients were still alive after 5 years. In the group of patients who were treated with BCG, 80% were still alive.

Personal opinion: BCG generates fever which is known to have a healing influence on cancer. However only a few physicians use BCG, due to lack of knowledge, and due to the possible side effects.

Cartilage

Since 1998 the term of antiangiogenesis has appeared more and more frequently in the headlines. Angiogenesis is nothing more than formation of the blood vessels that supply the tumor with blood. Various substances have proven in the past that they can suppress formation of new blood vessels.

Two of these products are shark cartilage and cattle cartilage. In 1972 Professor John Fletcher under the supervision of the FDA successfully treated cancer patients with cattle cartilage (VitaCart). In the study, cases were listed which showed stabilization of the tumor, reversal, or complete remission. Interesting, and unfortunately quite a problem in this regard, is that the monthly cost of substance is only USD 175.00.

Dr. Charles Simone, the doctor who treated Ronald Reagan, is a well-known oncologist, founder of the Simone cancer center in Lawrenceville, and author (*Cancer and Nutrition and Breast Health*). He has conducted studies with conventional therapies and non-conventional therapies. One of these therapies involved shark cartilage. He was able to prove that in a certain dose this cartilage has positive effects on tumor growth. He also treated his patients under the supervision of the FDA and in accordance with the IND protocol (Investigational New Drug Permit).

Shark cartilage is "naturally" considered to be a quack remedy. At the same time however, in late 1999, the FDA attempted at great effort to prohibit Benefin (a preparation made of shark cartilage). On one hand the government issues studies that are supposed to prove that Benefin cannot have a positive effect on cancer disease, and on the other hand they use every effort to prohibit the sale of such a worthless product produced by Lane Labs in New Jersey. Why? The answer is easy! Benefin is also an angiogenesis inhibitor, i.e. it is a prodjct that is supposed to be able to suppress new formation of blood vessels. Angiogenesis however is currently the favorite subject of all cancer gene researchers. This is easily seen in the fact that there are more than 100! new patent applications for angiogenesis suppressors.

Naturally a product which has proven itself in practical application, is inexpensive, and which cannot be patented, is a great thorn in the flesh for these companies. Thus pressure is brought to bear so that at last the "proper" and naturally the angiogenesis inhibitors that are one hundred times more expensive can come on the market.

Personal opinion: Angiogenesis inhibitors have a legitimate place in oncology, because they can at least stop tumor growth, in theory. Thus a person could gain time and in parallel pursue the 3E program. Cancer patients however should not be deceived by the flamboyant promises made by the manufacturers. Angiogenesis inhibitors will never be able to cure cancer, and to this day there is not a single preparation which comes even close to justifying the large investments made in recent years.

Cancer vaccines

In order for our immune system to better detect cancer cells, cancer cells are "loaded" with antigens in the laboratory, and returned to the body. Basically this is not any different than what is done with every other vaccine. And this is also precisely the problem which is associated with every other vaccine. We do not know how our immune system deals with these vaccines produced in the lab. Theoretically this manner of thinking is correct, but if you look closely at the history of vaccination, then you quickly start to doubt the whole theory, because everyone can find out that many of the "successes" which today are attributed to vaccines, in reality do not function at all, and have never functioned. What was considered to be scientifically recognized a few years ago, is being questioned more and more every day.

Although I was initially excited about the theory of cancer vaccination, the studies available today do not convince me. Naturally you can read about the success of dendrite cells everywhere today, but let's be realistic. Where are the proofs with human beings – and not in the lab. Here I still see great discrepancies. Nobody seems to want to discuss the risk of what it means when cancer cells are injected into the body Everyone says that these cells have been "neutralized" in the lab and thus they are no longer dangerous. But how much do we really understand about cancer cells? When are they "neutralized"? How good is the lab and its personnel?

Basically there are two different types of vaccines:

1. In the *ASI* (active specific immunotherapy) four to
   five grams of tumor mass are required. By the way this is
   a lot and naturally can only be obtained in major operative

intervention. The cells are then "loaded" in a laboratory and are injected usually 1-2 times a month.

2. The production of *dendrite cells* is the newer procedure. Here a few cancer cells suffice to produce the vaccines.

To point 1:

After studies from Göttingen University on dendrite cells were shown to be falsified, criticism on the studies produced by Professor Dieter Jocham and Dr. Christian Doehn from the University of Lübeck on the tumor vaccine has been increasing. The daily newspaper "Die Welt" called it a "Breakthrough in the fight against kidney cancer, and the "Tagesspiegel" even asked the question whether cancer "could certainly be conquered".

Such flamboyant statements are nothing new in the field of oncology. Thus Prof. Jocham said among other things: "Our study results show that the new vaccine reduces the relative risk of recurrence by app. 30% and thus could increase the life expectancy of the affected patients". However the writings of biometricians Professor Hans Joachim Trampish and Dr. Stefan Lange at the Ruhr University in Bochum are totally differently in this regard. They see such serious deficiencies in the study that these studies "cannot be considered as proof for the effectiveness of the vaccine".

But why? Between January 1997 and September 1998 doctors from 55 German clinics divided a total of 558 patients with already advanced renal cell cancer into two groups. All patients had the kidney removed but only one group received six injections of the tumor vaccine in monthly intervals. Success was monitored every six months over an observation period of more than five years. The result: During the first five years metastasis occurred in 23 of 100 patients treated with the vaccine, on the other hand of 100 patients who were not vaccinated, 32 had a relapse. The magazine Lancet evaluated this as: "immunological breakthrough" - once again!

What the average doctor does not know is that the study was NOT accepted in the register by the Study Group on Urologic Oncology (Arbeitsgemeinschaft Urologische Onkologie or AUO). Acceptance criteria were ignored: "Acceptance of tumors of the former tumor size category T2 (2.5 – 5 centimeter diameter) did not seem practical, as the risk of metastasizing in general is viewed at app. 10%", this means that even without therapy the tumor is so small that the vaccine can hardly have an effect. Or it came out in the case of 89 patients that they did not have a renal cell carcinoma in the intended stage. In total, even 174 patients – almost a third – were **subsequently** taken out of the evaluation. And by the way: The costs for this therapy are app. 18,000 Euro!

About point 2:
Dendrite cells were first described in 1973 by Steinman and Cohn, (first in mice), as highly potent antigen presenting cells. They have a characteristic morphology in certain differentiation stages, which is characterized by long membrane offshoots – thus the name (Gr. dendron = tree). Ontogenetically they originate from haemopoetic CD34 positive stem cells from bone marrow. As immature progenitor cells they emigrate from the bone marrow into the blood channel and here they form the monocytes. After maturation the monocytes leave the blood vessels and wander into the adjacent tissue. Here these cells differentiate further into histiocytes or macrophages and immature dendrite cells.

After contact with foreign antigens and activation, probably through cytokines that are produced by surrounding cells or macrophages, the dendrite cells start to wander and mature in the direction of regional lymph nodes, the spleen, or other secondary lymphatic tissues. When entering into the lymph nodes they come into contact with T-cells which give an additional maturation signal to the dendrite cells. At the same time the dendrite cells stimulate and activate the lymphocytes as well. If the T-cell receptor of the lymphocyte recognizes the peptide presented by the dendrite cell then the lymphocytes are stimulated to cell division. This is the theory, which scientists believe explains how dendrite cells (could) function.

Personal opinion: What was initially viewed as the great hope of oncology, has long since returned to the hard ground of reality. Cancer vaccinations have never established themselves, and a study published in 2000 in *Nature Medicine* undertaken by the Universities of Göttingen, Tübingen, and Humboldt University in Berlin on the treatment of metastasizing renal cell cancer using a vaccination composed of cell hybrids of tumor cells and dendrite cells had to be retracted later because: "not enough had been done to ensure the scientifically necessary precaution" – as it was expressed by the University of Göttingen. Others have not been so polite in their expressions and have called the professors money grubbing criminals.

Nor should it be forgotten that the costs of the therapy (which must be paid privately), are usually between 2,000 and 30,000 Euros. Although I have not yet dismissed the theory of cancer vaccination, and I still am interested in it, you must be very well informed relative to who is recommending which therapy, and why.

Fetal cell therapy

The use of fetal stem cells has been researched for decades in Russia and China. Currently this therapy is again in the media naturally due to the global discussion about stem cells and human clones. While politicians discuss the issue, these cells however have been used for decades, because in theory, fetal cells are capable of changing into almost any cell that is required in the body. For instance if people have too few immune cells, then stem cells help to re-stimulate the immune system. In studies the immune system was increased by a factor of 22 over the normal, in some cases. In one study there was even a clear increase in 86% of all participants. Moreover examinations have shown that fetal stem cells are capable of inhibiting the side effects of chemotherapy and irradiation.

Currently I only know of one company outside of Germany which manufacturers fetal cell vaccines, and one doctor in Germany who injects fetal cells. Unfortunately I am personally aware of only one successful cancer case so that there is little I can about possible successes. However what I do know for certain is that it is not just in China and Russia where extensive research is underway with fetal stem cells, and it is entirely possible that we are on the threshold of great innovations in medicine. This is based on the prerequisite that the theory really is correct which posits that fetal cells can travel through our bodies "like policemen and helpers".

By the way, currently the therapy is used more in the area of anti-aging than it is for cancer. In this process the rich and beautiful of this world who have fetal cell injections are also really milked, since between 8,000 and 15,000 Euro is charged for one injection. Whether this is right or not remains to be seen. In any case this theory proves that bone marrow transplant is not the only therapy with which a lot of money can be earned.

Personal opinion: When we discuss fetal stem cells, we must also deal the issue of ethics. At this point I have not made a decision as to whether I should consider this therapy direction good or not. On one hand I am against it because I do not believe that we should intervene so deeply in genetic processes, and on the other hand I understand desperate cancer patients and parents who say: The main thing is to get healthy again. Since an incredible amount of money is charged for a single injection, I consider the therapy only appropriate if, (A) you are very rich, and (B) you have come to grips with the issue that cells from other people are being used in your body.

Xenogenetic peptides

Xenogenetic means: coming from individuals of different species, and peptides are short amino acid chains. Xenogenetic peptides (the best known is certainly thymus) stimulate the activities of all types of lymphocytes (e.g. helper cells), and cause the release of cytokines (immunological messenger substances). Often they are also used in reconvalescence, so that patients more quickly recover from chemotherapies or irradiation. The most frequently used preparations are:

Thymus preparations:
Thymoject, Thym-Uvocal, Thymophysin, Zellmedin-Thymus and THX.

Peptide preparations:
Factor AF 2 (spleen, liver), polymer (spleen) an organ extract from the spleen and liver of new-born sheep.

Peptide-lysate combination:
NeyTumorin is a protein preparation produced from different organs of cattle and pigs. Unfortunately NeyTumorin is very expensive to manufacture and very expensive to buy.

Personal opinion: It is very difficult for me to evaluate xenogenic peptides because the statements about their successes exclusively come from the manufacturers, or from doctors who get money for such studies. On the other hand, I have had many very positive reports from doctors and patients e.g. about NeyTumorin or Polyerga, so that it is quite difficult for me to correctly assess the value of these preparations, which often are very expensive.

Enzymes

The cradle of modern enzyme therapy is Vienna, where the researchers Freund and Kaminer worked with cancer cells. The found out that cancer cells were destroyed by the blood of healthy people, however cancer cells were not destroyed by the blood of cancer patients. Freund's student, Max Wolf, was the first to prove that hydrolases (special enzymes) were the reason for this. Together with the biologist, Benitez, he then proved that it was primarily combinations of plant and animal enzymes that successfully killed cancer cells. Today these are known under the name WOBE (e.g. Wobe-Mucos or Wobenzym).

Enzymes like those cited above, (naturally from other manufacturers as well), can influence tumor growth in many different ways, for example: Neutralizing the blocking factors, such as mucins or cytokine polymers. Removal of the so-called sheath substances like fibrin. Reducing the bonding capability of cancer cells, and much more.

Personal opinion: Certainly enzymes play a major role in a holistic cancer therapy today, and there are only a few therapists who do not work with them. If the financial aspect is not a major issue for you, then integration would probably be worthwhile. Particularly chemotrypsin in high doses could be worthwhile for cancer patients. I wish that there was more research in this area particularly. Instead, in most cases health insurance companies have stopped paying for enzymes.

Carnivora

Carnivora is the pressed juice from the carnivorous plant, Venus fly trap (Dionaea muscipula). For more than 20 years the physician Dr. Helmut Keller has been researching this field. In Germany many doctors are familiar with carnivora, either through the press or because they have used it themselves. In 1983 the German Federal Health Office (Bundesgesundheitsamt) prohibited carnivora. Although Dr. Keller was able to prove that he could prevent contamination through endotoxins (fragments of bacterial membranes) in future production, Carnivora was never properly marketed again.

In his book: *Handbook of Holistic Cancer Therapy*, Dr. Keller, ascribes this to his own naiveté in dealing with government agencies. This is certainly a sad story, because Dr. Keller spent a lot of money in order to prove how successfully Carnivora can kill cancer cells, without having the same side effects as chemotherapy.

In one study it was shown that Carnivora T406 and GW27 can prevent tumor cells (glioma cells) from growing. In an additional study an antiproliferative effect (anti-tumor effect) was demonstrated for sarcoma 180 cells. In August 1995 Professor D.K. Todorov from the university of Sofia in Bulgaria was even able to prove that Carnivora had a tumor inhibiting effect for 0-342/DDP cells, which were immune to Cisplatin. Here you must know that Cisplatin for instance is the standard medication for fallopian tube cancer and has extremely serious side effects. However Carnivora was prohibited because slight chills and fever were produced with this therapy. In this case as well we can clearly see what a difference there is if a pharmaceutical company is behind an approval process, or whether just a "simple oncologist" is behind the approval process. While the list of Cisplatin's side effects is pages long and extremely serious irreversible side effects must be taken into account, this medication is not only approved, but it is considered to be the standard treatment for different types of cancer – while Carnivora was prohibited due to light side effects.

Personal opinion: I first became acquainted with Dr. Keller when he started work as senior physician with Dr. Douwes in the St. Georg Clinic. From there he moved to the Winnerhof Clinic, which was closed at the end of 1999. Today he works in Mexico and is trying to establish Carnivora in North America. In recent years I have personally become acquainted with many of Dr. Keller's patients who have all assured me that they would not be alive without Dr. Keller. Here however you must be aware that Dr. Keller usually employs many therapies, and not just Carnivora.

More information is available at:
www.carnivora.com

Photodynamic Therapy and Cytoluminescent Therapy

The idea of photodynamic therapy is basically quite simple and has been known for more than a century. Neils Finsen even won a Nobel Prize for his light therapy, and Hermann von Tappeier published his work in 1904. But it was not until the 1960s when laser research was being advanced that people remembered this work. The idea however stayed the same. (Cancer) cells are enriched with a dye and then these cells are radiated with light. Enrichment can occur through salves (aminolevulinic acid) or through orally administered photo-sentizers.

But what sounds so ingenuous in theory, unfortunately is anything but a successful cancer therapy. Determining the correct photosensitizer in combination with the right wavelength, or the determination of which light is even the proper light, will continue to provide issues for discussion in the future. Although there have been frequent smaller studies for different types of cancer, which seemed entirely hopeful, to this point no team has been successful in producing significantly better chances for survival. And this will never happen, because the therapy focuses on fast destruction of the tumor.

Even cytoluminescent therapy which was so highly praised in 2002, and which was used intensively first in Ireland, and then even in a clinic in Germany, has proven itself to be anything other than successful. In this therapy a fast-acting photosensitizer (photoflora) is used with the promise that it better and more quickly enriches in cancer cells. Not only the fact that both clinics today distance themselves from the therapy, even all of the great promises have quickly dissolved into thin air, and in 2005 there are not very many people talking about this therapy.

Personal opinion: I believe that the photodynamic therapy has a future as a selectively effective therapy for fast tumor destruction. Even if we are quite far the goal today, this could certainly be an area of considerable progress in the future. However I discount some of the extravagant promises which do not have the well-being of the patient in mind.

Vitamins

There is not a day that goes by when I am not asked about vitamin C, or the importance of vitamins, enzymes, amino acids, like lysine etc. in general. For example Particularly in Germany Dr. Rath is very well known through his presence in the media. My first answer relative to vitamins is always the same: Yes they are important, but they are certainly not the most important factor in a cancer therapy. Only after I have made this statement do I then discuss the details such as, which vitamins in which doses, from which company. I also consider the question of oral or intravenous administration to be very important. But here I am happy to repeat myself. I do not believe that artificial vitamins, particularly those taken orally are as important as they are always made out to be in discussions.

Even if I do not make any friends in the unconventional scene with the following lines I would still like to say: "It is absolute nonsense to believe that you can compensate for that which you otherwise are doing wrong with artificial vitamins (and those are all vitamins in pill or tablet form!)." It is not just in America where many people are of the opinion that they can compensate for their poor nutrition, by taking synthetic vitamins, minerals and enzymes. Other arguments, that are put forth include that our food today is a lot worse in terms of quality, and that we must compensate for this deficit, or that we have more stress etc. Some of the arguments are even correct, however it is incorrect to then conclude that this is why we must take artificial vitamins, these arguments primarily serve those parties who present them. There is a reason why so many vitamins are sold in MLM (multi-level marketing) structures.

In this case as well please do not misunderstand me. Basically I am not against artificial vitamins, absolutely not. I just consider all the discussion in this regard to be exaggerated. Instead of dealing with the really important changes, here things are discussed that not nearly as important. Often vitamins are preferred for reasons of convenience, as it is really not all that difficult to swallow a few pills a day – instead of changing your diet, having enemas, etc. And this is precisely what I consider to be extremely dangerous. Cancer patients are not the only ones who are only too happy to talk about "that which is not so important in life", instead of dealing with the really important issues. If you think I am exaggerating, then just look checkout a cancer forum on the Internet and you will see how thousands of cancer patients discuss in detail everyday, all of these matters that are third or fourth in terms of importance.

Therapeutically there must be a distinction between orally administered and intravenous applications. Thus in several studies, vitamin C administered intravenously has been able to demonstrate that it certainly has a legitimate place in oncology (L. Benade and D. Burk, C. Maramag and M. Menon, NH and HD Riordan, and many more). Logically the important influence on the blood pH value is different if vitamins are administered intravenously, or if they are administered orally. On the other hand there are studies in which vitamin C has clearly increased the growth of cancer cells (Dr. Chan Park or Dr. Joel Schwartz). Now I am not impressed when laboratory studies are applied to people, but such studies are "overlooked" by proponents of Vitamin C, and instead other laboratory experiments are consistently overvalued without considering this side of the coin.

This one-sided view is not just limited to vitamin C, it is also evident in many studies in which individual substances in the laboratory react differently than they do in the human body. These studies are evaluated in different directions, depending on whoever then reads the study.

Personal opinion: I know just as little as does any other honest person about how much vitamin C or Selenium or... you require. Relative to cancer however my experiences have shown that vitamins taken orally are not nearly as important as others would have us believe, particularly those who directly or indirectly earn money with them. I repeat I have nothing against people believing that they must take artificial vitamins. However I find it tragic that I must experience almost daily that cancer patients spend more time thinking about how many, and which, tablets, they should take, instead of dealing with personal changes.

IPT (Insulin Potentiation Therapy)

The IPT therapy was developed by a Mexican physician, Dr. Perez Garcia, who used insulin to treat syphilis patients 1926. Years later, together with his son, he started to use IPT as cancer therapy as well. The basic theory of the therapy is that insulin followed by a sugar solution helps other medications get into the cells more effectively, and in a more concentrated form. Thus IPT is naturally not a classic cancer therapy, but rather it is used in different areas of medicine.

IPT is used in oncology for different reasons. First naturally to reduce the dose of a chemotherapy, or just to get the toxin into the cancer cells. But the literature also cites, breaking through the blood brain barrier, better detoxification possibilities, or use as an immunomodulator. My experiences with IPT in oncology however are limited to its use as a supporting, cell-destroying therapy. And this poses precisely the greatest challenge for me, because I am not of the opinion that cancer cells should always be destroyed, and certainly not too quickly. However since most patients desire a rapid tumor destruction, I am not surprised that a handful of doctors use this therapy in Germany.

There are many issues surrounding IPT that are still open for me. Thus through IPT greater angiogenesis (formation of new blood vessels) takes place, different growth hormones are stimulated, the insulin level, which is already high anyway, becomes higher, and particularly cancer cells become even hungrier for sugar. These are just a few of many other arguments that initially speak against IPT.

Personal opinion: My personal experiences with IPT are not very extensive. Also the few studies on IPT are not very meaningful for cancer patients, particularly relative to survival time. Nevertheless I see great potential in the direction of fast tumor destruction and I am sure that this therapy one day will also find access to university groups.

Additional information: Do not confuse IPT with **IHT** (insulin induced hypoglycemic therapy). These are two completely different therapies with conflicting ideas.

Caesium chloride

Caesium is an alkaline metal (please do not confuse it with the artificially-manufactured and radioactive caesium 137) and caesium chloride is the salt thereof.

Cancer cells are known to have a far lower cell membrane potential. A result of this is that only a few substances can penetrate the cell. In addition to water, sugar, potassium and rubidium, caesium chloride is one of these, as can be read in the works of A. Keith Brewer. Doctors such as the famous Dr. Nieper in Hanover or the American Dr. Sartori have already used this knowledge many years ago, to offer their cancer patients therapy using caesium chloride. Above all, the study including 50 apparently hopeless cancer patients by Dr. Sartori in the 80's caused a minor sensation.

The reasoning behind the therapy is to supply increased amounts of the highly alkaline caesium to the cancer cells and thus, by an increase in the pH-value, to cause the death of the cancer cells. Additional therapies are often used in conjunction with this, such as e.g. laetril, high-dose vitamin C and vitamin A, EDTA etc., all with the aim of more effectively introducing the caesium into the cancer cell . The ultimate aim, however, is always to kill the cancer cells and not to convert them in any way. In addition, daily practice has shown that this therapy is often an excellent and very rapidly-working pain reliever.

Other aspects also make this therapy very interesting. In contrast to chemotherapy, caesium takes effect immediately and not only when cell division takes place. Also the blood-brain barrier is penetrated, thus theoretically pre-destining it for the treatment of brain tumours.

With regard to dosage and duration there is unfortunately a great challenge, which is perhaps why the therapy is still so little used. In addition to potassium loss, depending on the dose there can be increased nausea and diarrhoea. However, the most important fact is that there have not been any definitive studies which give the minimum dose which a patient should take. There are also discussions as to whether other caesium compounds, such as e.g. caesium carbonate would not be better and, above all, about how long caesium remains in the body. In any case, there are far too few studies with human subjects, which is a considerable obstacle to the widespread use of the therapy. Also, since the therapy can no longer be patented, the interest of the industry is predictably almost zero.

Personal opinion: In my view, caesium chloride makes sense as a tumour-destroying therapy. If there were not the „small problem of non-patentability", there would certainly be more to report here. However, this therapy thus continues to vegetate and "expensive" studies are not in view. Even if this therapy "only" destroys tumours, I think it is a shame that, at least officially, there is currently not a single researcher in this area who is publishing data.

Please note: Caesium chloride leads to a decline in potassium levels. For this reason, the treatment should be carried out by a qualified therapist.

Non-Conventional Cancer Therapies

Group 3

Cell Specific Cancer Therapy

CSCT is supposed to destroy cancer cells by using magnetic energy. Using an energy beamer cancer cells are supposed to be precisely homed in on and destroyed. After 8 years of research, Bob Scarbrough and Jim Claxton, both from Tennessee/USA, developed the CSCT device which consists of two circular rings in which their are two types of magnets. First, this is a permanent, low-strength magnet, which generates a permanent electromagnetic field. Second, there is a pulsing electromagnetic coil.

You can think of the whole thing as an egg-shaped energy field. If dynamic changing alternating current flows through the coil, then a dynamically changing electromagnetic field is induced around the coil. This dynamic field (which is also egg-shaped) acts with the static field of the permanent magnet. The result is a complex interactive electromagnetic field.

The CSCT-2000 theoretically has the job of identifying and then specifically attacking these cancer cells, by availing itself of the unique structure of the cancer cells. Cancer cells have an atypical metabolism. Each cell, including cancer cells, participates in a metabolic process (i.e. processing nutri-

715

ents into energy and water). In this process there are electrical activities, in which positive and negative ions flow in and out through the cell membrane in balance. While normal healthy cells require about 30 steps to conclude their metabolic process, cancer cells do it in 4 steps.

In addition normal cells use at least 90% of their nutrients in this process, as opposed to cancer cells, which only use 20% of their materials. It could be that cancer cells release more iron than do normal cells, for this reason. And precisely this excessive ionization is supposed to be detected by the apparatus. A cancer cell is more strongly illuminated than is a normal cell. Physicists know that all matter is energy, with different vibration and frequency rates. A healthy liver vibrates with a certain, detectable frequency, just like cancer cells. This therapy is offered for about 25,000 USD in Santo Domingo (Dominican Republic), in Mexico, and in Switzerland.

Personal opinion: In 1999 I was personally in Santo Domingo and reviewed 11 cases. Although I feel that the theory is very illuminating, I cannot confirm the cases published in different magazines. Although the CSCT-2000 did not show any more cancer cells, for at least 2 patients the tumor continued to grow, and I could not find the proclaimed successes in the other cases that were submitted to me. Even the study, published in 2001 with 25 pancreatic cancer patients, and the evaluation that patients lived 3 times (332%) as long, is not impressive with close scrutiny. To demand 25,000 USD for a therapy that has not been proven to help, I consider to be unethical.

IHT

(Insulin induced hypoglycemic therapy)

With IHT cancer patients are given so much insulin under intensive monitoring that for one to two hours these patients have so little sugar in the blood that the internal milieu changes strongly, and cancer cells are not supposed to survive in this changed milieu.

The theory is that tumors cannot survive without sugar. This knowledge was discovered in 1957 in the US, however it has never been consistently implemented over a longer period of time under clinical conditions. At that time the physician Dr. Surgis Koroljow, maintained that in two of his patients treated with IHT due to psychological problems, the tumors disappeared completely under the treatment. He treated other patients, but however because Dr. Koroljow was a psychiatrist and not an oncologist, this knowledge was lost, until an American group reviewed his data in 1998 and started treating patients in Mexico and in the Germany with this treatment. In March 2001, the IHT clinic in Mexico was closed and IHT was prohibited. Months before the German clinic had stopped the IHT therapy.

Unfortunately IHT is a good example of how unsuccessful non-conventional therapies can establish themselves for a short time, if the financial interest behind them is large enough. The "success" of IHT was only possible because a company sold shares of the company to influential people who were capable of placing reports in alternative magazines, in order to promote this unsuccessful therapy for financial reasons from the outset. In my opinion this cost many people their lives.

Personal opinion: I basically do not consider the idea of using insulin in cancer therapy to be incorrect, and if we could find more money for intensive research, as has already occurred in the Ukraine or in Russia, then I could certainly imagine modified IHT as a successful therapy. However as long as therapies are in the hands of unscrupulous business people, there will always be „victims". Here it makes no difference whether these people are involved with illegal chemotherapies or perform IHT. This is another way to keep a promising therapy out of the market for ever.

Supporting Substances

On the following pages I would like to introduce plants or substances that are consistently associated with the word cancer. To what extent these statements are important for your cancer therapy, I would like you to decide for yourself. However because your therapist or other authors frequently speak or write about them, it is to your advantage if you have already heard something about these substances.

AHCC

AHCC is a monosaccharide from the mycel of the shiitake mushroom. In tests at several universities (Hokkaido University, Kyronin University, or Teikyo University) it was proved that it can contribute to an increase of the immune system, particularly cytokines like TNF, IFN, IL-1, or IL2 or IL12 responded well.

Carctol

Carctol is produced from 8 plants such as Jawanese pepper or caltrop, and unfortunately is presented as a cure-all for cancer patients like many other herbs. Patients are recommended to take Carctol as part of a special diet and to take it together with enzymes. In addition patients should drink three to five litres of water daily and undertake other detoxification measures. Naturally the question comes up here, as to what is really the therapy – the herbs or the additional recommendations?

Chaparral

Chaparral is a green plant and has been known to Indians as a remedy since prehistoric times. The healing effect is particularly ascribed to the NDG acid (nordihydroguairetic acid) which has an influence on the electron support in the mitochondria and on sugar metabolism (similar to hydrazine sulfate). Although there are promising studies from the University of Utah, unfortunately I know of no meaningful studies that have been able to prove an anti-cancer effect.

Curcumin

Curcumin is a major component of the Curcuma species, which is commonly used as a yellow coloring and flavoring agent in foods. Curcumin has shown anti-carcinogenic activity in animals. It has been considered by oncologists as a potential third generation cancer chemopreventive agent, and clinical trials using it have been carried out in several laboratories ein Europe and the USA.

D-Galactose

For colon cancer you can find certain Glycoproteins that enter into combinations with oligosaccharides (sugar). Tests have shown that particularly liver cells attract this sugar. With operations in which increased numbers of cancer cells get into the blood circulation system, patients get D-galactose prior to and after the operation to prevent these cancer cells from settling in the liver.

DHEA

DHEA stands for dehydroepiandrosterone, which is a hormone that our body produces less and less of with increasing age. Smart business people realized that, if older people were given DHEA then the aging process would at least be slowed down. This is a good business in America, in Germany free sale of this substance is prohibited.

There is no doubt that DHEA plays an important role in our body, certainly other hormones like estrogen, progesterone, or testosterone are produced with the help of DHEA.

DHEA appears to play a particular role for breast cancer, because studies have shown that women with low DHEA blood values more frequently got cancer.

The Mexican yam root (Dioscorea villosa) contains the natural preliminary stages of DHEA and is probably also capable of increasing the DHEA level in the blood.

DMSO

This is the abbreviation for dimethylsulfoxide. In body building circles or for models this is used in combination with substances that contain effedrine for rapid fat decomposition. Also it has been known for a long time as an infection-inhibiting medicine. But it was only through studies, such as the study by J.C. De la Torre, J.W. Stanley, or D.G. Volden, that oncologists became aware of the positive influence DMSO has on cancer cells. This substance was capable of normalizing degenerate cells, not just for bladder cancer, colon cancer, breast cancer, or skin cancer, but even for leukemias, as was proved by P. Marks, and R. Rifkind.

DMSO is capable of binding hydroxyl radicals, which explains many effects, particularly also the positive studies, which show limiting the side effects of chemotherapies or irradiations, as both therapies apparently release billions of hydroxyl radicals in the body. Because DMS makes cells "less impermeable", i.e. affects the cell membrane, there are also approaches in conventional medicine that give DMS concurrently with chemotherapies, in the hope that these toxins can more easily get into the cancer cells, or that through a reduced dose the side effects can be better limited. DMSO is an inexpensive substance and for this reason alone, it will never establish itself in oncology, because no one can earn enough money with it. In Germany DMSO cannot be purchased freely.

Escozul / Escocul

Escozul is a medication that is obtained from the blue Caribbean scorpion (Rhopalurus junceus) through electrical shock, and which is primarily used in Central and South America against infections, and also against tumors.

It is particularly well-known in Cuba, where to this day it has been given to more than 50,000 patients. Unfortunately those involved forgot to make studies before they gave it to the patients and the data which have been published, to this point are more than modest, or only come from the manufacturers.

Germanium

Organic germanium is obtained from coal and can also be found in almost all plants. In Japan the well-known physician Dr. Asai founded the Germanium Clinic in Tokyo whose main focus is on researching the cancer curing effect of germanium. In his view all illnesses are ascribed to a lack of oxygen in the body and according to his research germanium can contribute to resolving precisely this problem.

In solid form germanium is a crystal. Energies are ascribed to crystals, which can be effectively used for healing, because they absorb and give off electrons. Because the information flow in the body occurs though the flow of electrons, these play a very important role and release energies. Books: *Miracle Cure - Organic Geranium* – Dr. Kuzuiko Asai, and *Germanium – the health and life enhancer*, by Dr. Sandra Goodman.

Green tea

In green tea it is particularly the substance Epigallocatechin (EGC) which is demonstrably capable of suppressing the growth of cancer cells and at the same time, lowering the cholesterol level. EGC belongs to a group of polyphenol catechins that are known as antioxidants and have an effect that is significantly stronger than that of vitamins. Asians have been swearing by the positive effects of green tea for many years.

Hashish/cannabis

Doctors have been able to prescribe the active substance in hashish, Delta-9-THC, since 1998. I agree that this approach is correct because hashish has far fewer side effects than traditional pain killers, but it can effectively fight pain.

I3C

In 1991 researchers at the institute for hormone research in New York City reported that they succeeded in transforming the stronger estrogen (estradiol) into a weaker form (estrone 2-hydroxy). With a natural substance researchers were able to convert estradiol to weak estrogen by 50% in twelve healthy people.

The substance was indole-3-carbinol (I-3-C) a phytochemical preparation of vegetables like broccoli, cauliflower, red cabbage, beets, cabbage, spinach, etc. Today I-3-C has established itself as a replacement substance for tamoxifen.

IP6

The name IP6 stands for inositol hexaphosphate, which has 6 phosphate molecules. The patent holder is Dr. Abulkalam Shamsuddin from America. IP6 is found in rice, wheat or soy for instance. The main effect, which has been proven, through taking IP6 is an increase in NKC (natural killer cell) activity.

Jomol

Jomol is an extract of cell wall substances of the Nocardia opaca bacteria. In Germany it has mainly been researched by Dr. Udo Ehrenfeld. Jomol can also be used as diagnostic instrument, because it is capable of binding radionuclides or fluorescent dyes. Afterwards this combination can be observed with a gamma camera, or under the UV microscope, and can show cancer cells, as Jomol bonds to them.

Ozonide therapy
Ozonides are long-chained oxygen rich substances and are produced from natural fatty oils like olive oil or castor oil, and oxygen in the form of ozone. They have a germ killing effect against all types of anaerobes Like Candida yeasts, bacteria like clostrides, parasites, and also tumor cells, because these cells have few detoxification mechanisms against oxygen. Intravenous and oral administration of ozonides is possible.

Cats Claw or una de gato
The name cat's claw refers to the vine of the Uncaria tomentosa, which has very sharp thorns, like a cat's claw. In Peru this juice/wine has been known for all long time as a cancer medication or immune promoting medication. Its effect could possibly come from the many antioxidative components. Unfortunately there are few meaningful studies (such as P.N. Steinberg in TLFD 1995. p. 70-71.

KLH
KLH is the blood dye of the keyhole limpet. The company Biosyn in Fellbach Germany manufacturers the product Immucothel from this pigment. The product is currently only used for bladder cancer **after** an operation.

Kombucha
Kombucha is a very old and popular remedy in China. The fermented tea, Kombucha consists of a thick, gelatinous shiny membrane that occurs through a symbiosis of yeast cells and a several bacteria. As opposed to genuine yeast types it does not form any spores, the cells multiply exclusively through growth. The symbionts of the Kombucha ferment the sugar and form multiple metabolism products that go into the drink. In this way glucoronic acid, lactic acid, and acetic acid, are

formed. As a consequence Kombucha could be part of a very good detoxification process.

Lapacho
Lapacho, also referred to as pau d´arco in other countries, is produced from the bark of the Tabebuia tree, which principally grows in South America. Many studies showed that Lapacho could be used in a supporting role in oncology. Thus a study published in *Cancer Research* showed significant activities against special cancer cells (Walker 256). Another study conducted at the University of Hawaii showed higher activity against lung metastases, and in the Lapacho group, 5 times as many mice survived relative to the control group.

Marayuma Vaccine (SSM)
The vaccine consists of a polysaccharide, and according to the manufacturer's information it has been sold more than 300,000 times in Japan for immune stimulation. The SSM documentation reminds me quite a bit of the effects of a mistletoe therapy.

Megamin
Megamin is a zeolithic stone to which other minerals, which have a high proportion of calcium and magnesium have been added. Then it is ground and the partial destruction of the crystal structure on the surface of the particles effects a stabilization of negative charge on the surface and an increased ion exchange which makes it a strong antioxidant.

Melatonin
Melantonin is a hormone that is illegal to sell in Germany. In recent years it has been sold as a sleep hormone, as well as an anti-jetlag medication. Combined with DHEA in the mid-nineties it was the absolute top seller in America. In the field of oncology M. Carolea and B. Neri have shown that mela-

tonin is capable of increasing the activity of the T-helper cells, just as it increases the activity of natural killer cells or inter-leukin-2. In addition there are studies that show survival advantages for patients with metastasizing colon cancer, for stomach carcinomas, breast cancer, and for patients with brain tumors. DHEA and melatonin are sold in America as "Anti-aging products". However both are medications and belong in the hands of responsible therapists, and not on the supermar-ket shelves.

Microhydrin
According to information provided by its discoverer, Dr. Patrick Flanagan, Microhydrin is a combination of silicon and hydrogen atoms, which can give off large quantities of free electrons to the body. What is interesting for cancer patients is that the university of North Texas was able to prove in a study that the lactate value (lactic acid) could be lowered by taking microhydrin.

MGN3
In studies by Dr. M. Ghoneum, MGN3 likewise is supposed to have shown a clear increase of NKC (natural killer cell) activ-ity.

MTH 68
MTH 68 is a virus, or to be more precise the Newcastle Disease Virus which is fatal for chickens. The Hungarian Dr. Laszlo Csatary has been experimenting with the virus for many years, which for humans which may possibly produce positive results through its fever generating activity. He was able to demonstrate that his therapy was successful in double-blind studies. Most doctors are totally unfamiliar with MTH. For example in Germany the Physician Dr. Arno Thaller works with MTH 68.

Noni Juice

To this day I have no convincing data that this very expensive juice would be advantageous for cancer patients. With this statement I do not maintain that Noni juice is not beneficial for your health, but unfortunately the frequently-cited advantages for cancer patients are not confirmed.

Agaricus blazei murill

This mushroom from Brazil contains many proteins, including beta glucan. This protein has shown in several studies that it stimulates the natural killer cells and increases the count by over 300%.

Shiitake mushroom

Lentinan is a particularly interesting substance in the shiitake mushroom. Through increased formation of the body's own interferon, it activates the natural defense powers by stimulating production of lymphocytes and killer cells. In addition the shiitake mushroom also has the active substance, eritadenine. This substance can lower an excessively high cholesterol level.

Maitake mushroom

The maitake mushroom has also been able to demonstrate results that are similar to those obtained with shiitake mushrooms.

Other Japanese mushrooms

Currently there are three mushroom polysaccharides that have been approved for tumor therapy in Japan. These are lentinan, schizophyllan, and krestin. All three have proven in tests that they could clearly increase the survival time of cancer patients to some extent.

Selenium

Selenium was discovered in 1817 by Jöns Jakob Berzelius. Selenium is mostly bound in the soil and rocks but it also occurs in bodies of water and in the ocean. It functions as a component of enzymes and as such it protects the sensitive polyunsaturated fatty acids from oxidation. Many scientists, such as Dr. Schrauzer, also ascribe the preventative and protecting effect against cancer to the total antioxidizing action of selenium. Moreover Selenium is important in the metabolism of thyroid hormones. Selenium also has a detoxifying effect in that it helps free our bodies from harmful heavy metals, and it strengthens the immune system. Today many oncologists use high-dose selenium for detoxification, and naturally, as an easily digestible antioxidant.

Snake venom from Horvi

These products involve the DPN splitting enzymes (diphosphopyridinnucleotide) which occur in snake venom, because they inhibit glycolysis in the cancer cells. Here there is a distinction between the toxic groups and the fermentative groups. Dr. Waldemar Diesing was successful in lowering a so-called fermentative decomposition of the protein bridges, (the protein content) from 1.8% to 2%, without the venom decomposing and thus becoming ineffective.

Snake and spider venom in general

The German researcher Dirk Weidmann was successful in removing substances from snake and spider venom, which demonstrably can kill cancer cells. Peptide toxins are mixed with antagonistic acting substances. Unfortunately there are still no meaningful clinical studies. The theory of mixing both substances however is very interesting and could lead to positive results in the future.

Schliephake shortwave therapy
This therapy involves short-wave stimulation of the hypophyse, Dr. Erwin Schliephake, who by the way, lived to be over 100-years old, described very positive results for cancer patients with his therapy. Unfortunately there are only a few therapists who are familiar with this promising therapy. More information is available in the book *Cancer and Infection – treatment with high-frequency fields (short waves)*.

Incence/boswellic acid
Boswellic acid is mainly used primarily for brain tumors, to limit the edema. It has demonstrated its infection-inhibiting characteristics in many studies and this is its usual application.

Wheat grass
There is a lot of information about wheat grass in the literature. Particularly its high chlorophyll content, enzyme content, and vitamin content, play a significant role. Wheat grass can play also play an important role during detoxification therapies Chlorophyll plays a role for plants that is similar to the role that hemoglobin plays in people – it serves as a carrieor for oxygen. Also chemically it is almost identical (the only difference is that the atom consists of magnesium and not of iron). There are studies, such as the study from Dr. Y. Hagiwara, which show that chlorophll can be utilized in our body and that it participates in supporting the formation of hemoglobin. Dr. T. Kada was also able to show in his work that wheat grass can prevent chromosome damage. Other studies at the University of San Diego, and the M.D. Anderson Institute in Houston showed blocking of cancer cells in cell cultures.

Whoever has studied mitochondria therapy intensively and then investigates the enzymes that are present in wheat grass, readily understands why it is something special. Those enzymes that play a significant role in cellular respiration, are precisely those enzymes that we also find in wheat grass: Cytochromoxydase, lipase, protease, amylase, transhydrogenase, Pepsin and SOD (Superoxidismutase.) There is no doubt that wheat grass is something special for cancer patients.

Tributyrate

Tributyrate (PA und PB) is a preliminary stage of Dr. Burzynski's antineoplastons. Actually it was developed at John Hopkins University for a very rare disease (UCD, in which urea production does not function normally, due to an enzyme deficiency).

Therapists and clinics

In recent years I have naturally become acquainted with many clinics and doctors. When I started writing this book, I originally planned to also introduce some of these doctors or clinics. But I abandoned this idea and I would like to tell you why.

1. Many cancer organizations provide lists of alternative cancer clinics. However, these lists say absolutely nothing about the quality of the clinic, rather are put together for totally different reasons, membership in a certain organization, money, etc. However most patients are not aware of this and believe that the clinics on such a list are particularly suitable, or that they have been carefully selected. Patients do not know, that people gets money for writing "more positive" about a hospital in "independed reports".

2. I even used to "recommend" certain clinics myself, that I would never ever recommend today. But such lists are copied again and again over the years, and they are given out to people who are looking for clinics. Once such a list is in circulation it cannot be stopped.

3. I know some good clinics that are worth recommending. But like people, these clinics have their special characteristics which unfortunately change much too frequently. For a particular patient it can however be extremely important to become acquainted with the characteristics of a clinic in order to get the therapy that is optimal **for that individual**. Consequently in my capacity as a member of the executive board of *Menschen gegen Krebs e.V,* my policy is not just to give patients simple information about this clinic, or that clinic, but to always include what they should do on their own, as well, in order to be optimally treated there. I admit that often

it is only little things, but these little things often decide whether a person goes to a clinic or stays there. I am always up to date and know what is going on, naturally, because I have spend many hours talking with cancer patients on the telephone. This information has been very useful for a lot of people, and it is useful for a lot of people.

And now?

Where would I go now if I needed help? This is a legitimate question and one that is not so easy to answer, as I have already tried to explain in point three above. At *Menschen gegen Krebs e.V.* I try to answer this question several times a day, and believe me, often there is no pat answer. Particularly if cancer types are involved for which allopathy can show good statistics, but for which however allopathy did not help "for this patient in particular", then I don't know of any clinic either, because no clinic director wants to get his fingers burned for legal reasons with this patient. There are thousands of such patients in Germany and I wish there were chief physicians who were more courageous. Often a patient must make compromises and unfortunately it is necessary to know something about cancer, otherwise you are forced to accept too much on faith.

Thus get information from *Menschen gegen Krebs e.V.* or from another cancer organization that you trust. But regardless of which clinic you go to. You must understand the concept that is pursued there, so that you can organize for yourself the elements that are missing in that clinic. There is no clinic that can do everything, consequently your participation is strictly required.

There is also a lot of information on the Internet. However be very critical of all internet sites. Stay away from cancer forums. What is communicated in forums, so to speak from patient to patient, is often a catastrophe (to put it politely), and many patients are nothing other than purchased sysops (system operators), i.e. people who are paid for their comments. In my research I found many interesting sites, but then I later found out that even behind non-profit organizations, "free authors", or independent scientists, in reality, organizations like religious sects, or pharmaceutical companies were hidden through devious paths. These organizations only want one thing: Your money. **I always welcome it when people first test me**, to determine whether I am really independed. In any event maintain a critical attitude. The world needs people who are critical and who can still think positively. Naturally you can search for yourself.

Do not fall for the professionalism of the respective websites. The richer the company or the organization, the more expensive advertising companies they can buy. Even the "known seriousness" of an organization unfortunately does not have as much to say as you might like. This is the same as it is in politics. Just because a person is a member of a large party, does not necessarily means that he is telling the truth (most people have now come to realize this in the case of political parties).

Most web sites are either proponents of chemotherapies, or they are opponents of chemotherapies. Unfortunately there are only a few sites that deal constructively with the whole subject. Moreover there is a relatively high number of self-proclaimed judges who claim to know everything about alternative cancer therapies, which really means that they are all bad. I have personally asked many therapists whether one of these "experts" ever requested a look at the files. All the therapists who I asked answered this question with **no**. At this point any thinking person would immediately ask the question, how these experts know so much about therapists/therapies, who they have never visited on-site, or examined on site, in their life. At the same time however conventional therapies are always represented as being good. Be very careful of anybody who has never been to Mexico, or who did not know Dr.

Budwig personally, writes something about Gerson, or the oil protein diet.

The progress of "modern" oncology

Often I am told that modern oncology has finally made a little progress in recent years and thanks to this progress fewer patients have to die of cancer today. The statement that fewer people have to die of cancer is not true at all, and regarding the second statement about progress, I say let's take a closer look to see if there has been any.

Basically I would like to say that in my opinion, there can be no significant progress in oncological allopathy as long as genes alone are held to be responsible for cancer. Nevertheless I would like to introduce a few projects to you that oncologists around the world are focusing on.

A: Gene therapies
The idea here is that we introduce new genes into old structures, and thus we can cure cancer. Whatever you hear in this regard, be aware that this theory is bound to fail from the very beginning. First, after concluding the genome project, we still do not know which gene means what, and second, how can a gene repair induce a cure, if a gene is not even the cause of cancer? Moreover, in reality it is not so easy to cut out tiny particles like genes, and to insert others in their place. We are still light years away from this technology; we not on the threshold of it, as many publicly-traded companies constantly tell us.

B: Laboratory and human being
Most allopathic "modern cancer therapies" are developed in laboratories. Here the main priority is cell destruction. Naturally this presupposes that we have cells in our body that

734

must be destroyed. I also considered this allopathic approach to be wrong in 99% of all cases. We don't have any degenerated, malignant cells, rather we have cells that behave differently. That is a significant difference. I do not kill any "entire" person because he cannot fit into the community. Precisely in the same manner we must consider very carefully whether it is correct to kill cells, just because they currently cannot fit into the community correctly.

There is no doubt that what is being discovered in the laboratories around the word is genuinely interesting. These include the latest chemotherapies, with which the patient's hair does fall out immediately, modern angiogenesis inhibitors, which are supposed to cut off the tumor's blood supply, active substances which block ATP production of the cancer cell (methylglyoxal), preparations which are only effective for certain cancer types like CML (glivec), and many more. However what all of these developments have in common is that they are designed to kill cells, instead of returning cells to normal growth. Another thing that they all have in common is that the great successes that the media reports to us every day, in reality are only a few individual cases, and that these successes usually only serve the shareholders.

What is interesting in this regard is also the fact that allopaths always snicker at non-conventional doctors, when they introduce individual cases, instead of a large, randomized, double-blind study. But when the task at hand is to establish new therapies, then every single case of a tumor reduction is hailed as "pioneering", "sensational", or "the future direction of oncology". After you have heard or read this a hundred times, you cannot take such reports seriously, even with the best intentions.

C: Goal-specific therapies

To an increasing extent, even allopathy recognises that chemotherapies are not the final solution. But instead of approaching this problem openly, more and more the trend is to develop therapies that are more "goal-specific". These involve either active vaccines, which are supposed to help an individual's own cells to better recognize cancer cells, or toxins, which unfold their toxic effect only in the target cells, i.e. the cancer cells.

Here as well, I consider the approach to be false because once again it involves killing cells. Moreover vaccines are bound to fail because logically they can only be "armed" for a certain type of cancer cell. However cancer cells are extremely intelligent cells, like all of our cells, and laboratories are trying to match the cells to cancer cells, that may have changed a long time ago. I have nothing against toxins, which only develop their effect at the event location. They could be particularly helpful in life-threatening situations. But we must be careful of going too far. What has been announced for years has only functioned in the laboratory to this day. We are still far away from this technology, and I will only believe in all of the fairy tales which we can read today in all scientific magazines, when these fairy tales are true for human beings, and not for mice.

D: General

If we look at the study protocol of the EORTC (European Organization for Research and Treatment of Cancer) then we can see (May 2002 – but it will not change in 2005 or 2010!) that the 675 current studies are categorized as follows:

1. Chemotherapy (415 studies)
2. Radio therapy (85 studies)
3. Surgery (53 studies)

Approximately 82% of all studies involve the comparison of new and old allopathy therapies, and over 61% involve the comparison of different toxins. The rest mainly involve hormone therapies and immune therapies.

Now ask yourself: How in heaven's name can allopathic oncology make real progress? All the research is based on shareholders and people who earn money on the status quo, and on changes. The reports in the newspapers are always the same: "In two or three years we will have a marketable medication against cancer." Naturally most patients do not know that all these reports in 99% of all cases only serve shareholders and stabilize share prices, they do not help cancer patients. Whoever still believes that **genuine** progress is being made here, does not sail on the ocean because he believes he will fall off the horizon.

3E-Emergency Program

I think that you will agree that this book reports comprehensively on cancer. But this information also confronts many people with the problem: **What do I do first, and what do I do if I don't have time to read such a big book?**

I do not want to leave you alone with this question, in the next three pages I summarize what you should do in any case, regardless of which therapy you finally decide for. But there is one point that I would still like to discuss in detail, because in my work, I see daily that it causes the greatest difficulties for many patients. This point is called **discipline**. If there is one thing that I have learned in recent years, it is that cancer patients, particularly those in an advanced stage, can only become healthy if they are capable of living in a disciplined manner.

Discipline here does not mean no fun and no enjoyment, it means the complete opposite. Discipline her means first and foremost: be active and live. But the last two words represent the greatest challenge: to live. "I have cancer" is the preferred excuse to no longer to have fun, no sex, no party frame of mind etc. I repeat this often in this book, but you must understand that fun and joy in life can do more to stabilize your immune system, indeed your health in general, then any medication can.

If I tell you that you should now have fun, then I say this not because I believe that you will die soon, but because I know that only active and disciplined people can become healthy again in an advanced stage of cancer. And the same applies to people who only have one tumor and otherwise are quite healthy, if they want to stop the growth of the tumor. Naturally this group of cancer patients has more time, but nevertheless it is important that you also start living disciplined in a disciplined manner so that the tumor does not continue to grow.

Many people unfortunately have many nonsensical thoughts going through their heads has if there were an irrevocable law: Tumor = no fun. Please believe me this is absolutely incorrect! Start today thinking about what would be the most fun for you, or what you believe would bring you the most joy in life. I recommend to every person, not just cancer patients, that before going to sleep, to think about what was nice today, what was fun today, or what brought you closer to making your dreams reality, today. And every evening plan enough life time for the following day. This is time in which you laugh, live your dreams and in which you are totally satisfied. However you need a high level of discipline for this. It is particularly easy for cancer patients to be overtaken by daily life; the day is gone, and unfortunately again it was not a fantastic, beautiful day. If they were not sick then I would say OK, tomorrow is another day. But if you have cancer, then you cannot afford this type of thing.

You may not consider this to be not as important as "proper therapies" – and I can readily understand this idea. But since you have almost read my entire book, and if you believe, that I understand something about cancer, then I would like to ask you something. Trust me. Trust me please, when I say to you that in future modern cancer therapy, the first thing will be to create a basis. Similar to when building a house. First the foundation, then the walls, then the wallpaper. The foundation is your joy in life, the walls are nutrition, detoxification, and energy work, and only after these are in place should you discuss a wallpaper, by the name of mistletoe, hyperthermia, laetril, vitamins, etc. I am always sad at heart when I see how much energy and money disappears to purchase wallpaper for a house that will never be built, because the owner dies before it is done. Do not make this mistake, follow my suggestions on the next pages. Believe me it will be worth it.

1.	Clarify the diagnoses again. You would not be the first person who has had a life-changing therapy prescribed on the basis of a false diagnosis.

2.	Take 1-2 weeks to find your therapy. Nobody dies immediately after the diagnosis of cancer.

3.	Do not succumb to a "Why me" depression. Cancer is not nearly the terrible illness that you perhaps have considered it to be until today. This point is very important because in the days to come you must make many vital decisions. This is only possible if you are thinking rationally.

4.	Speak with a holistic-thinking therapist even if in your heart you have already decided on a conventional therapy.

5.	Verify all of the percentage-based information supplied by your therapist. **Never** accept statements like "If you undergo this therapy then you have chances that are ?? percent better". My experience is that many more lies than truthful statements are in circulation in this area.

6.	After reading this book, you have certainly understood that cancer is a systemic illness and consequently it must be treated holistically. **Always** start with the 3E program. This particularly includes:

*	*The Oil protein diet as developed by Dr. Budwig*

*	*Detoxification measures:*
	Colon cleanse through colon hydrotherapy and

Baking soda enemas.
Liver support through coffee enemas.
Removal of amalgam. Particularly dead teeth (teeth
that have had a root canal).
Attention: With few exceptions do NOT REMOVE
AMALGAM as long as tumors are present.
Balance the acid/alkaline balance through
daily baking soda baths.

* ***Visualization training, meditation, prayer***

Create a plan **today,** of what you need for this.
This includes a tumor contract. Please do not make the
mistake and believe, there is still time for this. Later is
perhaps too late.

7.   Get help. Give this book to a person you trust
so that they can read it. It is important that you have
somebody who supports you on **your** path, and not
someone who wants to force you onto **his**
path. If there is not such a person in your environment,
then it is better to proceed alone on your path than it is
to permanently waste all your energy explaining to
other people what you want and why.

8.   Many therapies not only cost a lot of energy, but they
also cost money. Consider carefully whether you want
to spend money for your therapy and how much
money you want to spend for your therapy. If you have
money now is the time to spend it - or do you know of
a better opportunity? If you do not have money, or if
you only have a little money then still create an
extensive therapy plan. Indeed it takes more effort, but
it is 100% possible

9.   This is for you, it is not for your partner or for your children. Explain this to your family. This has nothing to do with egoism, rather it makes it easier for you to make decisions and to get support. Do not allow yourself to be pitied. While this is pleasant in the short-term, what you need now are rational people around you.

10.   You have developed this tumor / these cells and only you are responsible for seeing that everything gets back on the right track. Take the responsibility for this and do not let it get out of your hands.

11.   Ensure that your life brings you joy. I am totally aware that at first this sentence will sound paradoxical to you. But this is really an important point which will contribute to your healing. Thus make the necessary decisions so that your life is fun (again) and ask yourself when you stopped living your dreams.

12.   Healing occurs inside of you. No medication in the world can heal you. Once you have internalized this sentence you are already on the way to healing.

The future of oncology

I do not want to conclude this book without sharing with you what I hope for the oncology of the future. The following lines are not written to all readers of this book, namely because most of the readers of this book are interested in learning how they can help themselves, or other people with cancer. That is my main reason for writing this book.

However there is another reason for this book, and that is to make a contribution towards changing the current oncology. With all my heart I am convinced that we need profound changes not only in oncology, but in medicine in general. Changing this or changing that is inadequate in this regard, we need major steps. If the citizens of German Democratic Republic had discussed changes to their laws instead of demonstrating in the streets, and believing in the dream of a life without the wall, or visualizing this dream – the wall would still be there.

Nothing will change to a significant degree as long as parties accept donations, and politicians and doctors need not fear punishment. Since I consider it utopian to believe in such changes, I call on all people to make the necessary changes in smaller steps. If all doctors who do not prescribe chemotherapies for their families would stop prescribing them for their patients then we would be a step further. If more doctors had the courage to publicly state what they often state in small groups, that would represent yet another step further.

There are still many such steps to list, but I simply maintain that many people have known the steps, that we must take for a long time, unfortunately they do not take them. My book is designed to also give the courage to finally take these steps. If we do not do it, then who will? Our children? Let's not count on that, rather let us start to usher in the necessary steps today. Consider what **you** can do, so that things go better for all of **us**. And if you are doing well, and you do not see any need, then I can only say, that your child or your partner may need help tomorrow, and then you will happy if there are people who can show you paths that can be taken.

It is possible to convince insurance companies that they can also make their member's money available for nutrition therapies and detoxification therapies. It is possible that we can build or set-up completely alternative houses of healing, where the only important is to create healing fields. It is possible to show pharmaceutical companies and shareholders that they can earn money with things other than disease. It is possible to start healing processes in people in just a few days. It is possible ...!

Just think that if all the available money in the world were distributed "fairly", we would all be millionaires. I know (not believe!) that cancer can be healed in every stage, and that many people, too many people, have to die due to bureaucracy, ignorance, and "system errors". It remains in our hands to finally execute the necessary changes. One thing is certain, a few changes here and a few changes there will not be enough. Please do not leave your future and the future of your children to other people. Be courageous, and finally do that which earlier you only dreamed about. Today is the right time for this, not tomorrow. Not every person is born to be Gandhi or Spartacus. But every person can live his dreams and thus contribute to a better world.

If you believe that you cannot contribute anything, then I can only say that **everybody** can contribute. You can recommend this book to others, you can say no, and you can take time to do something for others. Regardless of whether the framework is large or small. We can all do something for a better future. Even if it "only" visualizing a better world daily, and thus contribute to this vision soon becoming a reality. I do it daily and you can do it too. Let's tackle this together, God certainly does not want us to sick and unhappy on this world.

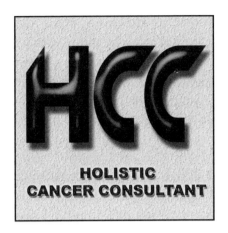

HOLISTIC CANCER CONSULTANT

An introduction to a new vocational profile

Independent, holistic cancer consulting

Sooner or later all those who are involved intensively with non-conventional cancer therapies, are confronted with the same problem: The majority of all patients only turn to biological therapies when conventional therapies have failed. Unfortunately the starting point at which a biological therapy is employed is totally different than it was when chemotherapy or irradiation was administered, because our body is no longer the same after irradiation or chemotherapy, not even if "objective data", such as hemograms, stabilize after several weeks.

In 99.9% of cases cancer is diagnosed by conventionally trained physicians, and consequently most patients are also treated conventionally. However, since doctors are only slightly familiar (or not at all familiar) with non-conventional therapies (mistletoe, thymus, enzymes, vitamins, etc.), and often they still have a large information deficit concerning the statistics on conventionally used therapies, patients usually can only choose between an operation, chemotherapy, and irradiation.

The greatest deficit however with those directly affected, and this also includes family members, who usually are not in a situation where they can make rational decisions immediately after the diagnosis. The emotional involvement does not permit this. This is unfortunately the reason why far too many rash decisions are still being made; decisions that many patients later regret. This is understandable, because when people have cancer, they almost always believe that they do not have any time to consider things, or to research the issues.

But let's be honest:

* what doctor provides his patients with copies of studies about the chemotherapy or the irradiation that will be administered?

* What doctor is even capable of describing a conventional approach AND a non-conventional approach?

* what patient can pose THE questions to his doctor that are really important (due to the patient's lack of knowledge and the emotional impact of the patient's diagnosis)?

However it particularly these three points that are the most important after a diagnosis of cancer. Unfortunately there are only a few people who have the good fortune to be able to sit across the table from a doctor who is familiar with both important directions of oncology. Another major challenge is to determine whether the therapy offered would help just the patient, or whether it also helps others. For a number of very different reasons many patients are "directed into studies" and thus they lose forever the chance that is afforded by non-conventional, successful, therapies. On the other hand others pay for expensive non-conventional therapies and only determine much too late that the therapies offered do not even come close to being worth the money. Unfortunately the issues of money, career, and therapies are almost always related and thus it is very difficult for a lay person (and often for experts as well) to understand whether the therapies offered are independent from other – mostly financial – interests. This is the reason why other teachers and I started offering career training to those interested in becoming a holistic cancer consultant.

FAQ

How do we do this?

We train people to be consultants, not therapists (consultants are people who only advise cancer patients verbally; they do not perform any therapy, not even psychological therapy. Therapists are people who use therapies on patients, or with patients). We consider separation between treating specialist/therapist and consultant to be absolutely necessary so that conflicts of interest do not even occur. This is the only that a patient can be 100 % certain that he is being advised independently. A consultant earns money with his work, but ONLY with his verbal work, he does not earn "supplemental income" which unfortunately is the status quo today. Naturally we make all of our knowledge available to our consultants, this particularly includes which doctors and clinics offer holistic treatment, or successfully treat cancer.

May I request money for my consulting later?

Of course. Every holistic cancer consultant can and should advise people based on his personal life context (self-help group leader, former patient, physician, psychologist, naturopath, etc.), and naturally he should also be paid for this advice. The only difference between a treating specialist and the consultant is that the consultant does not perform any therapy on his own, for which he receives money from patients.

How long is the training course?

A total of 2 years, which is divided into 4 blocks each lasting 5 days. The blocks do not just facilitate the usual transmission of course content, (this primarily occurs at home), rather they are designed to provide more depth on the material, to answer open questions, and to aid the personal development of the consultant, and the exchange of experience among participants.

What does the training course include?

An extensive curriculum in which the minimum knowledge required to holistically advise people with cancer is presented. Naturally this also includes the entire 3E program (Eat healthy, Eliminate toxins, Energetic work) and the knowledge of different cancer therapies, standard allopathic therapies, and diagnosis, and most importantly, knowledge of which conventional and non-conventional therapies are demonstrably successful for which types of cancer. The training enables each consult to create a consulting offering for his work. We do not think that each consultant should work in the same manner. Just as each patient is a unique individual, so each consultant must identify for himself the best way that he can advise and accompany people who are ill. We regard this point as the greatest challenge of the training course.

Do I need basic medical knowledge?

Yes and no. Basically we say that natural medical training will be quite helpful in learning the material, however it is not a necessity, if the person being trained is prepared to acquire the necessary knowledge.

Who are the instructors?

Mr. Lothar Hirneise, and others who can contribute to achieving the learning objective.

Please describe the activity of a holistic cancer consultant in practical terms?

Naturally the answer to these questions depends on the context of the individual, the professional experience of the individual, or the profession in which the individual would like to work. Basically the consultants offer accompaniment on the patient's path – regardless of whether the patient wants to pursue a conventional path, or a non-conventional path. The consulting can take a few hours (3E program, accompanying the patient to the oncologist etc.) or it can extend over a longer period. Also close collaboration with the treating therapist is possible.

Where can I be trained and how much does it cost?

Up to this point the training was only available in German. Currently in Europe there are trained cancer consultants, or cancer consultants in training, in Germany, Austria, France, Holland, Slovenia, and in Spain. Those interested in English language training can register now for England and for the USA.

Start England / London: **Summer 2006.**

Start USA / New York or maybe in California: **Summer 2006**.

More information about costs and precise dates is available here: www.hcc-uk.com and www.hcc-usa.com or write to: mgk@krebstherapien.de.

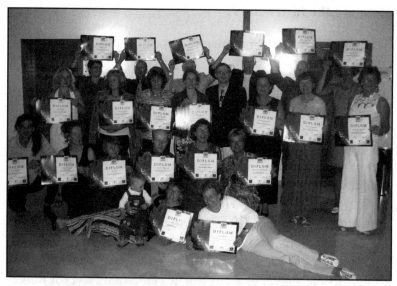

HCC graduating class 2005 in Mallorca / Spain

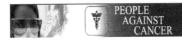

People Against Cancer

People Against Cancer is a grassroots, non-profit, public benefit organization dedicated to „New **Directions in the War On Cancer.**" We are a democratic organization of people with cancer, their loved ones, and citizens working together to protect and enhance medical freedom of choice.

USA
604 East Street - P.O. Box 10
Otho, Iowa 50569 USA
Tel: 515-972-4444 + Fax: 515-972-4415
www. PeopleAgainstCancer.com
info@PeopleAgainstCancer.net

Germany, France, Italy, Switzerland, Austria, Netherland, Slovenia, Spain
Menschen gegen Krebs
Cannstatter Str. 13 * 71394 Kernen, Germany
Tel: 49-715-191-0217 + Fax: 49-715-191-0218
www.krebstherapien.de * mgk@krebstherapien.de

United Kingdom
PO Box 56
Twickenham TW2 7UA
United Kingdom
Tel: 01784 885120 24/7

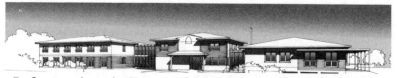

A new dimension

starts in spring 2006

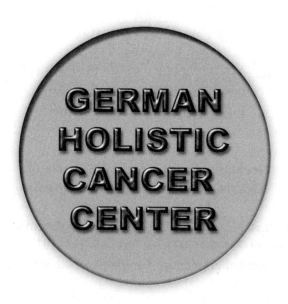

GERMAN
HOLISTIC
CANCER
CENTER

www.dgk-buoch.com

THE SUMMARY OF
50 YEARS CANCER
RESEARCH AND THERAPY

FINALLY AVAILABLE
IN ENGLISH!

DR. JOHANNA BUDWIG`S
LAST WORK

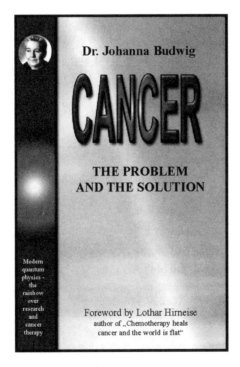

www.nexus-book.com

1% hurdle 121
2nd liver ,84
3E exercise ,553
3E Program ,30,32,34,80,294,305,379,411,417,531,587,673,695,748,749
3E-Emergency Program ,738
5FU ,159,161,162,163
5-FU
,160,161,162,204,207,213,237,238,239,251,252,255,269,282,314,324,32
9,356,357,371
714X ,661,662
A
ABBI ,128
ABCD rule ,276
Abel, Ulrich ,168
ABVD ,286
Acid base theory ,106
ACNU ,159,258
ACTH ,123,633
Acute lymphatic leukemia ,192,193,382
Acute Myeloic Leukemia ,196,231,306
Adler ,92
adriamycin ,165,272,286,293,344,357,371,400,408
adriblastin ,165
AFP ,123,124,125,359
aftercare ,144,145,148,149,151
Agaricus blazei murill ,727
AHCC ,719
AIDS ,31,42,78,384
Alcohol therapy ,241,273
Alexan ,162
Alkeran ,158
Alkylates ,158
Alloplant ,629,630
amalgam ,43,142,445,446,447,448,636,741
Amalgam removal program ,447
AMAS ,137
AML ,193,195,196,197,200,299,386
Anal carcinoma ,201
Antibodies
,101,190,195,200,204,209,214,221,229,233,241,244,252,256,260,264,27
0,278,282,286,294,300,306,307,310,316,321,327,328,330,335,341,352,3
57,361,368,373,377,386,402,409,602,606,620,648,668,690,691

Antimetabolites ,159
Antineoplaston therapy ,390,394,588
antinomycin ,164,392
Anus praeter ,203,204,236,237
Aquatilis ,242,265,274,576
Ara-C ,193,197,198,285,299
Aromatase ,223
Aromatase inhibitors ,223
asparaginase ,193,384
Astaldi ,180
Astrocytoma ,79,205,207,208,245,257,260,389,390,590
ATP-TCA-Test ,137
Avastatin ,242
Ayurveda ,110,437,444

B

Bach Blossoms ,679
Bacillus Calmette-Guérin ,693
Baking soda ,453,741
balance theory ,97,98,100,582
balance-sheet technique ,511,516
Basalioma ,211,328
Basel Bone tumor Reference Center ,119
BCG ,288,337,640,693
BCNU ,159,258,277,285
bendamustine ,159
Berne ,92
Bessis ,53,54,459
Bio Pro ,690
Bio-Electro-Therapy ,609
biofield test ,624,625,626
biological decoding ,94
Biopsies ,113,127,128,205,246,257,272,281,298,390,405
biopsy ,127,128,211,212,217,250,254,276,285,290,313,327,328,331,332,340,350,355,365,370,399
Black, Jack ,532
bladder cancer ,253,254,255,256,369,372,373,615,620,674,693,721,724
bleomycin ,251,277,286,329,360
Blood crystallization test ,141
Blumenschein, Willy ,149
Bone marrow therapies ,194,199,385,400
Bone marrow transplant ,177,194,199,200,219,232,285,293,299,304,385,

chlorambucil ,158,320
Chronic Myeloic Leukemia ,231
Cisplatin
,159,187,207,213,228,229,247,251,252,269,277,282,309,314,320,324,32
9,344,356,357,371,372,376,400,406,704
Cladribine ,162
Clark, Hulda ,103,636,670
Cluster Medicine ,583,584
CML ,231,232,233,735
Coffee enemas ,263,414,416,449,455,597,598,599,741
Coley ,352,410,591,592,594,693
Coley's toxin ,352,410,591,693
Colon cancer
,204,235,237,238,239,240,241,242,608,674,675,684,720,721,726
colon carcinoma ,235
Colon-hydro therapy ,448
Compresses ,454,455
COPP ,286
CoQ10 ,412,671,672
Corpus carcinoma ,243
Cousmine ,86,87,88,107
Curcumin ,672,720
cyclophosphamide
,158,193,207,218,240,247,282,285,286,292,305,309,320,344,345,351,36
9,376,384,406,408,633
Cyrotherapy ,215
Cytarabine ,162,207
Cytokine
,195,264,270,278,279,321,330,347,352,373,377,386,396,409,644,645,70
3
Cytoluminescent Therapy ,706
D
dacarbazine ,286
dark-field ,132,133,139
daunorubicin ,193,197,384
Decoder dermography ,141
demand switch ,461
Dendrite cells ,279,644,696,697,698,699
D-galactose ,204,237,720
DHEA ,720,721,725,726
Di Bella Protocol ,631,632
DMSO ,721

G

GALAVIT ,676
Gall bladder cancer ,253,254,255,256
Gallis ,53,54
Galvano Therapy ,609
Gautherie ,140
gemcitabin ,163,282
gemcitabine ,162,218,324,344,674
Gemzar ,162,163,164,324
Gene therapies ,200,209,248,341,347,393,407,734
German holistic cancer center ,18
Germanium ,722
Gerson, Max
,163,164,213,277,325,326,436,437,439,449,573,597,598,599,643,657,73
4
Glioblastoma ,79,205,209,246,257,258,259,389,565
Glivec ,233,234,735
glutathione ,78,412,622,623,648,692
Gonzales, Nicholas ,163,325,326,426
Govallo's VG 1000 ,612
Green tea ,722,723
Grossarth Maticek ,92
Growth factors ,300

H

Hackethal, Julius ,117,223,333,337,571,686
Haken, Hermann ,578
HAM ,197,550
Hamer, Geerd Ryke
,84,89,90,91,92,93,94,98,117,146,387,388,404,651,667
Hannigan ,228,229,375
Hashish/cannabis ,723
HCG ,123,125,359
healing field ,547,550,551,552
HECKER, E. ,184
Heine ,110,444
Heitan ,133
Herceptin ,221,241
Herrmann, Prof. ,169,170,171,172
High-dose chemotherapy ,194,200,219,278,285,292,299,304,385,401
Hirneise, Lothar ,20,25,188,564,749
HITT ,242,265,274
HLB ,133

Holistic cancer consultant ,745,747,748,749
Holo-Medicine ,94
holoxan ,158,240
Hölzel, Prof. ,219,334
Homeopathy ,64,455,583,604,605,679
Horwin, Michael ,394
house on the right bank ,534,536,537
Hoxsey Therapy ,638,639
HPLAP ,123
Hübener ,173,174
Hydrazine Sulfate ,687,688,689,720
hydroxycarbamide ,232
Hydroxylamine ,138,646
Hyperthermia
,209,248,352,393,407,410,593,594,595,596,663,664,674,739
I
I3C ,723
IAT ,283,564,606,607,608
idarubicin ,197,218,292
ifosfamide ,158,293,324,351,360,376,400,406,408
IHT ,712,717,718
Illmensee, Karl ,68
Imatinib ,233
Immune status ,126,145
Incence/boswellic acid ,729
Indian*Essence ,683,684,685
Intercalants ,164
Interferon
,42,195,214,233,264,270,277,278,279,294,301,307,316,330,373,386,457,
620,644,727
Interleukin ,42,264,270,278,300,316,330,347,373,396,402,644,691,726
IP6 ,723
IPT ,614,711,712
Iressa ,310
Issels Therapy ,641
Ixoten ,158
J
J.P. van Netten ,113
J.SEGAL ,183
Jefferson technique ,484,490
Jomol ,723,724
Joschko, Bernd ,578

Jung ,92,116,549

K

Kappis ,54,55

Kemnitz ,129,130

Kingsley, Patrick ,47

Klehr, Nikolaus ,644,645

Klemke, Erich ,646

KLH ,724

Koch ,103,603,680

Kombucha ,724,725

Kremer, Heinrich ,78

Kushi, Michio ,655

L

Laetril ,616,617,713,739

LaGarde ,133

LAK ,127,402,621

Lapacho ,725

Laryngeal carcinoma ,266

law of order ,36,550

Le Shan ,92

Lebedewa ,103

Leibowitz ,336

Leibowitz, Robert ,336

leucoverin ,237,238

leucovorin ,159,161,162,239,240,255,314

Leukeran ,158

Leustatin ,162

levamisol ,237,238

Leydig cell tumors ,358,361

Light
,23,28,35,36,37,39,95,96,101,103,110,132,134,145,167,178,211,214,254,
327,337,341,344,356,373,394,420,425,429,432,442,455,456,460,461,462
,525,527,575,634,635,665,679,680,705,706,734

Lindemann ,172

Link ,143,158,464

LITT ,242,265,273,274

liver cancer ,274,590,630,677,678

Liver tumor ,71,271

Livingston Therapy ,652

Lomustine ,159

M

M2PK ,124,125

TPA ,124,125
Trampoline ,455
Transfer Factors ,264,347,620,621,693
transferin ,123
trastuzumab ,221,241
Tributyrate ,730
trofosfamide ,158
tumor contract ,150,503,517,741
TUMORSPECIFIC IMMUNO-THERAPY ,644
Tumosterone ,646,648,649
TUR ,370,371

U

Ukrain ,326,373,404,674,675
Urea & Creatine Therapy ,677
Urtherapy ,650
Uterine cancer ,244,374,376,377
uterine carcinoma ,374

V

vinblastin ,263,286,371
vincristin
,193,207,232,247,258,277,286,293,305,329,344,351,376,384,392,400,406,408
VIP ,123
Visualization ,28,49,150,381,468,530,531,532,537,741
vitamin C
,19,33,36,169,412,421,438,457,565,610,631,632,658,672,675,689,708,709,710,713
VP16 ,197

W

Warburg, Otto ,106,179,182,424,425,600,665
Weber, Alfons ,104
What Doctors Don't Tell You ,46
Wheat grass ,729,730
Wiewel, Frank ,151,633,674

X

Xenogenetic peptides ,702

Y

Yeast Cells ,692,724
Yperite ,158,159

Z

Zabel, Erich ,179